AUDIOLOGY

THE FUNDAMENTALS

SECOND EDITION

AUDIOLOGY

THE FUNDAMENTALS

SECOND EDITION

FRED H. BESS
Division of Hearing and Speech Sciences
Vanderbilt University School of Medicine
and Bill Wilkerson Center
Nashville, Tennessee

LARRY E. HUMES
Department of Speech and Hearing Sciences
Indiana University
Bloomington, Indiana

Williams & Wilkins

BALTIMORE • PHILADELPHIA • HONG KONG
LONDON • MUNICH • SYDNEY • TOKYO

A WAVERLY COMPANY

Editor: John P. Butler
Managing Editor: Linda Napora
Copy Editor: John M. Daniel
Designer: Ann R. Feild
Illustration Planner: Ray Lowman
Production Coordinator: Charles E. Zeller

Accurate indications, adverse reactions, and dosage schedules for drugs are provided in this book, but it is possible that they may change. The reader is urged to review the package information data of the manufacturers of the medications mentioned.

Printed in the United States of America

First Edition 1990

Library of Congress Cataloging in Publication Data

Bess, Fred H.
  Audiology : the fundamentals / Fred H. Bess, Larry E. Humes.—2nd ed.
    p.   cm.
  Includes bibliographical references and index.
  ISBN 0-683-00620-7
  1. Audiology.   I. Humes, Larry.   II. Title.
  [DNLM: 1. Audiology. WV 270 B557a 1995]
RF290.B44 1995
617.8—dc20
DNLM/DLC
for Library of Congress   94–11556
                                                      CIP

96 97 98
3 4 5 6 7 8 9 10

To our wives,
Susie and Marty;
our children, Danny, Amy, Andy, and Lauren;
and the memory of our parents,
Helen and Samuel H. Bess
and Mary L. Humes

PREFACE

The second edition of *Audiology: The Fundamentals* continues to offer a contemporary treatment of the profession of audiology at the introductory level. Although audiology is a relative newcomer to the health care professions, it is a dynamic discipline that has undergone rapid change and growth since its inception during World War II. Because of these transformations, and space limitations, we continue to find ourselves forced to choose among areas of audiology to include in this text. As in the first edition, we have chosen to discuss the topics considered most important to the beginning student rather than provide a cursory review of the broad scope of the profession.

Initially, this book was written for three reasons. First, we saw a need for an introductory book that provides a contemporary approach to audiology: one that strikes a balance between the traditional concepts and newer developments in the profession. Second, we believed that there is a place for an introductory book that considered the type of student typically enrolled in a beginning audiology course. Our experience suggested that most students taking an introductory course in audiology were planning careers in either speech-language pathology or special education. With this in mind, we have tried to emphasize material on auditory pathology in children, especially middle ear disease, and we have included chapters on screening auditory function and education for the hearing impaired. It was our hope that such information would be of value to students when they begin practicing their chosen profession. The widespread acceptance of the first edition of this text reaffirmed our belief in the need for a new introductory book in audiology.

The second edition updates the previous edition and provides greater detail in several chapters. For example, we have tried to expand on the material offered in those chapters concerned with the nature of sound, the structure and function of the auditory system, and audiologic measurement. At the end of each of these chapters, advanced material is provided for students who wish to pursue given topic areas in greater depth. We have also tried to maintain the easy-to-read, easy-to-understand style. As before, references are intentionally omitted from the body of the book with the exception of a few direct quotations. A popular component of the first edition was the Vignettes designed to enhance interest, to illustrate ideas, and to crystalize definitions of difficult-to-grasp concepts. Numerous additional Vignettes have been added throughout the book. All figures have been redrawn, and numerous additional figures have been added. It is our sincere hope that the second edition will demonstrate to the student our enthusiasm for audiology and, more importantly, the challenges and rewards of this health-related discipline. We sincerely hope that this book will enhance enthusiasm and motivate students to pursue a career in audiology.

The book is divided into three sections. The first section provides background information on the profession of audiology and a basic review of the underlying principles of acoustics and the anatomy and physiology of the auditory system. A general understanding of Part I is essential to the practice of the profession of audiology. Part II is concerned with the principles of audiologic measurement and the general application of audiologic procedures. Toward this end, Part II focuses on basic measurement of auditory function, auditory pathologies and their associated audiologic manifestations, and screening for hearing loss in middle ear disease. Part III provides a general understanding of rehabilitative approaches used with children and adults with hearing loss and the status of education for the hearing impaired.

This book could not have been prepared without the generous help and support of many individuals. Kathy Hollis expertly and cheerfully prepared drafts on a timely basis, as well as the final version of the book. Several individuals reviewed the book or portions of the book and offered insightful analysis and suggestions for improvement. They included Gene W. Bratt, Thomas Klee, Michael J. Lichtenstein, Freeman E. McConnell, J. W. Sanders, and four anonymous reviewers whose constructive comments strongly influenced the content of this book. In this second edition, we are grateful of the comments of Gus Mueller, Rebecca Fischer, David Chandler, David Cieliczka, and Barry Freeman. John Butler, our editor, provided support and encouragement throughout the revision process. The staff and faculty of the Bill Wilkerson Center, Vanderbilt University School of Medicine (Division of Hearing and Speech Sciences), and Indiana University (Department of Speech and Hearing Sciences) offered continued support and facilities. To all of these individuals we offer our sincere appreciation.

Finally, in the first edition we took the opportunity to express our love and gratitude to our parents, Helen and Samuel H. Bess, and Mary and Charles E. Humes, for their confidence, direction, and continual support. Since then, each of us has experienced the loss of one or both parents. Therefore, this second edition is dedicated to the memory of Helen and Samuel H. Bess, and Mary L. Humes.

F.H.B.

L.E.H.

CONTENTS

Part II
ASSESSMENT OF AUDITORY FUNCTION

Chapter Four
Audiologic Measurement

Chapter Five
Pathologies of the Auditory System

Chapter Six
Screening Auditory Function

PART III

MANAGEMENT STRATEGIES

Chapter Seven

AMPLIFICATION AND REHABILITATION FOR THE HEARING IMPAIRED

Chapter Eight

EDUCATION FOR THE HEARING IMPAIRED

PART I

INTRODUCTION

AUDIOLOGY AS A PROFESSION

Following completion of this chapter, the reader should be able to:

- Discuss the prevalence of hearing loss and the complications associated with hearing impairment.
- Define the profession of audiology.
- Appreciate the lineage of the profession of audiology.
- Describe the employment opportunities available to the audiologist.
- Understand the academic and clinical requirements needed to become an audiologist.
- Appreciate the essential accreditations and professional affiliations important to clinical audiology.

The purpose of this opening chapter is to offer a general discussion and review of the profession of audiology. The discussion focuses on several areas. First, statistics on the total number of cases of hearing loss, or the prevalence of hearing loss, are reviewed. The impact of hearing loss on the well-being of the individual is also briefly described. These two areas are reviewed to give the reader some sense of the magnitude of the problem, both on a national scale and as it is experienced by the affected individuals themselves. Next, the definition and historical evolution of audiology are reviewed. Various employment opportunities in this health-related discipline are surveyed. The chapter concludes with a summary of typical graduate training programs in audiology and a description of some of the professional affiliations that audiologists find worthwhile.

PREVALENCE AND IMPACT OF HEARING IMPAIRMENT

Before discussing audiology as a profession, it is helpful to develop some understanding of the nature of hearing loss in the United States. The estimated prevalence, or total number of existing cases, of hearing loss varies according to several factors. These factors include (*a*) how hearing loss was determined (i.e., questionnaire vs. hearing test), (*b*) the criterion or formula used to define the presence of a hearing impairment (severe vs. mild hearing loss), and (c) the age of the individuals within the population sampled (adults vs. children). Regardless of the methods used to determine prevalence, hearing loss is known to affect a very large segment of the population in the United States. Estimates of the prevalence and prevalence rates of hearing loss for the population as a whole, and for different age groups, are summarized in Table 1.1.

It may be noted that the total number of persons with hearing impairment in the United States is slightly more than 22 million. It also can be seen that there are some 1,053,000 young people under the age of 18 years with hearing losses reported in either one or both ears. Other studies focusing on the population under 18 years of age have estimated that there are about 56,000 children under the age of 6 years with significant hearing impairment in both ears. This means that these children exhibit a hearing deficit in both ears, with the better ear exhibiting some difficulty in hearing and understanding speech. It has also been estimated that one of every 1000 infants is born with a severe to profound hearing loss. If young children with the milder forms of hearing loss are included, the prevalence rate is thought to involve 20–30 times more children. The above data should be viewed in light of the fact that elementary-school enrollment is expected to jump 10% in the next decade as the "baby boomlet" continues to swell the school-age ranks. The number of children in kindergarten through eighth grade should grow to 38.5 million in 2003 from 35 million now.

Returning to the statistics shown in Table 1.1, notice that the prevalence rate for hearing loss increases with increasing age. For example, in the age category of 18–44 years, the prevalence rate is 49.7/1000, whereas for the age groups 65–74 years and 75 years or older, the prevalence rates are 266.2/1000 and 403.6/1000, respectively. These statistics confirm what many of us with living grandparents and great-grandparents already know: hearing loss is commonly associated with old

Table 1.1.

Prevalence and Prevalence Rates, According to Age, for Hearing Loss in the United States[a,b]

Age Group	Prevalence	Prevalence Rate (per thousand)
All ages	22,630,000	91.2
Under 18 years	1,053,000	16.1
18–44 years	5,252,000	49.7
45–64 years	6,666,000	141.3
65–74 years	4,871,000	266.2
75+ years	4,839,000	403.6

[a]Data were obtained from household interviews and reflect the prevalence of hearing loss in either one or both ears.

[b]Adapted from Adams PF, Benson V: Current estimates from the National Health Interview Survey, 1991. Vital and Health Statistics, Series 10 (184). National Center for Health Statistics.

age. This is particularly important when one considers the current number of elderly persons in the United States and the projected growth rates of the aged population. The number of individuals over the age of 65 presently exceeds 23 million, and that figure is expected to increase to more than 55 million by the year 2030. This substantial increase in longevity has stemmed from the medical profession's improved success in controlling infectious and chronic diseases.

The preceding paragraphs have established that many Americans of all ages have significant hearing problems. Although statistics such as these are important, they provide little insight into the devastating impact that a significant hearing impairment can have on the individual. Children who are born with a severe or profound hearing impairment experience the greatest hardship and, under most circumstances, exhibit a significant lag in educational progress. This is because the hearing impairment interferes with the child's speech perception ability which, in turn, may result in impairment of speech and language development, reduction in academic achievement, and disturbances in social and emotional development. Because the development of our language system depends heavily on auditory input, a reduction or elimination of auditory input drastically curtails the ability to learn speech and language. To illustrate, it has been noted that the average high-school graduate from a state school for the deaf has the equivalent of an eighth-grade education. Even children with hearing losses in only one ear or very mild losses in both ears may experience difficulties in speech or language development, speech recognition under adverse listening conditions (e.g., classroom noise), educational achievement, and psychosocial behavior.

Children are not the only ones affected negatively by the presence of a significant hearing loss. Hearing loss in the adult can produce a number of psychosocial complications. For the elderly adult, the deterioration in hearing sensitivity and the associated problems with understanding speech are known to affect the quality of the individual's daily living activity. That is, the elderly who are hearing impaired are more likely to have poor general health, reduced mobility, fewer excursions outside the home, fewer interpersonal contacts, more depression and anxiety, and increased tension.

Hearing impairment also imposes a significant economic burden; relatively few deaf individuals are employed in professional, technical, and managerial positions. The lifetime economic cost of congenital deafness is estimated currently to exceed 1 million dollars. Other, less tangible costs borne by affected individuals and by their families derive from emotional stress, breakdowns in family communication, and isolation from peer and educational systems.

In summary, hearing loss occurs in large numbers of people and affects both children and adults. In addition, the prevalence rate of hearing loss increases markedly for the elderly population. Finally, the overall impact of hearing loss is significant, causing retardation in the educational progress of children and producing serious psychosocial consequences for those who acquire hearing loss later in life.

AUDIOLOGY DEFINED

Audiology is a new health care profession concerned with the study of both normal and disordered hearing. It evolved as a spin-off from such closely related fields as speech-language pathology, medicine, special education, psychology, and hearing aid instrumentation. In the most literal sense, the term *audiology* refers to the science of hearing. A much broader definition of audiology is *the discipline involved in the prevention, identification, and evaluation of hearing disorders, the selection and evaluation of hearing aids, and the habilitation/rehabilitation of individuals with hearing impairment.* Although these definitions represent commonly accepted descriptions of the profession, they in no way reflect adequately the breadth of the field or the challenges, rewards, and self-fulfillment that can result from a career in audiology. Whether your interest centers on serving people or producing new knowledge through inquiry and study, a career in audiology has much to offer.

The profession is typically subdivided into different specialties according to the nature of the population served or the setting in which the audiologist is employed (Vignette 1.1). For example, a common area of specialization is pediatric audiology, in which the focus is placed on the identification, assessment, and management of the hearing-impaired neonate, infant, and school-age child. The pediatric audiologist develops special knowledge in such areas as the causes of childhood deafness, the development of audition in children, child development, the audiologic screening and evaluation of children of different age groups, and parent counseling.

Another common specialty area is medical audiology. The medical audiologist is typically employed in a medical center and assists the physician in establishing an accurate diagnosis of an auditory disorder. Toward this end, the audiologist employs highly sophisticated and specialized tests to help pinpoint the location and cause of the hearing problem. The medical audiologist spends much of his or her time determining whether hearing loss is due to a problem in the middle ear, the inner ear, or the higher centers of the auditory system within the brainstem and cortex.

Rehabilitative audiology is a third area of specialization that is gaining widespread popularity and acceptance. The rehabilitative audiologist is concerned with the appropriate management of an individual with a hearing deficit. It is common for the rehabilitative audiologist to specialize even further by limiting the service population to either adults or children. The rehabilitative audiologist is interested in fitting the individual with appropriate amplification, such as a personal hearing aid, to help compensate for the hearing loss. This specialist also provides the individual with information on the use and care of the hearing aid. Other services offered might include speechreading, speech remediation, auditory training, and individual and family counseling. If the audiologist specializes in the rehabilitation of children, his or her activities might also include conducting special parent-infant

Illustration of various specialty areas in audiology.

The profession of audiology is categorized into a number of specialty areas based on the population served or the employment setting. The **pediatric audiologist** concentrates on the audiologic management of children of all ages. The pediatric audiologist is often employed in a children's hospital or a health care facility primarily serving children. The **medical audiologist** works with patients of all ages and is more concerned with establishing the site and cause of a hearing problem. Medical audiologists are typically employed in hospitals as part of either a hearing and speech department or a department of otolaryngology (i.e., ear, nose, and throat). The **rehabilitative/dispensing audiologist** focuses on the management of children or adults with hearing impairment. Rehabilitative audiologists are often seen in private practice and specialize in the direct dispensation of hearing aids. Rehabilitative audiologists are also employed by a variety of health care facilities (e.g., hospitals, nursing homes). The **industrial audiologist** provides consultative hearing conservation services to companies whose workers are exposed to high noise levels. The industrial audiologist may be in private practice or work on a part-time basis. Finally, the **educational audiologist** serves children in the schools and is employed or contracted by the educational system.

PEDIATRIC AUDIOLOGIST

MEDICAL AUDIOLOGIST

REHABILITATIVE/DISPENSING AUDIOLOGIST

EDUCATIONAL AUDIOLOGIST

INDUSTRIAL AUDIOLOGIST

training programs, teaching speech and language, counseling parents, and readying the child for school.

Some audiologists practice exclusively in an industrial setting. These audiologists are referred to as industrial audiologists. Noise is a common by-product of our highly industrialized society. As we'll learn later, high levels of noise can produce permanent loss of hearing. Because many industries have work areas that produce high noise levels, audiologists are needed to develop programs that will protect employees from noise. Audiologists organize hearing conservation programs. These programs are designed to protect the worker from hearing loss by reducing the noise levels produced by noisy equipment, monitoring the hearing of employees, teaching employees about noise and its damaging effects, and providing ear protection to those workers placed in high-noise areas.

Finally, some audiologists specialize in educational audiology and are employed by the public schools. Recall that the prevalence of hearing loss among school-age children is considerable. Educational audiologists are involved in identification, assessment, and monitoring of all school-age children with temporary or permanent hearing problems. The educational audiologist also selects and maintains hearing aids for children with hearing impairment and assists regular teachers with educational programming.

HISTORICAL DEVELOPMENT OF AUDIOLOGY

Although instruments (audiometers) used to measure hearing date back to the late 1800s, the discipline of audiology essentially evolved during World War II. During and following this war, many military personnel returned from combat with significant hearing impairment resulting from exposure to the many and varied types of warfare noises. Interestingly, it was a prominent speech pathologist, Robert West, who called for his profession to expand their discipline to include the area of audition. West stated: "Many workers in the field of speech correction do not realize that the time has come for those interested in this field to expand the subject so as to include . . . problems of those defective in the perception of speech. Our job should include . . . aiding the individual to hear what he ought to hear." Although a term had not yet been coined for this new field proposed by West, there was evidence that activity and interest in hearing disorders was present as early as 1936.

There has been considerable debate over who was responsible for coining the term *audiology*. Most sources credit Norton Canfield, an otolaryngologist (ear, nose, and throat physician) and Raymond Carhart, a speech-language pathologist, for coining the term independently of one another in 1945. Both of these men were intimately involved in planning and implementing programs in specialized aural rehabilitation hospitals established for military personnel during World War II. Today, Carhart is recognized by many as the Father of Audiology (Vignette 1.2).

**VIGNETTE 1.2.
Raymond Carhart (1912–1975),
"Father of Audiology."**

The contributions of Dr. Raymond Carhart to the development of audiology from its earliest origins were so numerous and so significant that many think of him today as the "Father of Audiology." A young professor in the School of Speech at Northwestern University when World War II broke out, he was commissioned a captain in the Army to head the Deshon General Hospital aural rehabilitation program for war-deafened military personnel at Butler, Pennsylvania. Deshon was named as one of three Army general hospitals to receive, treat, and rehabilitate soldiers who incurred hearing loss as a result of their military service. These three Army hospitals, together with the Philadelphia Naval Hospital, admitted and served some 16,000 hearing-impaired enlisted personnel and officers during the war.

This wartime mobilization effort served as the basis for the development of the new discipline that is now audiology. In 1945 Carhart and otologist Norton Canfield were credited with coining the word *audiology* to designate the science of hearing. From the outset, Carhart recognized that the strong interprofessional relationships between audiology and otology must be maintained. The military program was modeled on this concept, which determined its direction for the future. As a leader in the American Speech Correction Association, Carhart was instrumental in changing the name to the American Speech and Hearing Association soon after the close of World War II. He was, moreover, one of the Association's most effective liaisons between audiology and otology, over the years, when potentially divisive issues arose.

Returning to Northwestern as professor of audiology at the close of the war, Carhart set about immediately to develop a strong audiology graduate program and a clinical service center, placing Northwestern at the forefront of this field nationally. Many of his graduates became prominent in other universities across

VIGNETTE 1.2—*continued*

the country as teachers, research scientists, and clinical specialists. They, as well as his many professional associates in audiology and medicine, remember him for his brilliant and inquiring mind, which provided many of the research findings still undergirding the field today; for his scholarly publications; for his masterful teaching and speaking ability; and for his skill in the management of controversial issues within his national association, now the American Speech-Language-Hearing Association. But most of all, his former students and associates remember him as a warm human being and a mentor who was first of all a friend.

PROFESSIONAL OPPORTUNITIES

As shown in Figure 1.1, the modern-day audiologist has the opportunity to work within a wide variety of employment settings. The largest number of audiologists are shown to be employed in hospitals and physicians' offices, followed by speech pathology or audiology offices and university or college-based clinics. A growing number of audiologists are finding employment in military-based programs (not shown in the figure). Perhaps the most rapid increase, however, is seen in private practice. The following discussion is a more detailed presentation of the professional opportunities in audiology.

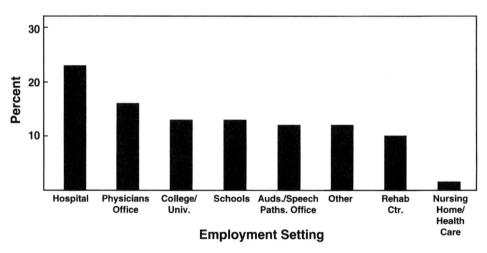

FIGURE 1.1.
Bar graph illustrating the distribution of employment settings for audiologists. Private practitioners are most typically seen in two employment settings, the "physician's office" and the "speech pathology or audiology office." (Adapted from Demographic Profile of ASHA Membership. American Speech-Language-Hearing Association, Research Division, 1993.)

Community Hospitals and Health Care Facilities

Most hospitals in the United States employ between one and four audiologists. Currently, the demand for audiologic services in hospitals, long-term care facilities, and home health agencies is increasing steadily. The increased demand for audiologists in this type of setting, especially since the mid-1980s, may be attributed to several factors. First, there is a growing trend for hospitals to develop or enhance their rehabilitation programs because the government's reimbursement systems (e.g., Medicare) now emphasize short-term hospital stays and subsequent outpatient rehabilitative services. Audiologic services are one form of outpatient rehabilitative service. Second, there is an increased awareness of the overall value of audiology and its contributions to health care. Finally, as was mentioned, the number of elderly individuals in the United States is growing, with at least one-third seeking health care, including audiologic services in many cases.

Predictably, the audiologic services provided in the hospital setting tend to be medically based. These audiologic services usually focus on providing information about the identification and location of an auditory disorder. The audiologist utilizes sophisticated auditory tests to evaluate the middle ear, the inner ear, the nerve pathways to the brain, and the auditory portions of the brain. This information is then pooled with diagnostic data obtained from other disciplines, such as otology (ear specialists), neurology, pediatrics, and psychology, to obtain a final diagnosis. In the hospital setting, the audiologist often works as part of a multidisciplinary team of both medical and nonmedical professionals.

Assisting the team in determining the diagnosis, however, is not the only service the audiologist provides in the hospital environment. Other services might include dispensing hearing aids, managing patients with other nonconventional hearing devices, and monitoring the hearing of patients who are treated with drugs that could damage hearing.

Audiology as a Private Practice

Certainly the fastest growing and perhaps most exciting employment setting is that of private practice. No other subgroup within the profession has shown such accelerated growth. In the 1970s, very few audiologists were in private practice. Today, 24.5% are employed full-time in private practice and another 13.3% are employed on a part-time basis. In fact, the private practice phenomenon has created an excellent market for professional opportunities in other areas of the profession. Many audiologists are leaving the traditional employment settings, attracted by the lure of a small business practice. The focus of these practices is on the sale of hearing aids, although many audiologists in private practice offer a wide array of audiologic services. Some audiologists may operate their businesses in medical clinics, hospitals, speech-language pathology offices, or otolaryngology practices; others may set up their own free-standing operation. There is, of course, a substantial risk involved in setting up a small business: the Small Business Administration estimates that about 60% of all new businesses fail during the first 5 years. There are today, however, more and more successful businesses in audiology started each year.

Why is it that private practice has become so popular, and why is it growing at such a fast pace? There are several reasons. First, small businesses provide an opportunity for financial independence and entrepreneurial expression and, perhaps most importantly, an opportunity to work for oneself. Second, private practice is growing because the opportunities it provides are becoming much more visible to those audiologists working in other settings. There is a dramatic increase in the memberships of organizations that are concerned with private practice and hearing aid dispensing and in the number of publications that serve the field. We are also beginning to witness the concept of franchises, or regional and national "chains," in the hearing aid dispensing business. Third, we find that the sale of hearing aids continues to increase on an annual basis and that the number of unserved hearing-impaired Americans is about 10 million, suggesting considerable potential and promise for future growth. The accelerated growth of hearing aid sales since the mid-1980s is shown in Figure 1.2.

Note that the sale of such devices remained relatively stable throughout most

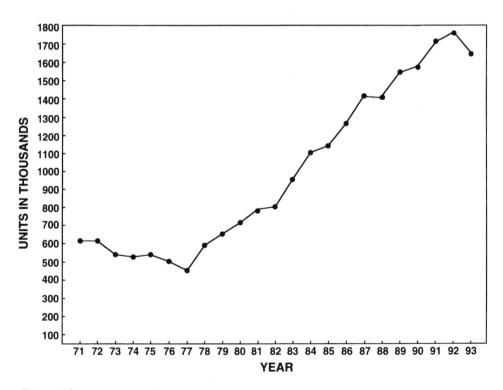

FIGURE 1.2.
Annual hearing aid sales from 1971 to 1993. (Adapted from Kirkwood DH. The economy + FDA + the media add up to an off year for hearing aid sales. *The Hearing Journal,* 46:7–14, 1993.)

of the 1970s. Since 1977, however, the sale of hearing aids has been substantial, exhibiting more than a three-fold increase in less than 20 years. With the increased public awareness of hearing loss and hearing aids, the improved acoustic performance and cosmetic appeal of these instruments, and the projected increases in the number of elderly persons with hearing impairment, the observed growth rate in hearing aid sales is likely to continue for some time.

College and University Settings

Most major colleges and universities offer undergraduate and/or graduate training in audiology. Many audiologists with doctoral degrees assume academic positions in the university and become involved in teaching, service, and research. In order to train a clinical audiologist adequately, the university must offer appropriate clinical training experiences. Accordingly, audiologists, many without doctoral degrees, are employed by the university to service hearing-impaired patients from the community and to supervise students in training for a graduate degree in audiology. Audiologists working in this setting have frequent opportunities to participate in research and to train students.

Audiology in the Schools

The advent in 1975 of the Education of All Handicapped Children Act (PL 94-142), a federal law designed to assure all handicapped children a free and appropriate public-school education, resulted in an increased awareness of the need for audiologic services in the schools. In 1990, this act became known as the Individuals with Disabilities Education Act (IDEA). In general, the act specified that each local educational system must provide, at no cost to the child, a wide range of audiologic services. These services included hearing evaluations, auditory training, speechreading, language training, and the selection and fitting of both personal and group-type amplification units. Needless to say, such a mandate required that audiologic services be offered in the schools. In 1986, PL 99-457 was passed, which authorized the extension of PL 94-142 to infants and toddlers, 0–2 years of age. Additional factors, such as the emergence of mainstreaming, have further increased the demand for educational audiology. Within the context of audiology, mainstreaming refers to the practice of placing hearing-impaired children in regular classrooms, rather than in special classrooms containing only hearing-impaired children. As more hearing-impaired children are integrated into regular classroom settings, the need to provide these children with special audiologic assistance increases. Another important variable has been the general recognition that many hearing-impaired children within the schools are not being adequately served. It has been reported, for example, that less than 50% of the hearing-impaired children in the educational system are receiving adequate services. To be sure, the introduction of PL 94-142 and PL 99-457, along with mainstreaming and an awareness of the audiologic needs of a larger group of children, has created a market for educational audiology. It is expected that this market will continue to grow as audiology continues to demonstrate how it can contribute significantly to the needs of hearing-impaired children in the schools.

The responsibilities of the school audiologist include many shared by most audiologists, such as hearing screening, hearing assessment, selection and evaluation of hearing aids, and direct provision of rehabilitative services. Additional services specific to the educational setting include maintenance of personal and group hearing aids; parent counseling; in-service education to teachers, special educators and administrators; consulting for educational placement; and serving as a liaison to the community and other professional agencies.

Community Hearing and Speech Centers/Rehabilitation Centers

A common setting for the practice of audiology has been the community-based hearing and speech center. Such programs can be implemented as a free-standing hearing and speech center or a component of a larger rehabilitation center. Today, the majority of metropolitan communities with populations greater than about 100,000 maintain community hearing and speech centers. These facilities provide comprehensive diagnostic and rehabilitative services to individuals with disorders of hearing, speech, or language. These centers receive much of their financial support from the community through individual contributions and through organizations such as the United Way and civic clubs. It is because of this type of support that such centers are able to serve substantial numbers of low-income patients. Audiologists are typically employed by these centers to provide a wide array of hearing services, such as hearing assessment, hearing aid selection and evaluation, hearing aid orientation, and aural rehabilitation for both children and adults with hearing impairment. Some of the larger community hearing and speech centers in the United States are also involved in conducting hearing research and in training future professionals in audiology.

Military-Based Programs

Hearing health care services are currently available in all branches of the armed forces (Army, Navy, and Air Force). As noted earlier, the military services played a key role in the historical development of the profession of audiology. In fact, immediately after World War II, the Army set up and staffed three hospitals, and the Navy one; each of these hospitals was devoted entirely to the rehabilitation and care of military personnel with hearing impairment or other disorders of communication acquired in the military service.

Audiologic services are still an important and growing need in the armed forces. In 1975, it was reported that as many as 50% of all service personnel exposed to combat arms suffer measurable hearing loss. Such documentation led to the recognition of a great need for military audiologists. For example, in 1967 there were only 11 audiologists employed in the Army, whereas in 1985 there were more than 70. A recent prevalence study of hearing loss among Army combat-arms personnel showed (*a*) a systematic relationship between increased hearing loss and increased time in service and (*b*) a larger percentage of soldiers (19%) with normal or near-normal hearing in 1989 than in 1974. Such data may be the result of an increased presence of Army audiologists and subsequent increased awareness of hearing conservation over the past 15 years.

The most dramatic change over the past several years for the employment of audiologists in the military setting has been the rapid increase in the number of female audiologists. Presently, one-third of Army audiology officers are women. The other branches of the military have similar percentages of female audiology officers.

Because of the overall reduction of troop strength in the past several years, the number of active-duty officers in the military has been reduced significantly. Nevertheless, many audiologists have attained the prestigious rank of Colonel and serve as managers of large health care commands. In fact, several of today's prominent audiologists started their careers in the military.

The military audiologist provides a typical range of audiologic services, although there is considerable emphasis on hearing conservation, audiologic screenings and assessments, diagnostic evaluations, hearing aid evaluations, and aural rehabilitation. Military hearing conservation programs must include such components as noise measurement analysis, the use of caution signs and labels warning of hazardous exposures to noise, noise reduction measures, the selection and fitting of personal hearing protection devices, education in hearing health care, audiometric testing, and audiologic record keeping. Finally, the military audiologist also has the opportunity to participate in research activity, primarily in the areas of aural rehabilitation and hearing conservation.

Department of Veterans Affairs Medical Centers and Other State and Federal Agencies

Most Department of Veterans Affairs (VA) Medical Centers maintain programs in speech-language pathology and audiology. In an effort to provide veterans with all the patient services that might be needed, the VA has grouped medical centers into geographic regions. Each region has a cross-section of different-sized medical centers. To receive audiologic services, the veteran typically attends the closest hospital offering an audiology program within his or her medical district.

The number of audiology and speech-language pathology programs within the VA system is growing rapidly, and this growth is expected to continue over the next several years. A recent survey revealed that between 65 and 75% of veterans exhibit significant hearing impairment. When one considers this high prevalence rate of hearing disorders, as well as the increased numbers of elderly veterans that will be expected over the next several years, it appears that the market for employment in this type of setting will be excellent.

A number of other federal agencies and state agencies also employ audiologists. At the state level, there is typically a department responsible for insuring the hearing health care needs of young children, usually associated with the Department of Public Health. Departments of public health employ audiologists to perform the full range of audiologic services and to serve as advocates for hearing-impaired children and their parents. Similarly, state departments of education and of vocational rehabilitation often employ audiologists to meet the audiologic needs of the populations their agencies are charged with serving. At the federal level, most opportunities for audiologists are administrative and are not concerned with direct service delivery. Their function is usually to assist the states and regions in implementing or improving programs for hearing-handicapped citizens.

EDUCATIONAL PREPARATION FOR AUDIOLOGY

For several decades, the entry-level degree required for the practice of clinical audiology had been the master's degree. In 1993, however, the American Speech-Language-Hearing Association (for historical reasons, generally referred to as the ASHA instead of ASLHA), the primary accrediting body for training programs in audiology, endorsed the professional doctorate as the entry-level credential required for the practice of audiology. Moreover, ASHA supported the Doctor of Audiology (Au.D.) as the preferred designation for the professional doctorate in audiology. Presently, we have two doctoral degrees available, the clinical Ph.D., which has been in existence for several years, and now the new Au.D. In 1993, the first Au.D. program was established at the Baylor College of Medicine in Houston, Texas, and its first group of six students entered the program in January of 1994. The 1990s will be a very significant period of transition in the type of education required to practice audiology as the field moves from 2-year master's degrees to 4-year doctoral degrees. At present, however, the prevailing educational model for the practice of audiology remains the master's degree.

Preparation for a career in audiology, however, should begin at the undergraduate level with basic courses that provide a strong foundation for subsequent graduate or professional study. Courses in physics, biology, statistics, mathematics, computer science, anatomy and physiology, psychology, child development, human behavior, and education can provide meaningful preparation for graduate or professional study in audiology.

Students who have pursued graduate work in audiology have come from a variety of backgrounds. In a typical large graduate master's degree program (10–15 students), it is not unusual to find students with diverse undergraduate majors, including speech-language pathology, psychology, education, and special education. Students with undergraduate majors in the basic sciences and the humanities have been less frequently encountered. With the advent of the Au.D., however, it is hoped that more students will come with undergraduate degrees in basic or life sciences, much like other pre-professional health care disciplines (e.g., pre-medicine, pre-dentistry, pre-optometry, etc.)

It is estimated that over 300 colleges and universities in the United States provide training in speech-language pathology and audiology. Of these, 116 offer master's degrees in audiology, approximately 25 offer clinical Ph.D. degrees in audiology, and 2 offer the Au.D. (although many more Au.D. programs are being developed). Selecting the most appropriate institution for a given student is sometimes difficult. Students interested in pursuing an advanced degree in audiology are encouraged to obtain the booklet, *Guide to Graduate Education in Speech-Language Pathology and Audiology,* published by ASHA.

What is master's degree training in audiology like? Table 1.2 details a graduate training profile for an audiology student enrolled in a five-semester master's degree program. Both the probable academic content of the program and the parallel practicum experiences are shown. Note that, in the first semester of study, most of the course work focuses on basic science and background information. Furthermore, the practicum during this first semester is more observation than participation. In the second semester, the applied courses are introduced, and the student becomes much more involved in practicum experiences, especially in case management. Hence, it is seen that the program progresses from basic to applied science, and that specialization increases during the later stages of the training program. In this example, the program offers an externship that allows the student to obtain work experience during the final semester of study. That is, a student will arrange for an 8- to 10-week practicum experience outside the university's training program. The purpose of the externship is to help the student make the transition from academic to professional life.

The 4-year doctoral degree programs are primarily expanded versions of the 2-year master's degree programs. They allow for additional coursework, both in basic and applied aspects of audiology, and for much more extensive clinical experience. In general, formal coursework is heavy and clinic practicum light during the initial semester. The time spent in formal coursework steadily decreases throughout the first 3 years, and clinical experiences increase. Clinical experience includes short-term externships and intensive clinical clerkships in a variety of areas. The final year is typically devoted to full-time clinical practicum in most Au.D. models or to clinical research in the clinical Ph.D. model. Table 1.3 outlines a graduate training profile for an audiology student enrolled in an Au.D. program (Baylor College of Medicine).

Receiving an advanced degree in audiology is just the first step toward becoming a clinical audiologist certified by the ASHA. For the majority of audiologists, certification by the ASHA is the desired clinical credential. In the current educational model, once the student receives the master's degree, the second step toward certification is to complete an internship known as the Clinical Fellowship Year (CFY). This means that the student must spend the first year of salaried practice under the supervision of an experienced and certified audiologist. It is anticipated

TABLE 1.2.

Typical Graduate Training Profile for an Audiology Student

Semester	Academic Content[a]	Practicum
1	*Basic science and normal background courses*: Child Development, Psychoacoustics, Physiology of Hearing, Phonetics, Psychoacoustic Instrumentation, Hearing Science, Measurement of Hearing, Research Methods	Introduction to practicum opportunities; supervised observation of diagnostic and rehabilitative techniques
2	*Case management study*: Pathologies of the Auditory System, Amplification for the Hearing Impaired I, Pediatric Audiology, Speech and Language Development	Beginning diagnostic and therapy practicum; participation in community and hospital diagnostic clinics; development of case management skills under close supervision
3	*Advanced study of communication disorders:* Speech and Language Development of the Acoustically Handicapped, Language Disorders in Children, Avanced Audiologic Evaluation, Amplification for the Hearing Impaired II, Parent Counseling, Electives	Full participation in supervised diagnostic and therapy practicum; broad experience in all types of auditory disorders; introduction to private practice, schools, and hearing aid dispensing; observation and study of normal family development and educational processes; experience in parental group counseling sessions
4	*Concentration in special topics*: Central Processing Disorders, Assistive Hearing Aid Devices, Pediatric Audiology, Medical Audiology, Auditory Electrophysiology, Aural Rehabilitation, Business Issues in Audiology	Development of independent skills in adult and child management; major responsibility for patients; written reports, professional interaction, conferences with allied professionals
5	*Externship (10 weeks)*: Preselected sites commensurate with trainees' interests and aspirations	Examples: (*a*) community hospital, (*b*) hospital associated with a research university, (*c*) private practice, (*d*) community hearing and speech center, (*e*) private or public schools

[a]Academic content represents topics covered during a given semester. Typically, a student will take 3–5 courses each semester.

TABLE 1.3.
Sample Student Program for Au.D. (Baylor College of Medicine)

Year	Term
1	1

Structure and Function of the Auditory System (3 hrs)
Clinical Instrumentation (3 hrs)
Pediatric Audiology (3 hrs)
Amplification (3 hrs)

2

Psychoacoustic Principles in Clinical Audiology (3 hrs)
Physical Acoustics (3 hrs)
Seminar in Audiology (3 hrs)
Physiology (2 hrs)

3

Medical Neuroscience I (6 hrs)
Selected Readings in Audiology (Speech Pathology) (1 hr)
Hearing Impairment and Linguistic Behavior (3 hrs)
Physiology (2 hrs)

4

Medical Neuroscience II (6 hrs)
Seminar in Audiology(3 hrs)
Pharmacology (3 hrs)
Physiology (2 hrs)

5

Sensory Systems (3 hrs)
Evaluation of the Peripheral Auditory System (3 hrs)
Selected Readings in Audiology (Peripheral Auditory Disorders) (1 hr)
Clinical Clerkship: Audiologic Assessment—Peripheral Auditory Disorders
    (2 hrs)
Pharmacology (3 hrs)

2   1

Principles of Counseling (3 hrs)
Ethics in Health Care Delivery (3 hrs)
Selected Readings in Audiology (Counseling of Hearing-Impaired Patients) (1 hr)
Clinical Clerkship: (Counseling of Hearing-Impaired Patients) (2 hrs)
Seminar in Audiology (3 hrs)

2

Auditory Perceptual Organization (3 hrs)
Evaluation of the Central Auditory System (3 hrs)
Selected Readings in Audiology (Central Auditory Disorders) (1 hr)
Clinical Clerkship: Audiologic Assessment—Central Auditory Disorders (2 hrs)
Seminar in Audiology (3 hrs)

TABLE **1.3**—*continued*

Year	Term
	3

Clinical Neuropsychology (3 hrs)
Introduction to Research Methods (3 hrs)
Selected Readings in Audiology [(Neuro)Psychology of Hearing Impairment] (1 hr)
Clinical Clerkship: Neuropsychologic Aspects of Hearing Impairment (2 hrs)
Seminar in Audiology (3 hrs)

4

Pediatric Audiology (3 hrs)
Ethics in Health Care Delivery (3 hrs)
Selected Readings in Audiology (Vestibular Disorders) (1 hr)
Clinical Clerkship: Overview of Vestibular Disorders and Evaluation (2 hrs)
Seminar in Audiology (3 hrs)

5

Quantitative Methods (3 hrs)
Special Project (3 hrs)
Selected Readings in Audiology [(Re)habilitative Audiology] (1 hr)
Clinical Clerkship: (Re)habilitative Audiology (2 hrs)
Seminar in Audiology (3 hrs)

3   1

Special Project (3 hrs)
Selected Readings in Audiology (Pediatric Audiology) (1 hr)
Clinical Clerkship: (Pediatric Audiology) (1 hr)
Practicum: Texas Children's Hospital (6 hrs)

2

Special Project (3 hrs)
Selected Readings in Audiology (Electrophysiologic Audiology) (1 hr)
Clinical Clerkship: (Electrophysiologic Audiologic Applications) (2 hrs)
Practicum: The Methodist Hospital (6 hrs)

3

Amplification (3 hrs)
Selected Readings in Audiology (Amplification Systems) (1 hr)
Clinical Clerkship: (Amplification Systems) (2 hrs)
Practicum: Houston School for Deaf Children (6 hrs)

4

Special Project (3 hrs)
Selected Readings in Audiology (Geriatric Audiology) (1 hr)
Clinical Clerkship: (Geriatric Audiology) (2 hrs)
Practicum: V.A. Medical Center (6 hrs)

5

Special Project (3 hrs)
Selected Readings in Audiology (Electroacoustic Audiologic Applications) (1 hr)
Clinical Clerkship: (Electroacoustic Audiologic Applications) (2 hrs)
Practicum: Ben Taub General Hospital (6 hrs)

TABLE 1.3—*continued*

Year	Term
4	1
	Clinical Clerkship: Basic Electronics (2 hrs)
	Practicum: The Methodist Hospital (6 hrs)
	2
	Clinical Clerkship: Overview of Otology (2 hrs)
	Practicum: Texas Children's Hospital (6 hrs)
	3
	Clinical Clerkship: Speech Pathology (2 hrs)
	Clinical Neurotology (3 hrs)
	Practicum: Ben Taub General Hospital (6 hrs)
	4
	Research Project (6 hrs)
	Practicum: V.A. Medical Center (6 hrs)
	5
	Research Project (6 hrs)
	Practicum: The Methodist Hospital (6 hrs)

Note: Program requires bachelor's degree, or its equivalent, from a U.S. accredited college or university. Undergraduate course work is required in the following areas: 1 year of Biology, including laboratory; 1 year of English; 1 year of Mathematics (through calculus); 1 year of Physics; 2 years of Psychology; Chemistry. Undergraduate course work is recommended in the following areas: Statistics; Humanities; Social Sciences; Foreign Language(s).

that many of the doctoral-level programs will build this internship into the final year of their doctoral programs so that an additional CFY will not be required. The third step toward certification by the ASHA, which can be completed at any time, is passing a national written examination in audiology.

Some students prefer to continue their study of audiology and obtain a doctoral degree in research, the Ph.D. This program usually takes 3–4 years beyond the master's degree or 1–2 years beyond the Au.D., and the student concentrates on theoretical and research aspects of the profession. Common employment opportunities for the Ph.D. include college and university teaching, research, and administration.

PROFESSIONAL AFFILIATIONS

Like all professionals, audiologists should maintain affiliations with their respective professional organizations. A primary professional organization for the audiologist is the ASHA. As mentioned above, the ASHA decides on standards of competence for the certification of individuals in the area of audiology (also speech-language pathology). The ASHA also conducts accreditation programs for colleges and universities with degree programs in speech-language pathology and audiology and for agencies that provide clinical services to the public. Among the many services that the ASHA offers its more than 70,000 members, of whom approximately 10,000 are audiologists, is an extensive program of continuing education. This program includes an annual national convention, national and regional conferences, institutes, and workshops. The Association also publishes professional and scientific journals, public information material, reports and position statements, monographs, and many other special publications.

An important new professional organization for the audiologist is the American Academy of Audiology (AAA). Now comprising more than 10,000 practitioners, the profession of audiology has reached a level of size and maturity that requires a separate organization of, by, and for audiologists. With this in mind, the AAA was developed in 1988. The academy, which has more than 5000 members, is dedicated to providing quality hearing care to the public. The academy is also committed to enhancing the ability of its members to achieve career and practice objectives through professional development, education, research, increased awareness of hearing disorders, and audiologic services. The academy typically focuses on issues related to the practice of audiology, such as standards and ethics, publications, training, standardization of methods, professional meetings, and professional scope. Also, the AAA publishes a professional and a scientific journal, public information material, and position statements.

The Academy of Dispensing Audiologists (ADA) is an organization of around 1000 members designed to meet the professional needs of audiologists in private practice, especially those who directly dispense hearing aids. Most members of the ADA also hold membership in the AAA; in fact, the two organizations collaborate on a number of activities of mutual interest. Similar to other professional organizations, the ADA publishes a professional journal, sponsors an annual meeting, offers continuing education, and promotes public awareness of hearing loss.

Another professional affiliation for the audiologist is the American Auditory Society, an organization encompassing numerous disciplines concerned with hearing and deafness. The membership roster includes practitioners of such professions as audiology, otolaryngology, education of the hearing impaired, pediatric medicine, and psychology, as well as members of the hearing aid industry. The society sponsors an annual convention and publishes a journal, *Ear and Hearing*. The purpose of the journal is to promote conservation of hearing and to foster the habilitation and rehabilitation of the hearing impaired.

Audiologists may associate with many other professional organizations depending on their areas of interest and specialization. There are professional organizations for the pediatric audiologist, the rehabilitative audiologist, the military audiologist, and the audiologist employed in the educational setting.

SUMMARY

Hearing loss affects a large segment of the population of the United States, and this figure is expected to grow over the next several years. Furthermore, hearing impairment in both children and adults can be a significant handicapping condition. The profession of audiology evolved in an attempt to help individuals with hearing impairment overcome these handicaps. Audiology has been described as a profession that is concerned with the prevention of hearing impairment and the identification, evaluation, and rehabilitation of children and adults with hearing loss. The audiologist has numerous employment opportunities and can work in a variety of employment settings. Audiology is a young, dynamic, and challenging profession that provides a wide range of exciting opportunities for a rewarding career.

REFERENCES AND SUGGESTED READINGS

Adams PF, Benson V: Current estimates from the National Health Interview Survey, 1991. Vital and Health Statistics, Series 10 (184). National Center For Health Statistics.

American Academy of Audiology: The professional doctorate. *Audiology Today*, August:3, 1989.

Bunch CC: *Clinical Audiometry*. St Louis, CV Mosby, 1943.

Cherow E: The practice of audiology—a national perspective. *ASHA* 28:31–38, 1986.

Commission on Education of the Deaf: *Toward Equality: Education of the Deaf. A Report to the Congress of the United States*. Washington, DC, U.S. Department of Health, Education, and Welfare, 1988.

Herbst KRG: Psychosocial consequences of disorders of hearing in the elderly. *In* Hinchcliffe R (ed): *Hearing and Balance in the Elderly*. Edinburgh, Churchill Livingstone, 1983.

Kirkwood, DH. The economy + FDA + the media add up to an off year for hearing aid sales. *The Hearing Journal*, 46:7–14, 1993.

Matkin ND: Early recognition and referral of hearing impaired children. *Pediatrics in Review* 6:151–158, 1984.

Northern JL, Downs MP: *Hearing in Children*, ed 4. Baltimore, Williams & Wilkins, 1991.

Sedge RK: Administration of a military-based program of speech-language pathology and audiology. *In* Oyer H (ed): *Administration of Programs in Speech-Language Pathology and Audiology*. Englewood Cliffs, NJ, Prentice-Hall, 1987.

Walden B, Prosek R, Worthington D: *The Prevalence of Hearing Loss Within Selected U.S. Army Branches*. Interagency No. 1A04745. Washington, DC, Army Medical Research and Development Command, 1975.

Weintraub FJ, Abeson AR, Braddock D: *State Law and Education of Handicapped Children: Issues and Recommendations*. Arlington, VA, Council for Exceptional Children, 1971.

West R: The mechanical ear. *Volta Review* 38:345–346, 1936.

CHAPTER TWO

THE NATURE OF SOUND

Following completion of this chapter, the reader should be able to:

- Describe the nature of a sound wave in terms of a series of events happening to air particles.
- Describe acoustic signals in terms of their amplitude, frequency, and phase.
- Understand the dual representation of acoustic signals in the time domain (waveform) and frequency domain (spectrum).
- Define the measure of sound level known as the decibel.

In this chapter, we will explore some of the fundamentals of acoustics that are essential to the understanding of audiology. The chapter begins with a discussion of selected characteristics of sound waves, which is followed by a section on the representation of sound in the time domain (its waveform) and the frequency domain (its spectrum); it concludes with a brief description of the measurement of sound.

SOUND WAVES AND THEIR CHARACTERISTICS

The air we breathe is composed of millions of tiny air particles. It is the presence of these particles that makes possible the production of sound. This is made very clear by the simple yet elegant experiment described in Vignette 2.1.

It is clear from the aforementioned experiment that air particles are needed for the production and transmission of sound in the atmosphere. There are approximately 400 billion air particles in every cubic inch of the atmosphere. The billions of particles composing the atmosphere are normally moving in a random fashion. These random continual movements of air particles make up what is known as Brownian motion. These random movements, however, can for the most part be ignored in our discussion of sound waves. It is sufficient to assume that each particle has an average initial or resting position.

When an object surrounded by air particles vibrates, the air particles adjacent to that object also vibrate. That is, when a sufficient force is applied to the air parti-

VIGNETTE 2.1.

Importance of a medium for generating sound.

The equipment shown in the accompanying figure can be used to demonstrate the importance of air particles, or some other medium, to the generation of sound waves. An electric buzzer is placed within the jar. The jar is filled with air. When the buzzer is connected to the battery, one hears a buzzing sound originating from within the jar. Next, a vacuum is created within the jar by pumping out the air particles. When the buzzer is again connected to the battery, no sound is heard. One can see the metal components of the buzzer striking one another, yet no sound is heard. Sound waves cannot be produced without an appropriate medium, such as the air particles composing the atmosphere.

cles by the moving object, the air particles will be moved or displaced in the direction of the applied force. Once the applied force is removed, a property of the air medium known as its elasticity returns the displaced particle to its resting state. The initial application of force sets up a chain of events in the surrounding air particles. This is depicted in Figure 2.1. The air particles immediately adjacent to the moving object (labeled *A* in Fig. 2.1) are displaced in the direction of the applied force. They then collide with more remote air particles once they have been displaced. This collision displaces the more remote particles in the direction of the applied force. The elasticity of the air returns the air particles to their resting position. As the more remote particles are colliding with air particles still further away from the vibrating object, force is applied to displace the object in the opposite direction. The void left by the former position of the object is filled by the adjacent air particles. This displaces the adjacent particle in the opposite direction. It is important to note that the vibration of air particles is passed on from one particle to another

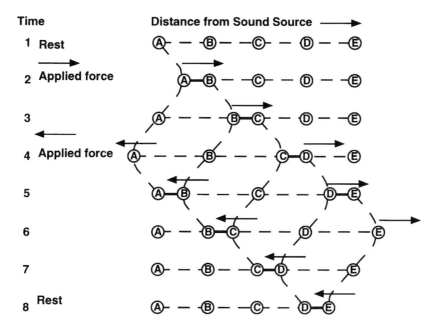

FIGURE 2.1.
The movement of air particles (*A* through *E*) in response to an applied force at time = 2 and time = 4. The *arrows* indicate the direction of the applied force and the direction of particle displacement. Notice that each of the particles goes through a simple back-and-forth displacement. The wave propagates through the air, so that back-and-forth vibration of particle *A* eventually results in a similar back-and-forth vibration of particle *E*.

through this sequential series of collisions followed by a return to resting position. Thus, the displacement pattern produced by the object travels through the air particles via this chain of collisions. Although we could measure this vibration in particles that are a considerable distance from the source of vibration, such as the particle labeled *E* in Figure 2.1, each particle in the chain of collisions has only moved a very small distance and then returned to its initial position. The air particles thus form the medium through which the vibration is carried. If the air particles adjacent to the vibrating object could actually be labeled, as is done in Figure 2.1, it would be apparent that the vibration of air particles measured away from the vibrating object at point *E* would not involve the particles next to the object, labeled *A*. Rather, the particle labeled *A* remains adjacent to the object at all times and simply transmits or carries the displacement from resting position to the next air particle (*B*). In turn, *B* collides with *C*, *C* with *D*, *D* with *E*, and so on. A sound wave, therefore, is the movement or propagation of a disturbance (the vibration) through a medium, such as air, without permanent displacement of the particles.

Propagation of a disturbance through a medium can be demonstrated easily with the help of some friends. Six to eight persons should stand in a line, with the last person facing a wall and the others lined up behind that person. Each individual should be separated by slightly less than arm's length. Each person represents an air particle in the medium. Each individual should now place both hands firmly on the shoulders of the person immediately in front of him or her. This represents the coupling of one particle to another in the medium. Another individual should now apply some force to the medium by pushing forward on the shoulders of the first person in the chain. Note that the force applied at one end of the human chain produces a disturbance or wave that travels through the chain from one person to the next until the last person is pushed forward against the wall. The people in the chain remained in place, but the disturbance was propagated from one end of the medium to the other.

Vibration consists of movement or displacement in more than one direction. Perhaps the most fundamental form of vibration is simple harmonic motion. Simple harmonic motion is illustrated by the pendulum in Figure 2.2. Note that the pendulum swings back and forth with the maximum displacement of A. The direction of displacement is indicated by the sign (+ or −) preceding the magnitude of displacement. Thus, $+A$ represents the maximum displacement of the pendulum to the left, 0 represents the resting position, and $-A$ represents the maximum displacement to the right. An object that vibrates in this manner in air will establish a similar back-and-forth vibration pattern in the adjacent air particles. That is, the surrounding air particles will also undergo simple harmonic motion.

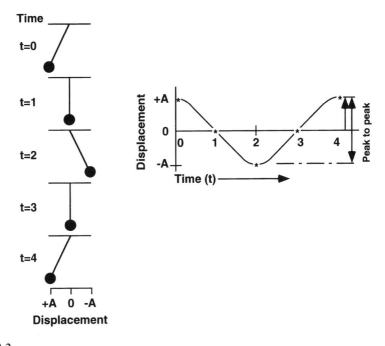

FIGURE 2.2.
Left, Illustration of the movement of a pendulum at five instants in time, $t = 0$ through $t = 4$. *Right,* Notice that the simple back-and-forth vibration of the pendulum results in a sinusoidal waveform when displacement is plotted as a function of time.

The five illustrations of the pendulum on the left side of Figure 2.2 illustrate the position or the displacement of the pendulum at five different instants in time ($t = 0, 1, 2, 3$ and 4). The plot in the right-hand portion of Figure 2.2 depicts the displacement as a function of time (t). Notice, for example, that at $t = 0$ the pendulum is displaced maximally to the left, resulting in a data point (*) at $+A$ for $t = 0$ on the graph in the right-hand portion of the figure. Similarly, at the next instant in time, $t = 1$, the pendulum returns to the resting position, or 0 displacement. This point is also plotted as an asterisk in the right-hand portion of Figure 2.2. The solid line connects the displacement values produced at each moment in time. If y represents the displacement, then this *solid line* can be represented mathematically by the following equation: $y(t) = A \sin (2\pi ft + \phi)$. The details regarding this equation are not of concern here. The term t in this equation refers to various instants in time. Note that displacement and time are related to one another in this equation via the sine function. It is for this reason that simple harmonic motion is often also referred to as "sinusoidal" motion.

Another common physical system that is used to represent simple harmonic or sinusoidal motion is a simple mass attached to an elastic spring. Such a system can be oriented horizontally or vertically. An example of a horizontally oriented mass-spring system is shown in Figure 2.3. The top panel illustrates the mass-spring system at rest. Next, at $t = 0$, force is applied to displace the mass to the right and to stretch the spring. When this applied force is removed, the elasticity of the spring pulls the mass toward the original resting position ($t = 1$). The inertial force associated with the moving mass, however, propels the mass beyond the resting position until it has now been displaced to the left of the original resting position ($t = 2$). This results in a compression of the spring. When the elastic restoring force of the spring exceeds the inertial force associated with the moving object, the motion of the object is halted and begins in the opposite direction ($t = 3$). As the moving mass reaches the original resting position, inertial forces again propel it past the resting position until it has once again been fully displaced to the right ($t = 4$). Notice that the displacement of the mass and the stretching of the spring at $t = 4$ is identical to that seen at $t = 0$. One complete cycle of back-and-forth displacement has been completed. The sinusoidal equation used previously to describe the back-and-forth motion of the pendulum can also be applied to this simple mass-spring system.

The mass-spring system, however, is often easier to relate to air particles in a medium. One can think of the mass in Figure 2.3 as an air particle, for instance, with the spring representing the particle's connection to adjacent air particles. In this sense, the movement of air particles described previously in Figure 2.1 can be thought of as a series of simple mass-spring systems like the one illustrated in Figure 2.3.

All vibration, including sinusoidal vibration, can be described in terms of its amplitude (A), frequency (f), and phase (ϕ). This is true for both the pendulum and the mass-spring system. The primary ways of expressing the amplitude or magnitude of displacement are as follows: (*a*) peak amplitude, (*b*) peak-to-peak amplitude, and (*c*) root-mean-square (RMS) amplitude. RMS amplitude is an indicator

A cube (mass) attached to a spring which is attached to a wall at its other end. The mass is sliding back & forth across a surface (like a table top).

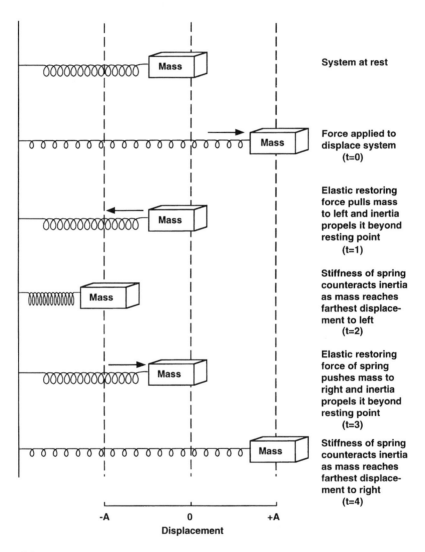

System at rest

Force applied to displace system (t=0)

Elastic restoring force pulls mass to left and inertia propels it beyond resting point (t=1)

Stiffness of spring counteracts inertia as mass reaches farthest displacement to left (t=2)

Elastic restoring force of spring pushes mass to right and inertia propels it beyond resting point (t=3)

Stiffness of spring counteracts inertia as mass reaches farthest displacement to right (t=4)

-A   0   +A

Displacement

FIGURE 2.3.
A simple mass-spring system in horizontal orientation is shown here to illustrate various stages of simple harmonic motion. The horizontal movement of the mass is depicted at five instants in time, $t = 0$ through $t = 4$. Notice that the simple back-and-forth vibration of this mass-spring system would result in a sinusoidal waveform of displacement as a function of time, just like the pendulum in Figure 2.2.

of the average amplitude and facilitates comparisons of the amplitudes of different types of sound waves. The peak and peak-to-peak amplitudes are illustrated in the right-hand portion of Figure 2.2. Peak amplitude is the magnitude of the displacement from the resting state to the maximum amplitude. Peak-to-peak amplitude is the difference between the maximum displacement in one direction and the maximum displacement in the other direction.

The period of the vibration is the time it takes for the pendulum to move from any given point and return to the same point. This describes one complete cycle of the pendulum's movement. Notice in Figure 2.2, for example, that at $t = 4$ the pendulum has returned to the same position it occupied at $t = 0$. The period in this case would be the difference in time between $t = 0$ and $t = 4$. For the mass-spring system in Figure 2.3, the time taken to progress from the system's state at $t = 0$ and to return to that state at $t = 4$ is the period or time required for one full cycle of displacement. If each interval in Figure 2.2 represented one-tenth of a second (0.1 s), the period would be 0.4 s. Hence, the period may be defined as the time it takes to complete one cycle of the vibration (s/cycle).

The frequency of vibration is the number of cycles of vibration completed in 1 s and is measured in cycles/s. Examination of the dimensions of period (s/cycle) and frequency (cycle/s) reflects a reciprocal relationship between these two characteristics of sinusoidal vibrations. This relationship can be expressed mathematically as follows: $T = 1/f$ or $f = 1/T$, where T = period and f = frequency. Although the dimensions for frequency are cycles/s, a unit of measure defined as 1 cycle/s has been given the name *Hertz,* abbreviated *Hz.* Thus, a sinusoidal vibration that completed one full cycle of vibration in 0.04 s (i.e., $T = 0.04$ s) would have a frequency of 25 Hz ($f = 1/T = 1$ cycle/0.04 s).

Finally, the phase (ϕ) of the vibration can be used to describe the starting position of the pendulum or mass (starting phase) or the phase relationship between two vibrating pendulums or masses. That is, two sinusoidal vibrations could be created that were identical in amplitude and frequency, but differed in phase, if one vibration started with the pendulum or mass in the extreme positive position (to the left) while the other began at the extreme negative displacement (to the right). In this case, the two pendulums or masses would be moving in opposite directions. This is called a 180° phase relationship. The two pendulums or masses could have the same amplitude of vibration (back-and-forth movement) and move back and forth at the same rate (same frequency), yet still have different patterns of vibration if they failed to have identical starting phases.

Figure 2.4 contrasts the various features used to describe sinusoidal vibration. In Figure 2.4A, the two displacement patterns shown have identical frequencies and starting phases, but the amplitude of vibration is about three times larger for wave X. The peak amplitude of the vibration pattern labeled X is A, while that of pattern Y is $0.3A$. In Figure 2.4B, on the other hand, amplitude and starting phase are equal, but the frequency of vibration for wave Y is twice as high as that for wave X. Notice, for example, that at the instant in time labeled T in Figure 2.4B, vibration

FIGURE 2.4.
Sinusoidal waveforms differing only in amplitude
(A), frequency (B), or starting phase (C).

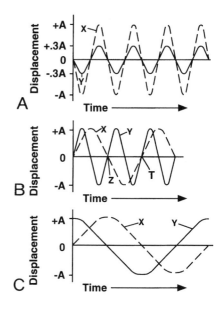

pattern X has completed one full cycle of vibration, while pattern Y has completed 2 cycles at that same instant. Interestingly, note that although these two functions start in phase (both beginning at $t = 0$ with 0 displacement), their phase relationship is very complex at other instants in time. At the point labeled Z in Figure 2.4B, for example, the phase relationship is 180°. That is, at the moment in time labeled Z, both function X and function Y are at 0 displacement, but one is moving in a positive direction and the other in a negative direction. Figure 2.4C illustrates two functions of identical amplitude and frequency that differ only in their starting phase. To fully describe sinusoidal vibration, all three parameters—amplitude, frequency, and starting phase—must be specified.

In the initial discussion of the vibration of air particles, a situation was described in which force was applied to an object that resulted in the object itself displacing adjacent air particles. When the force was removed, the object and the air particles returned to their resting positions. This was a case of forced vibration. Before describing the features of forced vibration in more detail, its counterpart, free vibration, deserves brief mention. In free vibration, as in the case of the pendulum or the mass-spring system described above, once the vibration was started by applying force, the vibration continued without additional force being required to sustain it. For free vibration, the form of the vibration is always sinusoidal, and the frequency of oscillation for a particular object is always the same. This frequency is known as the object's natural or resonant frequency (Vignette 2.2). The amplitude, moreover, can be no larger than the initial displacement. If there is no resistance to oppose the sinusoidal oscillation, it will continue indefinitely. In the real world, however, this situation is never achieved. Friction opposes the vibration, which leads it to gradually decay in amplitude over time. To illustrate this, imagine that

VIGNETTE 2.2.
Conceptual illustrations of mass, elasticity, and resonance.

You will be conducting a small experiment that requires the following materials: a yardstick (or meter stick), tape, 25 marbles, string (8 inches), and a small disposable cup with a lid (paper, plastic, or Styrofoam). (You may use sand instead of marbles or replace the cup altogether and use wooden blocks affixed to the yardstick with rubber bands. The following instructions, though, assume that you are using the cup and marbles.)

Place the string through two small holes in the top of the cup and tie a knot at each end. Tape the string (attached to the cup) to the 1-inch mark on the yardstick. Hold or clamp 3 inches of the other end of the yardstick firmly to the top of a table. Place 5 marbles in the cup. Apply a downward force to the far end of the yardstick (the end with the cup) to bend it down approximately 2–3 inches. (Don't push down too hard or the marbles may fall out of the cup when released.) Now release the far end of the yardstick and count the number of complete up-and-down vibrations of the far end over a 5-s period. Repeat the measurements three times, and record the number of complete cycles of vibration during each 5-s period. This is experiment A.

Now add 20 marbles to the cup so that all 25 are now in the cup. Repeat the same procedure as above, and record the number of complete cycles three separate times. This is experiment B. If the number of complete cycles of vibration in each experiment is divided by 5 (for the 5-s measurement interval), the frequency (f) will be determined (in cycles per second). How has the system's natural frequency of vibration changed from experiment A to experiment B? By adding more marbles to the cup in experiment B, the mass of the system was increased. How was the system's natural or resonant frequency changed by increasing the mass of the system?

Now hold 12 inches of yardstick firmly against the table and repeat experiment B (25 marbles). This is experiment C. This increases the stiffness of the system. How has the resonant frequency been affected by increasing the stiffness?

VIGNETTE **2.2.**—*continued*

The resonant frequency of an object or a medium, such as an enclosed cavity of air, is determined largely by the mass and stiffness of the object or medium. Generally, stiffness opposes low-frequency vibrations, whereas mass opposes high-frequency vibrations. In the figure on page 34, the opposition to vibration due to mass and stiffness is shown by the *solid lines*. The point at which these two functions cross indicates the resonant frequency of the system. The opposition to vibration due to either mass or stiffness is the lowest at this frequency. The vibration amplitude is greatest at the resonant frequency because the opposition to vibration is at its minimum value. The *dashed line* shows the effects of increasing the mass of the system. Note that the resonant frequency (the crossover point of the *dashed line* and the *solid line* representing the stiffness) has been shifted to a lower frequency. The frequency of vibration in experiment B (more mass) should have been lower than that of experiment A. Similarly, if stiffness is increased, the resonant frequency increases. The frequency in experiment C should have been greater than that in experiment B.

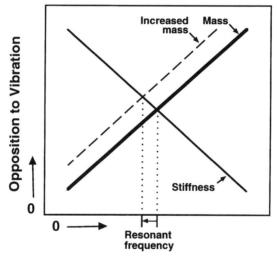

Frequency of Vibration (Hz)

the mass depicted in the mass-spring system in Figure 2.3 is a smooth wooden cube that is sliding back and forth on a smooth glass surface. If the smooth glass surface is now replaced with a sheet of coarse sandpaper, it is clear that there will be greater friction created to oppose the back-and-forth movement of the block. The increased friction associated with the sandpaper surface will result in a quicker decay of the back-and-forth movement of the block in comparison with the original glass surface that offered much less resistance to the motion of the mass.

If one wanted to sustain the vibration or to force the object to vibrate at other than its resonant frequency, it would be necessary to apply additional force. This is forced vibration. The amplitude of displacement that results when an external or driving force is applied to the object depends, in part, on the amplitude and frequency of the applied force. For a constant amplitude of the applied force, the vibration of the object is greatest when the frequency of vibration coincides with the resonant frequency of the object. An object that vibrates maximally when a force is applied, with the stimulating frequency of the applied force corresponding to the resonant frequency of the object, is said to be at resonance. Perhaps one of the most familiar examples of acoustic resonance is the shattering of a wineglass by the high-pitched voice of a soprano. When the frequency of the applied force (the singer's voice) coincides with the natural frequency of the air-filled cavity formed by the wineglass, the maximal amplitude of vibration exceeds the maximum amplitude tolerable by the glass structure, resulting in its shattering.

Having reviewed some general features of vibration, let us now return to the discussion of sound generation and propagation. Consider the following situation. The force applied to an object surrounded by air particles is sinusoidal, resulting in a sinusoidal back-and-forth displacement of the surrounding air particles. The object displaces adjacent air particles in one direction, causing a temporary build-up or increase in density of the air particles. As the object returns to resting position because of its associated elastic restoring forces, the momentum associated with the mass of the object forces it past the resting state to its point of maximum displacement in the opposite direction. The immediately adjacent air particles attempt to fill the void left by the object, resulting in a less dense packing of air particles in this space. In so doing, the air particles surrounding the vibrating object undergo alternating periods of condensation and rarefaction. That is, the density of air particles is alternately increased and decreased relative to conditions at rest (no vibration). The increased concentration (density) of air particles results in an increase in air pressure according to a well-known law of physics, the gas law. Thus, as the vibration propagates through the air medium, a volume of atmosphere goes through alternating periods of increased and decreased air particle density and, consequently, of high and low pressure. Waves of pressure fluctuations are created and travel through the medium.

Although the pressure variations associated with sound are small compared with normal atmospheric pressure, it is these small fluctuations in pressure that are important. The pressure fluctuations, moreover, can be described using the same features discussed previously to describe changes in displacement over time. That is, a sinusoidal driving force applied to an object vibrates the object and produces sinusoidal variations in pressure. These cyclic fluctuations in pressure, moreover, can be described in terms of their amplitude, frequency, and phase. Pressure is the parameter most often used to describe sound waves because most measuring devices, such as microphones, respond to changes in sound pressure.

The unit of sound pressure is the *Pascal* (abbreviated Pa). Recall that the term *Hertz*, rather than *cycles per second*, is used to describe the frequency of a sound.

The use of the term *Hertz* for frequency and the term *Pascal* for sound pressure reflects the contemporary practice of naming units of measure after notable scientists (Vignette 2.3).

Unfortunately for the student, this practice often obscures the dimensions of the quantity. Pressure, however, is force per unit area and has frequently been described in units of either N/m^2 or d/cm^2 (N = newtons, a unit of force named after yet another famous scientist; d = dyne, a unit of force).

Although sound pressure is the preferred quantity for depicting the amplitude of a sound wave, another commonly used quantity is acoustic intensity. *Acoustic intensity* and *sound power* are used synonymously in this book. It is possible to derive the acoustic intensity corresponding to a given sound pressure. For our purposes, however, suffice it to say that acoustic intensity (I) is directly proportional to sound pressure (p) squared. That is, $I \propto p^2$.

The sound wave propagates through air at a velocity or speed of approximately 330 m/s. This depends somewhat on the characteristics of the medium, including its elasticity, density, and temperature. For example, the speed of sound in air increases with temperature from 330 m/s at 0° C to a value of 343 m/s at 20° C.

Let us suppose that a vibrating object completes one cycle of vibration when the appropriate driving force is applied. As the first condensation of air particles, or local high-pressure area, is created, it travels away from the source. At the completion of one cycle, a new high-pressure area is created. By the time a second high-pressure area is completed, however, the first has traveled still further from its point of origin. The distance between these two successive condensations or high-pressure areas is called the wavelength of the sound wave. Now if the frequency of vibration is high, the separation between successive high-pressure areas is small. Recall that a high frequency implies a short period ($f = 1/T$). That is, the time it takes for one complete cycle is short for high frequencies. Consequently, the first high-pressure area is unable to travel far from the source before the second high-pressure area arises. Thus, the wavelength (λ), the separation in distance between successive high-pressure areas, is small. The wavelength (λ), frequency (f), and speed of sound (c) are related in the following manner: $\lambda = c/f$. Wavelength varies inversely with frequency; the higher the frequency, the shorter the wavelength.

To clarify the concept of wavelength and its inverse relationship to frequency, consider once again the human chain that represented adjacent air particles. Suppose that, once a force was applied to the shoulders of the first person, it took 10 s for the disturbance (the push) to travel all the way to the end of the human chain. Let us also say that the chain had a length of 10 m. If a force was applied to the shoulders of the first person every 10 s, the frequency of vibration would be 0.1 Hz ($f = 1/T = 1/10$ s). Moreover, 10 s after the first push, the second push would be applied. Because we have stated that 10 s would be required for the disturbance to travel to the last person in the chain, when the second push is applied, the last person in the chain (10 m away) would also be pushing forward on the wall. Thus, there would be a separation of 10 m between adjacent peaks of the disturbance or

VIGNETTE 2.3.
Units of sound named after famous scientists.

Hertz (*A*)

The unit of frequency, the Hertz (Hz), is named in honor of Heinrich Rudolph Hertz, a German physicist born in 1857 in Hamburg. Much of his career was devoted to the theoretical study of electromagnetic waves. This theoretical work led eventually to the development of radio, an area in which frequency is very important. Hertz died in 1894.

Pascal (*B*)

The unit of sound pressure, the Pascal (Pa), is named in honor of Blaise Pascal (1623–1662). Pascal was a French scientist and philosopher. He is well known for his contributions to both fields. As a scientist, he was both a physicist and a mathematician. In 1648, Pascal proved empirically that the mercury column in a barometer is affected by atmospheric pressure and not a vacuum, as was previously believed. Thus, his name is linked in history with research concerning the measurement of atmospheric pressure.

Newton (C)

The Newton (N), the unit of force, is named in honor of the well-known English mathematician, physicist, and astronomer Sir Isaac Newton (1642–1727), who spent much of his career studying various aspects of force. Of his many discoveries and theories, perhaps the two best known are his investigations of gravitational forces and his three laws of motion.

forward pushes. The wavelength (λ) would be 10 m. Now let us double the frequency of the applied force to a value of 0.2 Hz. The period is 5 s ($T = 1/f = 1/0.2 = 5$ s). Every 5 s, a new force will be applied to the shoulders of the first person in the chain. Because it takes 10 s for the disturbance to travel through the entire 10-m chain, after 5 s the first disturbance will only be 5 m away as the second push is applied to the shoulders of the first person. Thus, the wavelength, or the separation between adjacent "pushes" in the medium, is 5 m. Notice that when the frequency of the applied force was doubled from 0.1 to 0.2 Hz, the wavelength was halved from 10 m to 5 m. Frequency and wavelength are inversely related.

Another feature of sound waves that is obvious to almost anyone with normal hearing is that the sound pressure decreases in amplitude as the distance it travels increases. It would be fruitless, for example, to attempt to hail a taxicab a half block away with a soft whisper even on a quiet street. Because the amplitude of sound decays with increasing distance it would probably require high vocal effort to generate enough sound amplitude at the source so as to still be audible to the cab driver a half block away. That is, to be successful, one would have to yell "Taxi!" rather than whisper it.

Under special measurement conditions, in which sound waves are not reflected from surrounding surfaces and the sound source is a special source, known as a point source, the decrease in sound pressure with distance is well defined. Specifically, as the distance from the sound source is doubled, the sound pressure is halved. Similarly, because of the relationship between sound pressure and acoustic intensity described previously ($I \propto p^2$), it is apparent that the same doubling of distance would reduce the acoustic intensity to $\frac{1}{4}[(\frac{1}{2})^2]$ the initial value. This well-defined dependence of sound pressure and sound intensity on distance is known as the inverse square law.

So far, we have considered some of the characteristics or features of a single sound wave originating from one source. Moreover, we have assumed that the sound wave was propagating through a special environment in which the wave is not reflected from surrounding surfaces. This type of environment, one without reflected sound waves, is known as a free field. A diffuse field is the complement of a free field. That is, in a diffuse field, sound is reflected from many surfaces. The inverse square law that was just described holds only for free-field conditions. In fact, in a diffuse field, sound pressure is distributed equally throughout the measurement area, so that no matter how far we go from the sound source or where we are in the measurement area, the sound pressure is the same. The term *sound field* is sometimes used to describe a region containing sound waves. Free fields and diffuse fields, then, are special classes of sound fields.

Interference results when multiple sound waves encounter one another. Here, we will consider only the simplest case of interaction: *two* sound waves. The two sound waves referred to here may be two independent waves arising from separate sources (e.g., two loudspeakers or two people talking) or the original wave (usually called the incident sound wave) and its reflection off a wall, ceiling, floor, or other surface. The interference that results when two sound waves encounter one another may be either constructive or destructive. In constructive interference, the two sound waves add together to yield a resulting sound wave that is greater in amplitude than either wave alone. This is illustrated in the left-hand portion of Figure 2.5. In the case shown here, in which both waves are of equal amplitude, the maximum possible constructive interference would be a doubling of amplitude. Negative interference, on the other hand, occurs whenever the amplitude of the sound wave resulting from the interaction is less than the amplitude of either wave alone. The extreme case of negative interference results in the complete cancellation of the sound waves, as illustrated in the right-hand portion of Figure 2.5.

In addition to the interference that results when two sound waves interact, there are other interference effects that result when a sound wave encounters an object or structure of some kind. When a sound wave encounters an object, the outcome of this encounter is determined in large part by the dimensions and composition of the object and the wavelength of the sound. When the dimensions of the object are large relative to the wavelength of the sound wave, a sound shadow results. This is analogous to the more familiar light shadow in which an object in the path of light casts a shadow behind it. In the case of a sound shadow, the object

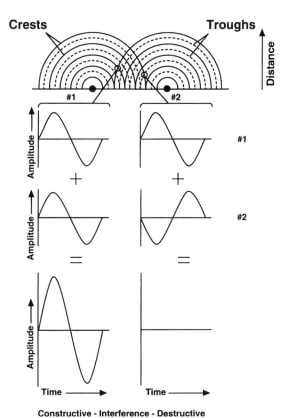

FIGURE 2.5.
Illustration of constructive and destructive interference of two sound waves (#1 and #2). The origin of each wave is represented by the *black circles* in the upper portion of the figure. The graph at the lower left illustrates the combination of waves #1 and #2 when the crests of each wave coincide. The two waves are in phase at this point, and the resulting sound wave is greater than either wave alone. This is constructive interference. The graph at the lower right illustrates the combination of the crest of wave #1 and the trough of wave #2. The two waves are 180° out of phase at this point, resulting in a complete cancellation of the two waves. This is destructive interference. (Adapted from Durrant JD, Lovrinic JH: Bases of Hearing Science, ed 2. Baltimore, Williams & Wilkins, 1984, p 41).

creates an area without sound, or a "dead area," immediately behind it. It is important to realize that all objects do not cast sound shadows for all sound waves. The creation of a sound shadow will depend on the dimensions of the object and the wavelength of the sound. For example, a cube having dimensions of 1 m × 1 m × 1 m will not cast a shadow for sound waves having a wavelength that is much larger than 1 m. Recall that wavelength and frequency vary inversely. In this example, a sound wave having a wavelength of 1 m has a frequency of 330 Hz ($f = c/\lambda$; $c = 330$ m/s; $\lambda = 1$ m). Thus, the object in this example would cast a sound shadow for frequencies greater than 330 Hz (λ 1 m). (See Vignette 2.4.)

Vignette 2.4.
Sound shadow created by the head.

As noted in the text, sound shadow occurs whenever the dimensions of the object in the sound field encountered by the sound wave are larger than the wavelength of the sound. Recall that wavelength is inversely related to frequency such that low frequencies have long wavelengths and high frequencies have short wavelengths. Consider the following three frequencies: 100, 1000, and 10,000 Hz. The corresponding wavelengths, calculated as described in the text, are: 3.3, 0.33, and 0.033 m, respectively.

Now, the human head can be grossly approximated by a sphere (or a cube for blockheads!) with a diameter of approximately 0.23 m (roughly 9 inches). When the head (preferably accompanied by the body) is placed in a sound field, therefore, it is capable of producing a sound shadow for wavelengths shorter than 0.23 m. Using the three frequencies from the preceding paragraph, for example, it is apparent that the average human head would create a sound shadow for 10,000 Hz, would possibly produce one at 1000 Hz, and definitely would not produce one at 100 Hz, where the wavelength is several times greater than the diameter of the head.

The figure on the next page illustrates how this so-called "head shadow" effect can be measured. In panel *A,* two microphones spaced about 9 inches apart are positioned in a free field (a sound field without any reflections) with a loudspeaker located to the right of the microphones at a distance of a few meters. The loudspeaker then presents a pure tone of 100 Hz and its sound level is measured at both microphones. This is then repeated for pure tones of 1000 and 10000 Hz. All three pure tones are presented at equal levels. Because the left microphone is farther from the sound source than the right microphone, the sound level is a little lower at the left microphone, consistent with the inverse-square law described in the text. The difference for these closely spaced microphones is small enough, however, that we can ignore it here and pretend that the sound levels are identical at both the left and right microphones.

In panel *B* of this figure, we have now inserted a head with a diameter of approximately 9 inches (0.23 m) between the two microphones. When we now repeat the measurements at 100, 1000, and 10,000 Hz, there is little change in sound level from panel *A* for 100 Hz and only a slight decrease in level at the left microphone for 1000 Hz. At 10,000 Hz, however, the sound pressure has been

VIGNETTE 2.4.—*continued*

reduced at the left microphone to a value that is only one-tenth of what it was in panel *A*. In terms of sound level in decibels (described later in the text of this chapter), the sound level has been decreased at the left microphone by about 20 dB with the head present for the 10,000 Hz signal. The head is blocking the 10,000-Hz sound wave from reaching the left microphone. Perceptually, the 10,000-Hz sound would be perceived as being much louder at the ear nearest to the loudspeaker and softer at the ear farthest from the sound source.

This difference in sound level at the two ears that results from head shadow is a very strong cue for the location of a sound in the horizontal plane. The sound is generally assumed to come from the side that has the highest sound level. Given the dimensions of the human head and the wavelength of sound in air for various frequencies, the sound level difference between the two ears helps locate sounds with frequencies above 1000 Hz. Below 1000 Hz, the size of the head does not create a sound shadow or a difference in sound level at the two ears. Cues other than the sound-level difference between the two ears are needed to locate low-frequency sounds (discussed in Chapter 3).

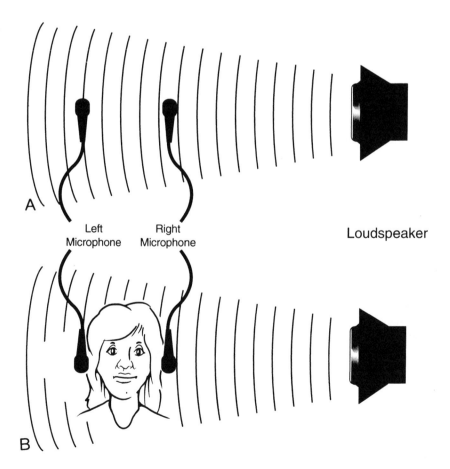

A

Left
Microphone

Right
Microphone

Loudspeaker

B

Finally, let us consider what happens when a sound wave encounters a barrier of some type. First, let us consider the case in which a hole is present in the barrier. In this case, as was the case for the sound shadow, the results depend on the wavelength (and, therefore, frequency) of the incident sound wave and the dimensions of the hole. For wavelengths much greater than the dimensions of the hole, the sound wave becomes diffracted. Diffraction is a change in direction of the sound wave. Thus, under these conditions the direction of the incident sound wave can be altered.

If the sound wave encounters a barrier that contains no holes, varying degrees of sound transmission, absorption, or reflection can occur. The proportion of the sound wave's energy reflected by the barrier and the proportion transmitted through the barrier depend on the similarity of the barrier's and the medium's impedance. Impedance may be thought of very generally as opposition to the flow of energy, in this case the advancement of the sound wave. If the barrier and the medium have the same impedance, 100% of the energy of the sound wave will be transmitted through the barrier. If the difference in impedances, often referred to as the "impedance mismatch," is large, then most of the incident sound wave will be reflected and little will be transmitted across the barrier (Vignette 2.5).

Aside from being reflected or transmitted, a portion of the sound wave may also be absorbed by the barrier. In the absorption of sound energy, the acoustic energy of the impinging sound wave is changed to heat. The materials out of which the barrier is constructed determine its ability to absorb sound.

WAVEFORMS AND THEIR ASSOCIATED SPECTRA

Many of the important features of a sound wave, such as its amplitude, period, and frequency, can be summarized in either of two common formats. One format, the waveform, describes the acoustic signal in terms of amplitude variations as a function of time. The sinusoidal waveform described previously for simple harmonic motion is an example of a waveform or time-domain representation of an acoustic signal. For every waveform, there is an associated representation of that signal in the frequency domain, called the amplitude and phase spectrum. Figure 2.6A illustrates the amplitude and phase spectrum for a simple sinusoidal waveform. Note that the x axis of the spectrum is frequency, while the y axis is either amplitude or phase. The amplitude scale can be peak-to-peak amplitude, peak amplitude, or RMS amplitude, as described previously. The phase spectrum in this case illustrates the starting phase of the acoustic signal. There can only be one possible waveform associated with the amplitude and phase spectrum shown in the right-hand side of Figure 2.6A. Similarly, there is only one set of amplitude and phase spectra associated with the waveform in the left-hand side of Figure 2.6A. Thus, both the time-domain and frequency-domain representation of the acoustic stimulus uniquely summarize its features. Furthermore, knowing one, we can derive

Vignette 2.5.
Discussion of impedance mismatch between air and water.

Consider the following situation. You and a friend are out on a boat in the ocean, scuba diving. Your friend is already underwater and you want to talk to him. He's only a few feet below the surface, yet, despite your yelling, he doesn't respond. Why not? The sound waves carrying your voice are traveling through an air medium. When the sound waves encounter the surface of the ocean water, a change in impedance is encountered. The impedance of ocean water is a few thousand times greater than that of air. As a consequence, only about 0.1% of the sound energy will be transmitted beneath the surface of the water to your friend. Approximately 99.9% of the airborne sound wave is reflected away from the surface. Thus, the impedance mismatch between the air and ocean water results in almost all of the airborne sound energy being reflected away from the surface.

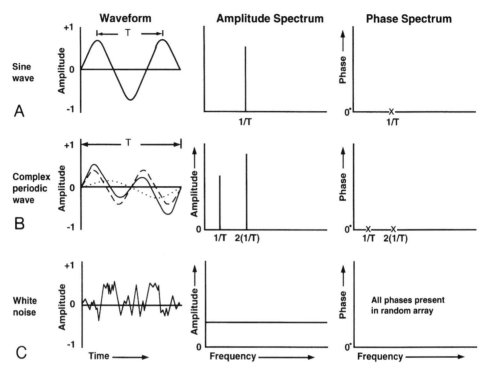

FIGURE 2.6.

Illustration of the waveforms and corresponding amplitude and phase spectra for a continuous sine wave (A), a complex periodic wave (B) (*solid line* is complex waveform, *dashed* and *dotted* lines are the two sine waves making up the complex sound), and white noise (C). All waveforms are assumed to be continuous, with only a brief "snapshot" of the waveform depicted here.

the other. For every waveform, there is one and only one amplitude spectrum and phase spectrum associated with it. For every amplitude and phase spectrum, there is one and only one possible waveform.

Simple sinusoidal sounds are more the exception than the rule in everyday encounters with sound. Over a century ago, however, a mathematician named Fourier determined that all complex periodic sounds consisted of a sum of simple sinusoids. A periodic sound is one in which the waveform repeats itself every T seconds. In the left-hand portion of Figure 2.6B, a complex periodic waveform is illustrated by the *solid line*. The *dashed* and *dotted* waveforms illustrate the two sinusoidal signals that, when added together, yield the complex sound. The spectrum of the complex sound then can be represented by the sum of the spectra of both sinusoidal components. This is illustrated in the right-hand portion of Figure 2.6B. Complex periodic sounds, such as that shown in Figure 2.6B, have a special type of amplitude spectrum known as line spectra. That is, the amplitude spectrum consists of a series of discrete lines located at various frequencies and having specified amplitudes. Each line represents a separate sinusoidal component of the complex sound. The component having the lowest frequency is called the fundamental frequency. The fundamental frequency corresponds to $1/T$, where T is the period of the complex sound. Additional components located at frequencies corresponding to integer multiples of the fundamental frequency are referred to as harmonics of the fundamental. If the fundamental frequency is 200 Hz, for example, the second and third harmonics of 200 Hz are 400 Hz ($2 \times$ 200 Hz) and 600 Hz ($3 \times$ 200 Hz), respectively. The first harmonic corresponds to the fundamental frequency. Additionally, the term *octave* means a doubling of frequency. Continuing the same example, 400 Hz would lie 1 octave above the fundamental frequency (200 Hz), whereas 800 Hz would be 2 octaves (another doubling) above the fundamental frequency.

Many acoustic signals in our environment are not periodic. Noise is probably the most common example. Noise is said to be an aperiodic signal because it fails to repeat itself at regular intervals. Rather, the waveform for noise shows amplitude varying randomly over time. This is illustrated in the left-hand portion of Figure 2.6C. The case shown here is an example of a special type of noise called white noise. White noise is characterized by an average amplitude spectrum that has uniform amplitude across frequency. That is, there is equal sound energy at all frequencies. ("White" noise derives its name from "white" light—light that is composed of all wavelengths of light at equal amplitudes.) This is depicted in the right-hand portion of Figure 2.6C. Note that the amplitude spectrum no longer consists of a series of lines. Rather, a continuous function is drawn that reflects equal amplitude at all frequencies. Aperiodic waveforms, such as noise, have continuous amplitude spectra, not discrete line spectra.

A variety of noises can be obtained from white noise using devices known as filters. Filters are typically electronic devices that selectively pass energy in some frequency regions and block the passage of energy at other frequencies. If we begin with white noise, an acoustic signal having energy at all frequencies, and send that noise through a filter called a low-pass filter, which passes only the low frequencies, the result is a low-pass noise that contains equal amplitude at low frequencies and little or no sound energy at high frequencies. A low-pass filter passes the low frequencies and filters out the high frequencies. Similarly, other noises, such as high-pass noise (sound energy at high frequencies only), can be generated. It should be noted that filters can be applied to a variety of acoustic signals, not just noise, to eliminate energy in certain frequency regions.

It has already been indicated that it is possible to represent an acoustic signal in both the frequency domain and the time domain. So far in our discussion of waveforms and spectra, it has been assumed that the acoustic signals are continuous ($\geq$ 1 s). Often, however, this is not the case. As a general rule, the shorter the duration of the signal, the broader the amplitude spectrum. Thus, a 1000-Hz pure tone that is turned on, and then turned off 0.1 second later, will have sound energy at several frequencies other than 1000 Hz. Approximately 90% of the sound energy will fall between 990 and 1010 Hz. If the duration of the pure tone is decreased to 0.01 second, 90% of the sound energy will be distributed from 900 through 1100 Hz. Hence, as the duration decreases, the spread of sound energy to other frequencies increases. The limit to the decrease in duration would be an infinitely short pulse or click-like sound. For this hypothetical sound, energy would spread equally to all frequencies. This is described in more detail in the Advanced Material at the end of this chapter.

SOUND MEASUREMENT

As mentioned previously, the amplitude of a sound wave is typically expressed as sound pressure (p) in Pascal units (Pa). Recall that one of the major reasons for this was that most measuring devices are pressure detectors. That is, devices such as microphones are sensitive to variations in air pressure and convert these pressure variations to variations in electrical voltage. In more general terms, the microphone can be referred to as an acousticoelectrical transducer. A transducer is any device that changes energy from one form to another. In this case, the conversion is from acoustical to electrical energy. (Usually, though, microphones are referred to as electroacoustical, rather than acousticoelectrical, transducers.)

Although the overall amplitude of sound waves is best expressed in terms of RMS pressure, the use of the actual physical units to describe the level of sound is cumbersome. In humans, the ratio of the highest tolerable sound pressure to the sound pressure that can just be heard exceeds 10,000,000:1! Moreover, the units dictate that one would be dealing frequently with numbers much smaller than 1. The lowest sound pressure that can just be heard by an average young adult with normal hearing, for instance, is approximately 0.00002 Pa (2×10^{-5} Pa) or 20 μPa.

Rather than deal with this cumbersome system based on the physical units of pressure, scientists devised a scale known as the decibel scale. The decibel scale quantifies the sound level by taking the logarithm (base 10) of the ratio of two sound pressures and multiplying it by 20. That is, the following formula is used to calculate the sound level in decibels (dB) from the ratio of two sound pressures (p_1 and p_2): $20 \log_{10} (p_1/p_2)$. Let us again use the range of sound pressures from maximum tolerable (200,000,000 μPa) to just audible (20 μPa) to see how this range would be represented in decibels. To do this, we begin by substituting 200,000,000/20 for p_1/p_2, which reduces to a ratio of 10,000,000/1. The $\log_{10}$ of 10,000,000 (or 10^7) is 7. When 7 is multiplied by 20, the result is 140 dB. This represents the maximum tolerable sound level. Now, for the just audible sound pressure of 20 μPa, the ratio of p_1/p_2 is 20/20, or 1. The log of 1 is 0, and 20×0 is 0. Thus, the just-audible sound pressure is represented by a sound level of 0 dB. We have taken a scale represented by a range of physical sound pressures of 200,000,000:20 and compressed it to a much more manageable range of 140 to 0 dB. The greatest sound pressure that can be tolerated is 140 dB greater than the sound pressure that can barely be heard. (See Vignette 2.6.)

Notice that the preceding statement only indicates that the sound pressure that is just tolerable is 140 dB above that which can just be heard, but does not indicate

Vignette 2.6.
Compressing effect of logarithms.

As noted in the text, one of the primary purposes of the decibel scale of sound level is to make the usable range of sound pressures more manageable. It would be inconvenient, and incomprehensible for many individuals, to use physical units of sound pressure to describe the range of sound amplitudes encountered in many everyday and clinical applications. For example, optimal hearing sensitivity of 0.00002 Pa can be more easily expressed as 0 dB, and painfully loud sounds of 200 Pa can be expressed as 140 dB using the same decibel scale of sound level.

Scientists frequently create different scales of measure to make working with the units of measure in the scale more convenient. A common example can be found in the various scales of temperature (Celsius, Fahrenheit, Kelvin). The Kelvin scale of temperature was designed to make it easier to work with low temperatures that became cumbersome in the Fahrenheit scale. For example, 0° in the Kelvin scale corresponds to −273.15° in the Celsius scale.

Societies and cultures have also attempted to make units of measure more practical and useful for the users of the measurement system. Often this has involved a system of conversion from one type of unit to another. The English system of length, for example, expresses length in units of inches when the lengths are small, feet when the lengths are intermediate, yards for still longer distances, and miles for very long distances.

Now, imagine that by imperial decree, everyone on planet Earth is required to express length in units of inches only. All other units of length have been abolished. Expressing the length of small objects in inches presents no major difficulty in everyday applications. Even the diameter of something as small as the period at the end of this sentence could be comfortably expressed as 0.01 inches. But what about the length of the playing surface on a football field (3600 inches), a 20-mile trip to Grandma's house (1,267,200 inches), or a trip around the world (1,584,000,000 inches)?!

If we were, in fact, confined to using inches as our sole unit of length, we could try to make the numbers more manageable by using logarithms. Logarithms essentially compress or squeeze a wide range of numbers into a smaller scale. Every tenfold change in our physical units results in an increment or decrement on the log scale of just one unit.

Let's see what happens when we compress our length scale by applying the logarithm to the set of length measurements from the preceding paragraph. We'll arbitrarily refer to this new scale of length based on the logarithm of length in inches as the "login" scale. The period with a diameter of 0.01 inches would have a new value of −2.0 logins ($\log_{10}$ of 0.01), the length of the football field would be 3.5 logins, the trip to Grandma's house would be 6.1 logins, and the trip around the world would be 9.2 logins.

Vignette 2.6.—*continued*

Wow! The logarithm function has really squeezed things together. The period at the end of this sentence has a diameter of −2.0 logins and a trip around the world (25,000 miles) is just 11.2 logins greater, or 9.2 logins! Now, if we were fairly certain that the diameter of this period was close to the smallest object we'd be interested in measuring, we could eliminate all negative numbers by taking the logarithm of ratios in which the denominator of the ratio is always 0.01 inches. This is just a way to make the zero point of the scale correspond to the smallest measurement that is likely to be made. In this new login scale, all values calculated previously simply increase by 2.0. Thus, our login values in this example range from 0.0 (period) ($\log_{10}$ of 0.01/0.01) to 11.2 (trip around the world).

Perhaps we've gotten a little carried away and have compressed our system of length measurement too much. We could *un*compress it by multiplying the logins by a factor of 10 (decilogins), 100 (centilogins), or 1000 (millilogins). In decilogins, our range of lengths would span from 0.0 decilogins (period) to 112 decilogins (trip around the world).

The preceding material should give you a better idea as to what transpires in the conversion from sound pressure in physical units of Pascals to sound level in decibels and why this system was developed. The use of logarithms compresses an unmanageable range of sound pressures into a more reasonable scale of numbers that is then expanded slightly through multiplication by a factor of 10. The logarithm function, however, was not chosen arbitrarily to perform this compression of the sound pressure scale. It was chosen both for its mathematical compression capabilities and because a similar type of compression was believed to be performed by the auditory system when presented with sounds covering a wide range of sound pressures.

---

what either of those sound pressures is in Pascal units. This is because a ratio of two sound pressures has been used in the calculation of decibels, and ratios are dimensionless quantities. That is, we are calculating the decibel increase of one sound relative to another. Sometimes all we are interested in is a relative change in sound pressure. Recall from the discussion of the inverse square law, for example, that as distance doubled from the sound source, the sound pressure was decreased to half its original value. The corresponding change in decibels associated with this halving of sound pressure can be calculated by using a ratio of 0.5/1. The $\log_{10}$ of 0.5 is −0.301, which, when multiplied by 20, yields a change in sound pressure of approximately −6 dB. We can restate the inverse square law by indicating that as the distance from the sound source is doubled, the sound pressure decreases by 6 dB. Again, this does not indicate what the values are of the two sound pressures involved in this change. The sound pressure may begin at 10 Pa and be halved to 5 Pa or may start at 10,000 Pa and decrease to 5000 Pa. Either of these cases corresponds to a halving of the initial sound pressure, which corresponds to a 6-dB decrease.

Often, an indication of the sound pressure level is needed that provides an absolute rather than a relative indication of the sound level. To accomplish this, it is necessary to evaluate all sound pressures relative to the same reference sound pressure. That is, the denominator of the decibel equation becomes a fixed value called the reference sound pressure. The reference sound pressure for a scale known as the sound pressure level (SPL) scale is 2×10^{-5} Pa, or 20 µPa ("twenty micropascals"). As noted above, this corresponds to the softest sound pressure that can be heard by humans under ideal conditions. Calculation of the sound pressure level (*SPL*) for a specific sound pressure (p_1) can be accomplished by solving the following equation: *SPL* in dB = 20 log $[p_1/(2 \times 10^{-5}$ Pa)]. Perhaps the simplest case to consider is the lowest sound pressure that can just be heard—that is, 2×10^{-5} Pa. If $p_1 = 2 \times 10^{-5}$ Pa, then the ratio formed by the two sound pressures is $(2 \times 10^{-5}$ Pa)/$(2 \times 10^{-5}$ Pa), or 1. The log of 1 is 0, which, when multiplied by 20, yields a sound level of 0 dB SPL. Consequently, 0 dB SPL does not mean absence of sound. Rather, it simply corresponds to a sound with a sound pressure of 2×10^{-5} Pa. Sound pressures lower than this value will yield negative SPL values, whereas sound pressures greater than this yield positive values.

Let us consider another example. A sound pressure of 1 Pa corresponds to how many decibels SPL? This can be restated by asking the reader to solve the following: *SPL* in dB = 20 log $[1.0$ Pa/$(2 \times 10^{-5}$ Pa)]. We begin by first reducing $1.0/(2 \times 10^{-5})$ to 5×10^4. The log of 5×10^4 is approximately 4.7, which, when multiplied by 20, yields a sound pressure level of 94 dB. Thus, a sound pressure of 1 Pa yields a sound pressure level of 94 dB SPL. This sound level is within the range of typical noise levels encountered in many factories.

Fortunately, laborious calculations are not required every time measurements of sound pressure level are required. Rather, simple devices have been constructed to measure the level of various acoustic signals in decibels SPL. These devices, known as sound level meters, use a microphone to change the sound pressure variations to electrical voltage variations. The RMS amplitude of these voltage variations is then determined within the electronic circuitry of the meter, and an indicator (e.g., needle or pointer, digital display) responds accordingly. In the case of 1 Pa RMS sound pressure input to the microphone, for example, the meter would either point to or display a value of 94 dB SPL.

Other measuring devices may be used to measure other features of the sound waves. Filters, for example, can be used in conjunction with the sound level meter to determine the amplitude of various frequencies contained in a sound. One can get at least a gross estimate of the amplitude spectrum of an acoustic signal by successively examining adjacent frequency regions of the signal. This can be accomplished with filters. For example, the filter might first be set to pass only low frequencies and the sound pressure level measured with the sound level meter. The filter could then be adjusted so as to pass only intermediate frequencies, then high frequencies, and so forth. This would provide a gross indication of how much sound energy was contained in various frequency regions. Very detailed and fine descriptions of the amplitude spectrum could be obtained by using narrow filters or by using a device known as a spectrum analyzer. This device essentially plots the amplitude spectrum associated with the waveform. The waveform itself may be examined in detail with a device known as an oscilloscope. An oscilloscope displays the waveform of the sound impinging on the microphone. Various means can be used to either "freeze" or store the waveform until all of its details (e.g., amplitude, period, phase) have been quantified.

Microphones, sound level meters, electronic filters, spectrum analyzers, and oscilloscopes are just a few of the basic tools utilized by the scientist and the clinician in the measurement of sound. The audiologist frequently uses these tools to check the equipment used in the testing of hearing. This equipment must be checked frequently to ensure that the results obtained with the equipment are accurate and that other clinics could obtain the same findings from a given patient.

SUMMARY

The fundamentals of acoustics were reviewed in this chapter. Simple harmonic motion, or sinusoidal vibration, was discussed. The effects of varying the amplitude, frequency, and starting phase of the sinusoidal waveform were examined. The relation between the representations of sound in the time domain, the waveform, and sound in the frequency domain, the amplitude and phase spectra, were reviewed. Resonance and its relation to impedance was also discussed. Finally, the measurement of sound levels in decibels (dB) was reviewed.

ADVANCED MATERIAL

Concepts of Impedance, Admittance and Resonance

In our discussion of the vibration and displacement of objects, whether the object was a pendulum, a mass-spring system, or an air particle, mass, elasticity, and resistance (friction) were mentioned repeatedly as critical factors affecting the vibration. The mass-spring system described previously in Figure 2.3 probably best illustrated the interplay between mass, elasticity, and resistance in the back-and-forth sinusoidal vibration of a mass. This was also illustrated in Vignette 2.2, in which a simple vibrating system was constructed from a yardstick and a cup of marbles.

Systems having mass, elasticity, and resistance can be forced to vibrate in response to applied forces of various frequencies. The frequency at which the system vibrates maximally for equal applied force is the resonant frequency of the system. The resonant frequency and the amplitude of vibration at that frequency are both determined by the impedance of the system. Impedance is the net opposition to vibration resulting from the mass, elasticity, and resistance of the system. Admittance is the reciprocal of impedance and indicates how easily energy is "admitted" by a system, rather than "impeded" by it.

Inertia is a force of opposition associated with objects having mass and one that opposes acceleration of the object (speeding up or slowing down its movement). Elastic restoring forces are associated with a system's elasticity and oppose the displacement of the object. When a spring is stretched, for example, its elastic restoring force opposes that displacement and attempts to restore it to its original (resting) position. Finally, friction is a form of resistance that opposes the velocity or speed at which an object is moving. The faster an object is moving, the greater the opposition to that movement due to friction. Frictional forces usually oppose the movement of an object by converting the kinetic energy associated with the moving object to heat. Rubbing the palms of your hands together, for example, will be opposed by frictional forces and will generate heat. The faster you rub them together, the greater the opposition due to friction and the greater the heat generated. Again, the net sum of the inertial, elastic, and frictional forces of opposition to motion is impedance. The higher the impedance, the greater the opposition to movement or vibration of the object, and the less the object moves or vibrates.

As noted previously in Vignette 2.2, the opposition to vibration associated with a system's mass increases with increase in frequency while the opposition associated with a system's elasticity or stiffness decreases with increases in frequency. The opposition associated with a system's mass is referred to as mass reactance (Xm), whereas that due to a system's elasticity is referred to as elastic reactance (Xe). Frictional forces, referred to as resistance (R), do not vary with frequency; they are frequency independent. For a system with mass M, the mass reactance can be calculated from the following equation: $Xm = 2\pi fM$. For a given mass, M, the forces of opposition associated with that mass increase with increase in frequency, f. In addition, the greater the mass (M) of an object, the greater the opposition to movement or vibration (Xm). For a system with elasticity E, the elastic reactance associated with that system can be calculated from the equation: $Xe = 1/2\pi fE$.

For a given E, the opposition due to elasticity (Xe) decreases as frequency (f) increases. In addition, as elasticity (E) increases (and stiffness decreases), the opposition due to elasticity, or elastic reactance (Xe), decreases.

Impedance, the combination of Xm, Xe, and R, is usually symbolized as Z. Impedance is a complex, vector quantity, as are Xm, Xe, and R. This simply means that it is a quantity with both magnitude *and* direction. Wind velocity is an everyday example of a vector quantity; a quantity in which both magnitude and direction are important. For example, a weather report might cite the wind at 25 miles per hour *out* of the southwest, rather than simply indicating its magnitude only (25 mph). Although impedance and its constituents are vector quantities with both magnitude and direction, we will focus here on the magnitude only. The magnitude of the impedance, Z, is calculated as follows: $Z = [R^2 + (Xm - Xe)^2]^{0.5}$. In words, the size of the impedance, Z, is equal to the square root of the sum of the resistance (R) squared and the net reactance ($Xm - Xe$) squared. Increases in R,

Xm, or *Xe* result in increases in the magnitude or size of the impedance. The greater the impedance or net opposition to vibration, the less the vibration or movement.

There exists some frequency, known as the resonant frequency, for which the impedance is at a minimum. Recall that *Xm* varies directly with frequency, whereas *Xe* varies inversely with frequency. As frequency increases upward from 0 Hz, *Xm* is increasing and *Xe* is decreasing. (The resistance, *R*, does not vary with frequency and remains constant.) At some frequency, *Xe* will equal *Xm*. At this frequency, the net reactance (*Xm* − *Xe*) will equal 0. According to the above equation for impedance, impedance will then be equal to the square root of R^2. That is, at the resonant frequency, the opposing forces associated with the system's mass and elasticity cancel each other, and all that remains to oppose the vibration is the resistance. At resonance, *Z* = *R*. This is the smallest amount of opposition to vibration possible, so the system will vibrate maximally at this frequency. At frequencies other than the resonant frequency, *Xm* will not cancel *Xe*, and the impedance will be greater than that at resonance. How much and how long the object or system vibrates will be determined by *R*.

The reciprocal of impedance (*Z*) is admittance (*Y*). Just as impedance (*Z*) represented the net sum of resistance (*R*) and reactance (*X*), admittance (*Y*) represents the net sum of conductance (*G*) and susceptance (*B*). Just as with reactance, there is a susceptance term associated with the system's mass (*Bm*) and one associated with the system's elasticity (*Be*). Similarly, the formula for the calculation of admittance, *Y*, is as follows: $Y = [G^2 + (Bm - Be)^2]^{0.5}$. In general, as impedance increases, admittance decreases, and vice versa. So, at the resonant frequency, *Z* is minimum and *Y* is maximum. Admittance and impedance are alternative, but equivalent, ways of describing the flow of energy through a system. Impedance summarizes the overall opposition to vibration, whereas admittance reflects the ease with which the system is set into vibration. It's akin to having the option to describe a 12-ounce glass filled with 6 ounces of water as being either half full or half empty. Either description is accurate.

Although admittance-based and impedance-based descriptions of a system are both equally appropriate, clinical measurement of the impedance or admittance of the middle-ear system (see Chapter 4) has evolved from an initial favoring of impedance terminology to more recent consensus for admittance measures and terminology. The choice, however, is not due to one being more accurate or better than the other, but has to do with the ease with which one can be measured validly with the equipment available in the clinic.

Finally, it should be noted that the impedance and admittance concepts described here are for mechanical systems. These concepts, however, have been applied to numerous types of systems, including electrical and purely acoustical systems. Although the details change from one type of system to another, the concepts remain the same. Table 2.1 illustrates some of the parallels among mechanical, acoustical, and electrical impedance.

TABLE 2.1.

Terms for Equivalent Components of Impedance (Z) for Mechanical, Electrical, and Acoustical Systems

Mechanical	Electrical	Acoustical
Mass reactance (Xm)	Inductive reactance (Xl)	Inertance (Xm)
Elastic reactance (Xe)	Capacitive reactance (Xc)	Elastic reactance (Xe)
Resistance (R)	Resistance (R)	Resistance (R)
Impedance (Zm)	Impedance (Ze)	Impedance (Za)
$Zm = [R^2 + (Xm - Xe)^2]^{0.5}$	$Ze = [R^2 + (Xl - Xc)^2]^{0.5}$	$Za = [R^2 + (Xm - Xe)^2]^{0.5}$

More on Waveforms and Spectra

Earlier in this chapter, the correspondence between a sound's representation in the time domain, referred to as its waveform, and its associated representation in the frequency domain, referred to as its spectrum, was briefly reviewed. A distinction was made between periodic and aperiodic waveforms and their corresponding amplitude spectra. The primary example used for aperiodic waveforms was white noise.

Recall that the definition of an aperiodic waveform is one that fails to repeat itself at regular intervals (every T seconds, where T is the period of the waveform). There are many other waveforms that meet this definition in addition to random noise. A type of aperiodic sound that is becoming increasingly common in clinical audiology is generally referred to as a transient signal. Transients in clinical audiology have typically been either brief bursts of a pure tone or clicks. As was noted earlier in this chapter, as the duration of a sound decreases, its amplitude spectrum becomes broader. Because of the increasingly common use of transient acoustic signals in audiology, this trade-off in the time and frequency domains will be examined in more detail here.

Figure 2.7A illustrates the waveform and amplitude spectrum for a continuous pure tone with a peak amplitude of A, starting phase of 0°, and a frequency of 1000 Hz. In principle, a "continuous" signal is one that is infinitely long. For practical purposes, however, acoustic signals having a duration, D, of 1 s or longer will be considered continuous. Note that the 1000-Hz waveform in this panel has a period, T, of 0.001 s, or 1 ms. The amplitude spectrum plotting peak amplitude as a function of frequency, therefore, consists of a line with amplitude A at 1000 Hz ($f = 1/T$).

In Figure 2.7B, the 1000-Hz pure tone has been abruptly turned on and off for a total duration, D, of 0.1 s, or 100 ms. It is now no longer considered a continuous periodic sound. Rather, it is a transient sound; one that occurs only once and for a duration of less than 1 s. As an aperiodic sound, the corresponding amplitude spectrum no longer consists of lines, but is a continuous function of frequency. The spectrum of this 100-ms, 1000-Hz tone burst has several key features, as shown in

FIGURE 2.7.
Illustration of the trading relation between representations of an acoustic stimulus in the time and frequency domains. The left column shows the waveforms for a 1000-Hz pure tone of various durations; the right column depicts the corresponding amplitude spectra. Duration of the 1000-Hz tone is infinite (continuous) in *A*, 0.1 s in *B*, 0.01 s in *C*, and 0.001 s in *D*. Note that as the duration is decreased from *A* through *D*, the amplitude spectrum becomes flatter and broader.

the right-hand portion of Figure 2.7*B*. First, notice that the spectrum is broader than it was for the continuous 1000-Hz pure tone shown in the top panel (Fig. 2.7*A*). That is, there is acoustic energy present at frequencies other than 1000 Hz for the tone burst, whereas this was not the case for the continuous pure tone. Second, although the peak in the amplitude spectrum is still located at 1000 Hz, the amplitude at that frequency has been decreased. In fact, the amplitude is now equal to the peak amplitude of the waveform (*A*) multiplied by the duration of the signal (*D*) in seconds (0.1), or 0.1 *A*. Reducing the energy present at 1000 Hz, however, is accompanied by a broader distribution of that energy across other frequencies, as noted above. Finally, the amplitude spectrum has several points at which the amplitude is 0 and the locations of these zero-amplitude regions occur at regular intervals above and below 1000 Hz. These points of zero amplitude are called "nodes" in the amplitude spectrum. They occur at frequencies above and below the pure-tone frequency and can be determined according to the following formula: n (1/D) and $-n$ (1/D), where n is 1, 2, 3, ... In the particular example shown in Figure 2.7B, D = 0.1 s; therefore 1/D = 10 Hz. The nodes or points of zero amplitude occur at 1000 + 10 Hz, 1000 − 10 Hz, 1000 + 20 Hz, 1000 − 20 Hz, 1000 + 30 Hz, 1000 − 30 Hz, and so on, as shown in Figure 2.7B. The frequency region between the first positive node (1010 Hz in Fig. 2.7B) and the first negative node (990 Hz) is referred to as the main lobe of the amplitude spectrum. The other adjacent regions between successive nodes are referred to as side lobes. When the pure tone is instantly turned on and off, as in these examples, 90% of the signal energy is contained in the main lobe; the remaining 10% is contained in the side lobes. As we've progressed from a continuous pure tone in Figure 2.7A to one lasting only 0.1 s in Figure 2.7B, the amplitude spectrum has started to broaden such that we've progressed from 100% of the acoustic energy at 1000 Hz to 90% spread from 990 to 1010 Hz.

In Figure 2.7C, the duration of the 1000-Hz pure tone has been decreased still further (D = 0.01 s, or 10 ms). The main lobe of the amplitude spectrum now stretches from 900 to 1100 Hz because 1/D is now 1/0.01, or 100 Hz. Thus, the first positive node occurs at 1000 + 100 Hz and the first negative node occurs at 1000 − 100 Hz. In addition, the peak amplitude at 1000 Hz has been reduced still further to 0.01 A ($D \times A$). Ninety percent of the signal energy in the main lobe of the amplitude spectrum for this brief tone burst is now spread over a range of 200 Hz.

If the duration of the 1000-Hz pure tone is shortened further by another factor of 10, as in Figure 2.7D, the corresponding amplitude spectrum continues to flatten and broaden. In this case, the duration of the pure tone is 0.001 s, or 1 ms, which corresponds to a single cycle of the 1000-Hz pure tone. Notice now that the main lobe containing 90% of the signal energy spans from 0 to 2000 Hz. We now have a signal that is very brief or compact in the time domain (short waveform), but very broad or spread out in the frequency domain (broad amplitude spectrum). Just the opposite was true for the continuous pure tone described in the top panel of this figure (Fig. 2.7A). For the continuous pure tone, the signal was very spread out in the time domain (a continuous waveform), but very compact in the frequency domain (all of the amplitude at just one frequency).

This broadening of the spectrum with decrease in signal duration is apparent perceptually as well. As the listener is presented with each of the pure tones in Figure 2.7 in succession, the perception begins with that of a clear tonal sensation and progressively sounds more and more like a click. In fact, the amplitude spectrum for an ideal click (one that is infinitely short), is flat throughout the entire spectrum.

It is clear that the spectrum of the shortest duration tone burst (Fig. 2.7D) is beginning to look more like that associated with a click than that associated with the continuous pure tone (Fig. 2.7A).

In summary, the amplitude spectrum of a pure tone varies with its duration such that the shorter the tone, the broader the spectrum. In general, the amplitude spectrum for pure tones less than 1 s in duration having a period of T seconds, a peak amplitude of A, and turned on and off abruptly for a duration of D seconds, will have a peak amplitude at $1/T$ Hz of $A \times D$ and a main lobe containing 90% of the signal's energy between the frequencies $1/T - 1/D$ and $1/T + 1/D$ Hz. In Figure 2.7, T was 0.001 s, which resulted in all the spectra being centered at 1000 Hz ($1/T$), but the general formulas noted above will allow this same analysis to be applied to pure tones of any frequency.

REFERENCES AND SUGGESTED READINGS

Beranek LL: *Acoustics*. New York, McGraw-Hill, 1954.

Berlin CI: Programmed Instruction on the Decibel. Kresge Hearing Research Laboratory of the South, Louisiana State University School of Medicine, 1970.

Cudahy E: *Introduction to Instrumentation in Speech and Hearing*. Baltimore, Williams & Wilkins, 1988.

Denes PB, Pinson EN: *The Speech Chain*. New York, WH Freeman, 1993.

Durrant JD, Lovrinic JH: *Bases of Hearing Science*, ed 2. Baltimore, Williams & Wilkins, 1984.

Small AM: *Elements of Hearing Science: A Programmed Text*. New York, John Wiley & Sons, 1978.

Speaks, C: *Introduction to Sound: Acoustics for the Hearing and Speech Sciences*. San Diego, Singular Publishing Group, 1992.

Yost WA: *Fundamentals of Hearing: An Introduction*, ed 3. New York, Academic Press, 1994.

CHAPTER THREE

STRUCTURE AND FUNCTION OF THE AUDITORY SYSTEM

====== OBJECTIVES ======

Following completion of this chapter, the reader should be able to:

- Recognize and identify some key anatomic features or landmarks of the auditory system.
- Understand the functional roles of the outer ear and middle ear.
- Understand the mapping of frequency to place (tonotopic organization) that occurs throughout the auditory system.
- Recognize the ability of the peripheral auditory system to code information in both a time-domain and a frequency-domain representation.
- Appreciate some basic auditory perceptual phenomena, such as loudness and masking.

This chapter is divided into three main sections. The first two deal with the anatomy, physiology, and functional significance of the peripheral and central sections of the auditory system. The peripheral portion of the auditory system is defined here as the structures from the outer ear through the auditory nerve. The central auditory nervous system begins at the cochlear nucleus and is bounded at the other end by the auditory centers of the cortex. The third section of this chapter details some fundamental aspects of the perception of sound.

PERIPHERAL AUDITORY SYSTEM

Figure 3.1 shows a cross-section of the peripheral portion of the auditory system. This portion of the auditory system is usually further subdivided into the outer ear, middle ear, and inner ear.

Outer Ear

The outer ear consists of two primary components: the pinna and the ear canal. The pinna is the most visible portion of the ear, which extends laterally from the side of the head. It is composed of cartilage and skin. The ear canal is the long, nar-

FIGURE 3.1.

A cross-section of the peripheral portion of the auditory system revealing some of the anatomic details of the outer, middle, and inner ear. (Adapted from Kessel RG, Kardon RH: *Tissues and Organs: A Text-Atlas of Scanning Electron Microscopy.* San Francisco, W. H. Freeman, 1979.)

row canal leading to the eardrum. The entrance to this canal is called the external auditory meatus. The deep bowl-like portion of the pinna adjacent to the external auditory meatus is known as the concha.

The outer ear serves a variety of functions. First, the long (2.5-cm), narrow (5- to 7-mm) canal makes the more delicate middle and inner ear less accessible to foreign bodies. The outer third of the canal, moreover, is composed of skin and cartilage lined with glands and hairs. These glands, known as ceruminous glands, secrete a substance that potential intruders, such as insects, find terribly noxious. So both the long, narrow, tortuous path of the canal and the secretions of these glands serve to protect the remaining portions of the peripheral auditory system.

Second, the various air-filled cavities composing the outer ear, the two most prominent being the concha and the ear canal, have a natural or resonant frequency to which they respond best. This is true of all air-filled cavities. For the ear canal of the adult, the resonant frequency is approximately 2500 Hz, while that of the concha is roughly 5000 Hz. The resonance of each of these cavities is such that each structure increases the sound pressure at its resonant frequency by about 10–12 dB. This gain or increase in sound pressure provided by the outer ear can best be illustrated by considering the following hypothetical experiment. Let us begin by using two tiny microphones. One microphone will be placed just outside (lateral to) the concha, and the other will be positioned very carefully inside the ear canal so as to rest alongside the eardrum. Now if we present a series of sinusoidal sound waves, or pure tones, of different frequencies, which all measure 70 dB SPL at the microphone just outside the concha, and if we read the sound pressure levels measured with the other microphone near the eardrum, we will obtain results like those shown by the *solid line* in Figure 3.2. Notice that, at frequencies less than approximately 1400 Hz, the microphone located near the eardrum measures sound levels of approximately 73 dB SPL. This is only 3 dB higher than the sound level just outside the outer ear. Consequently, the outer ear exerts little effect on the intensity of low-frequency sound. The intensity of the sound measured at the eardrum increases to levels considerably above 70 dB SPL, however, as the frequency of the sound is increased. The maximum sound level at the eardrum is reached at approximately 2500 Hz and corresponds to a value of approximately 87 dB SPL. Thus, when sound waves having a frequency of 2500 Hz enter the outer ear, their sound pressure is increased by 17 dB by the time they strike the eardrum. The function drawn with a *solid line* in Figure 3.2 illustrates the role that the outer ear serves as a resonator or amplifier of high-frequency sounds. The function shown is for the entire outer ear. Experiments similar to the one just described can be conducted to isolate the contribution of various cavities to the resonance of the total outer ear system. Again, the results of such experiments suggest that the two primary structures contributing to the resonance of the outer ear are the concha and the ear canal.

The resonance of the outer ear, which is represented by the *solid line* in Figure 3.2, was obtained with a sound source located directly in front of the subject at eye

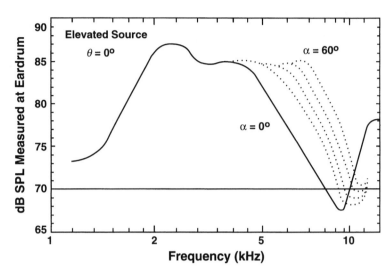

FIGURE 3.2.

The response of the head, outer ear, and ear canal for various angles of elevation (α) of the sound source. Zero degrees corresponds to a sound source at eye level and straight ahead (0° azimuth, ____) whereas 60° represents a source located straight ahead, but at a higher elevation. If the listener's head and outer ear had no influence on the sound level measured at the eardrum, a flat line at 70 dB SPL would result. This figure illustrates the amplification of high-frequency sound by the outer ear and the way that this amplification pattern changes with elevation of the sound source. (Adapted from Shaw EAG: The external ear. In Keidel WD, Neff WD [eds]: *Handbook of Sensory Physiology,* vol 5[1]. New York, Springer Verlag, 1974, p 463.)

level. If the sound source is elevated by varying amounts, a different resonance curve is obtained. Specifically, the notch or dip in the solid function that is located at 10 kHz in Figure 3.2 moves to a higher frequency and the peak of the resonant curve broadens to encompass a wider range of frequencies as the sound source is increased in elevation. This is illustrated in Figure 3.2 by the *dotted lines.* Each dotted line represents a different angle of elevation. An elevation of 0° corresponds to eye level, whereas a 90° elevation would position the sound source directly overhead. The response of the outer ear changes as the elevation of the sound source changes. This results from the angle at which the incident sound wave strikes the various cavities of the outer ear. The result is that a code for sound elevation is provided by the outer ear. This code is the amplitude spectrum of the sound, especially above 3000 Hz, that strikes the eardrum. Thus, the outer ear plays an important role in the perception of the elevation of a sound source.

Finally, the outer ear also assists in another aspect of the localization of a sound source. The orientation of the pinnae is such that the pinnae collect sound more efficiently from sound sources located in front of the listener than from sources originating behind the listener. The attenuation of sound waves originating from behind the listener assists in the front/back localization of sound. This is especially true for high-frequency sounds (i.e., sounds with short wavelengths).

In summary, the outer ear serves four primary functions. First, it protects the more delicate middle and inner ears from foreign bodies. Second, it boosts or amplifies high-frequency sounds. Third, the outer ear provides the primary cue for the determination of the elevation of a sound's source. Fourth, the outer ear assists in distinguishing sounds that arise from in front of the listener from those that arise from behind the listener.

Middle Ear

The middle ear consists of a small (2-cm^3) air-filled cavity lined with a mucous membrane. It forms the link between the air-filled outer ear and the fluid-filled inner ear (see Fig. 3.1). This link is accomplished mechanically via three tiny bones, the ossicles. The lateral-most ossicle is the malleus. The malleus is in contact with the eardrum or tympanic membrane. At the other end of the outer ear/inner ear link is the smallest, medialmost ossicle, the stapes. The broad base of the stapes, known as the footplate, rests in a membranous covering of the fluid-filled inner ear referred to as the oval window. The middle ossicle in the link, sandwiched between the malleus and stapes, is the incus. The ossicles are suspended loosely within the middle ear by ligaments, known as the axial ligaments, extending from the anterior and posterior walls of the cavity. There are other connections between the surrounding walls of the middle ear cavity and the ossicles. Two connections are formed by the small middle ear muscles, the tensor tympani and the stapedius. The tensor tympani originates from the anterior (front) wall of the cavity and attaches to a region of the malleus called the neck, whereas the stapedius has its origin in the posterior (back) wall of the tympanic cavity and inserts near the neck of the stapes.

We have mentioned that the middle ear cavity is air-filled. The air filling the cavity is supplied via a tube that connects the middle ear to the upper part of the throat, or the nasopharynx. This tube, known as the auditory tube or the eustachian tube, has one opening located along the bottom of the anterior wall of the middle ear cavity. The tube is normally closed but can be readily opened by yawning or swallowing. In adults, the eustachian tube assumes a slight downward orientation. This facilitates drainage of fluids from the middle ear cavity into the nasopharynx. Thus, the eustachian tube serves two primary purposes. First, it supplies air to the middle ear cavity and thereby enables an equalization of the air pressure on both sides of the eardrum. This is desirable for efficient vibration of the eardrum. Second, the eustachian tube permits the drainage of fluids from the middle ear into the nasopharynx.

What is the purpose of the elaborate link between the air-filled outer ear and the fluid-filled inner ear formed by the three ossicles? Recall from the example in Chapter 2 in which two people attempted to communicate, one underwater and one above the water, that the barrier formed by the interface between the media of air and sea water resulted in a "loss" of approximately 99.9% of the sound energy. That is, 99.9% of the energy in the impinging sound wave was reflected away, and only 0.1% was transmitted into the water. This loss amounts to a decrease in sound energy of approximately 30 dB. If the middle ear did not exist, and the membranous entrance of the fluid-filled inner ear (oval window) replaced the eardrum, sound waves carried in air would impinge directly on the fluid-filled inner ear. This barrier is analogous to the air-to-water interface described above. Consequently, if such an arrangement existed, there would be a considerable loss of sound energy.

The middle ear compensates for this loss of sound energy when going from air to a fluid medium through two primary mechanisms. The first of these, the areal ratio (ratio of the areas) of the tympanic membrane to the footplate of the stapes, accounts for the largest portion of the compensation. The effective area of the tympanic membrane (i.e., the area involved directly in the mechanical link between the outer ear and inner ear) is approximately 55 mm^2. The corresponding area of the stapes footplate is 3.2 mm^2. Pressure (p) may be defined in terms of force (F) per unit area (A) ($p = F/A$). If the force applied at the eardrum is the same as that reaching the stapes footplate, then the pressure at the smaller footplate must be greater than that at the larger eardrum. As an analogy, consider water being forced through a hose. If the area of the opening at the far end of the hose is the same as that of the faucet to which it is connected, the water will exit the hose under the same water pressure as it would at the faucet. If a nozzle is now attached to the far end of the hose and it is adjusted to decrease the size of the opening at that end of the hose, the water pressure at that end will be increased in proportion to the degree of constriction produced by the nozzle. The smaller the opening, the greater the water pressure at the nozzle (and the farther the water will be ejected from the nozzle). Applying the same force that exists at the faucet to push the water through a smaller opening created by the nozzle has increased the water pressure at the nozzle.

For the middle ear, given application of equal force at the tympanic membrane and the stapes footplate ($F_1 = F_2$), the pressure at the smaller footplate ($F_1/3.2$) is greater than that at the larger tympanic membrane ($F_2/55$). The ratio of these two areas is 55/3.2, or 17. Consequently, the pressure at the oval window is 17 times greater than that at the tympanic membrane for a given driving force simply because of their difference in area. An increase in sound pressure by a factor of 17 corresponds to a decibel increase of 24.6 dB. Thus, of the approximately 30 dB that would be lost if the air-filled outer ear were linked directly to the fluid-filled inner ear, almost 25 dB is recovered solely because of the areal ratio of the eardrum to the stapes footplate.

The other primary mechanism that might contribute to compensation for the existing impedance mismatch has to do with a complex lever system presumed to exist within the ossicles. The lever is created by the difference in length between the malleus and a portion of the incus known as the long process. This lever factor, however, recovers only approximately 2 dB of the loss due to the impedance mismatch. The assumptions underlying the operation of this lever mechanism, more-over, are not firmly established.

The middle ear system, therefore, compensates for much of the loss of sound energy that would result if the airborne sound waves impinged directly on the fluid-filled inner ear. Approximately 25–27 dB of the estimated 30-dB impedance mis-match has been compensated for by the middle ear. The ability of the middle ear system to amplify or boost the sound pressure depends on signal frequency. Specifically, little pressure amplification occurs for frequencies below 100 Hz or above 2000–2500 Hz. Recall, however, that the outer ear amplified sound energy by 20 dB for frequencies from 2000 to 5000 Hz. Thus, taken together, the portion of the auditory system peripheral to the stapes footplate increases sound pressure by 20–25 dB in a range of approximately 100–5000 Hz. This range of frequencies happens to correspond to the range of frequencies in human speech that are most important for communication.

Another, less obvious function of the middle ear also involves the outer ear/inner ear link formed by the ossicles. Because of the presence of this mechanical link, the preferred pathway for sound vibrations striking the eardrum will be along the chain formed by the three ossicles. Sound energy, therefore, will be routed directly to the oval window. There is another membranous window of the inner ear that also lies along the inner or medial wall of the middle ear cavity. This structure is known as the round window (see Fig. 3.1). For the inner ear to be stimulated appropriately by the vibrations of the sound waves, it is important that the oval window and round window not be displaced in the same direction simultaneously. This situation would arise frequently, however, if the sound wave impinged directly on the medial wall of the middle ear cavity where both the oval window and the round window are located. Thus, routing the vibrations of the eardrum directly to the oval window via the ossicles assures appropriate stimulation of the inner ear.

Finally, we mentioned previously that two tiny muscles are located within the middle ear and make contact with the ossicular chain. These muscles can be made to contract in a variety of situations. Some individuals can contract these muscles volun-tarily. For most individuals, however, the contraction is an involuntary reflex arising either from loud acoustic stimuli or from nonacoustic stimuli (such as a puff of air applied to the eyes, or scratching the skin on the face just in front of the external auditory meatus), or accompanying voluntary movements of the oral musculature, as in chewing, swallowing, or yawning. For acoustic activation, sound levels must gen-erally exceed 85 dB SPL to elicit a reflexive contraction of the middle ear muscles.

The result of middle ear muscle contraction is to compress or stiffen the ossicu-lar chain and to essentially pull the ossicular chain away from the two structures it links, the outer ear and inner ear. This results in an attenuation or decrease of sound pressure reaching the inner ear. The attenuation amounts to 15–20 dB and depends on frequency. Recall from the previous chapter that increases in a system's stiffness have the greatest effect on low-frequency vibrations. Consequently, the attenuation produced by the middle-ear muscles contracting and increasing the stiffness of the ossicles exists only for frequencies below 2000 Hz. The attenuation measured for acoustically elicited contractions, moreover, appears to apply only to stimuli of high intensities. That is, low-level signals such as those near threshold are not attenuated when middle ear muscle contraction is elicited, but high-level signals (> 80 dB SPL) may be attenuated by as much as 15–20 dB. The middle ear reflex is known as a consensual reflex, meaning that when either ear is appropriately stimulated, the muscles contract in both ears.

Inner Ear

The inner ear is a complex structure that resides deep within a very dense portion of the skull known as the petrous portion of the temporal bone. Because of the complexity of this structure, it is often referred to as a labyrinth. The inner ear consists of a bony outer casing, the osseous labyrinth. Within this bony structure is the membranous labyrinth. The osseous labyrinth, as shown in Figure 3.3, can be divided into three major sections: the *semicircular canals* (*superior, lateral, posterior*), the *vestibule,* and the *cochlea.* The first two sections house the sensory organs for the vestibular system. The vestibular system assists in maintaining balance and posture. The focus here, however, will be placed on the remaining portion of the osseous inner ear, the cochlea. It is the cochlea that contains the sensory organ for hearing. The coiled, snail-shaped cochlea has approximately 2¾ turns in human beings. The largest turn is called the basal turn; the smallest turn at the top of the cochlea is referred to as the apical turn. Two additional anatomic landmarks of the inner ear depicted in Figure 3.3 are the *oval window* and the *round window.* Recall that the footplate of the stapes, the medial-most bone of the three ossicles in the middle ear, is attached to the oval window.

The cochlea is cut in cross-section from top (apex) to bottom (base) in Figure 3.4. The winding channel running throughout the bony snail-shaped structure is

FIGURE 3.3.
Illustration of the osseous labyrinth and its landmarks. (Adapted from Durrant JD, Lovrinic JH: *Bases of Hearing Science*, ed 2. Baltimore, Williams & Wilkins, 1984, p 98.)

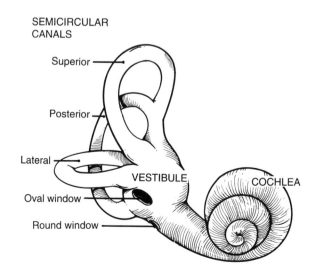

SEMICIRCULAR CANALS
Superior
Posterior
Lateral
Oval window
Round window
VESTIBULE
COCHLEA

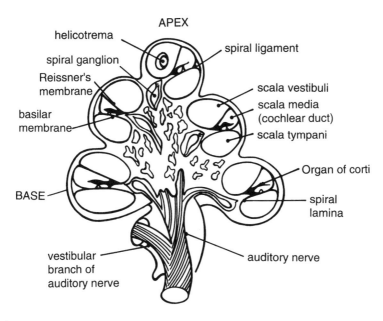

FIGURE 3.4.
Modiolar cross-section of the cochlea illustrating the scalae through each of the turns.
(Adapted from Zemlin WR: *Speech and Hearing Science: Anatomy and Physiology,* ed 2.
Englewood Cliffs, NJ, Prentice-Hall, 1988, p 464.)

seen to be further subdivided into three compartments. The compartment sandwiched between the other two is a cross-section of the membranous labyrinth that runs throughout the osseous labyrinth. All three compartments are filled with fluid. The middle compartment, known as the *scala media,* is filled with a fluid called endolymph. The two adjacent compartments, the *scala vestibuli* and *scala tympani,* contain a different fluid, called perilymph. At the apex of the cochlea is a small hole called the *helicotrema* that connects the two compartments filled with perilymph, the scala tympani and scala vestibuli. The oval window forms an interface between the ossicular chain of the middle ear and the fluid-filled scala vestibuli of the inner ear. When the oval window vibrates as a consequence of vibration of the ossicular chain, a wave is established within the scala vestibuli. Because the fluid-filled compartments are essentially sealed within the osseous labyrinth, the inward displacement of the cochlear fluids at the oval window must be matched by an outward displacement elsewhere. This is accomplished via the round window, which communicates directly with the scala tympani. When the oval window is pushed inward by the stapes, the round window is pushed outward by the increased pressure in the inner ear fluid.

When the stapes footplate rocks back and forth in the oval window, a wave is created within the cochlear fluids. This wave displaces the scala media in a wave-like manner. This displacement pattern is usually simplified by considering the motion of just one of the partitions forming the scala media, the *basilar mem-*

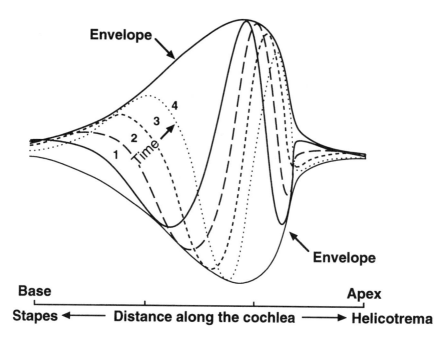

Base **Apex**

Stapes ← **Distance along the cochlea** → **Helicotrema**

Figure 3.5.
Illustration of the traveling wave pattern at four instants in time in response to a mid-frequency sound. The *thin solid lines* connect the maximum and minimum displacements at each location along the cochlea and for each instant in time. These lines represent the envelope of the displacement patterns. (Adapted from von Bekesy G: *Experiments in Hearing.* New York, McGraw-Hill, 1960, p 462.)

brane. The motion depicted for the basilar membrane, however, also occurs for the opposite partition of the scala media, *Reissner's membrane* (Fig. 3.4). Although we will be depicting the displacement pattern of the basilar membrane, the reader should bear in mind that the entire fluid-filled scala media is undergoing similar displacement.

Figure 3.5 illustrates the displacement pattern of the basilar membrane at four successive instants in time. When this displacement pattern is visualized directly, the wave established along the basilar membrane is seen to move or travel from the base to the apex. The displacement pattern increases gradually in amplitude as it progresses from the base toward the apex until it reaches a point of maximum displacement. At that point, the amplitude of displacement decreases abruptly. The *thin solid line* connecting the amplitude peaks at various locations for these four instants in time describes the displacement envelope. The envelope pattern is symmetrical in that the same pattern superimposed on the positive peaks can be flipped upside down and used to describe the negative peaks. As a result, only the positive or upper half of the envelope describing maximum displacement is usually displayed.

Figure 3.6 displays the envelopes of the displacement pattern of the basilar membrane that have been observed for different stimulus frequencies. Note that, as the frequency of the stimulus increases, the peak of the displacement pattern moves

Sound Frequency

25 Hz

50 Hz

100 Hz

200 Hz

400 Hz

800 Hz

1600 Hz

0   10   20   30

Distance from stapes - millimeters

Relative amplitude

FIGURE 3.6.

Envelopes of traveling wave displacement patterns illustrated for different stimulus frequencies. Notice that low frequencies (*top*) produce a maximum displacement of the basilar membrane in the apex (farthest distance from the stapes), whereas higher frequencies (*bottom*) produce maximum displacement in the basal portion of the cochlea (nearer to the stapes). (Adapted from von Bekesy G: *Experiments in Hearing.* New York, McGraw-Hill, 1960, p 448).

in a basal direction closer to the stapes footplate. At low frequencies, virtually the entire membrane undergoes some degree of displacement. As stimulus frequency increases, a more restricted region of the basilar membrane undergoes displacement. Thus, the cochlea is performing a crude frequency analysis of the incoming sound. In general, for all but the very low frequencies (50 Hz), the place of maximum displacement within the cochlea is associated with the frequency of an acoustic stimulus. The frequency of the acoustic stimulus striking the eardrum and displacing the stapes footplate will be analyzed or distinguished from sounds of different frequency by the location of the displacement pattern along the basilar membrane.

Because the pressure wave created within the cochlear fluids originates near the base of the cochlea at the oval window, one might think that this is the reason that the traveling wave displacement pattern appears to move from the base to the apex. On the contrary, experiments with models of the inner ear have shown that the source of vibration (oval window) can be located anywhere along the cochlea, including the apex, with no effect on the displacement pattern of the basilar membrane (Vignette 3.1). The primary physical feature of the inner ear responsible for the direction in which the traveling wave progresses is the stiffness gradient of the basilar membrane. The stiffness of the basilar membrane is greatest in the base and

VIGNETTE 3.1.
Discussion of the traveling-wave paradox.

As mentioned, regardless of where the vibration is introduced into the cochlea, the traveling wave always travels from base to apex. This phenomenon is known as the traveling wave paradox. The early tests of hearing that were routinely performed decades ago with tuning forks made use of this phenomenon. A tuning fork was struck, and the vibrating tongs were placed next to the outer ear. The tester asked the listener to indicate when the tone produced by the vibrating tuning fork could no longer be heard. Immediately after the listener indicated that the sound was no longer audible, the base of the tuning fork was pressed against the bony portion of the skull behind the ear known as the mastoid process. If the listener could now hear the tone again, it was assumed that the hearing sensitivity of the inner ear alone was better than that of the entire peripheral portion of the auditory system as a whole (outer ear, middle ear, and inner ear).

When the base of the tuning fork was placed on the mastoid process, the skull was vibrated. The cochlea is embedded firmly within the temporal bone of the skull, such that skull vibrations produce a mechanical vibration of the inner ear. Even though the vibration is not introduced at the oval window by the vibrating stapes, the tone produced by the tuning fork placed against the skull is still heard as though it were. The traveling wave within the inner ear behaves the same, regardless of where the mechanical vibration is introduced.

For normal listeners, the typical means of stimulating the inner ear is through the outer and middle ears. This is known as air conduction hearing. Sound can also be introduced by vibrating the skull at the mastoid process, forehead, or some other location. This is called bone conduction hearing. Whether the tone is introduced into the inner ear by bone conduction or air conduction, the traveling wave and the resulting sensation are the same.

Modern-day air conduction and bone conduction tests are described in more detail in Chapter 4. They are of great assistance in determining which portion of the peripheral auditory system is impaired in listeners with hearing loss.

---

decreases from the base to the apex. As we saw previously in Chapter 2, stiffness offers greatest opposition to displacement for low-frequency vibrations. Thus, the greater stiffness of the basilar membrane in the basal portion of the cochlea opposes displacement when stimulated by low-frequency sound and forces the wave to travel further up the cochlea toward the apex to a region having less stiffness and less opposition to low-frequency vibration.

A more detailed picture of the structures within the scala media is provided in Figure 3.7. The sensory organ of hearing, the organ of Corti, is seen to rest on top of the basilar membrane. The organ of Corti contains several thousand sensory

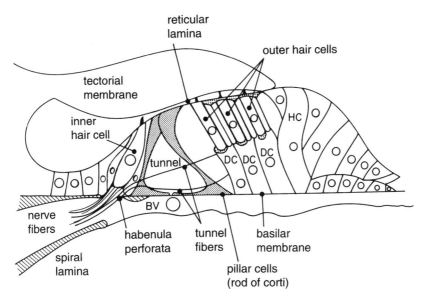

Figure 3.7.
Detailed cross-section of the organ of Corti. *BV*, basilar vessel; *DC*, Deiter cell; *HC*, Hensen cell. (Adapted from Pickles JO: *An Introduction to the Physiology of Hearing*, ed 2. London, Academic Press, 1988, p 29).

receptor cells called *hair cells*. Each hair cell has several tiny hairs or cilia protruding from the top of the cell. As shown in Figure 3.7, there are two types of hair cells within the organ of Corti. The inner hair cells make up a single row of receptors located closest to the modiolus or bony core of the cochlea. The cilia of these cells are free-standing (i.e., they do not make contact with any other structures). Approximately 90–95% of the auditory nerve fibers that carry information to the brain make contact with the inner hair cells. The outer hair cells are much greater in number and are usually organized in three rows. The cilia of the outer hair cells are embedded within a gelatinous structure known as the *tectorial membrane,* draped over the top of the organ of Corti.

Note that the organ of Corti is bordered by two membranes: the basilar membrane below and the tectorial membrane above. The modiolar or medial points of attachment for these two membranes are offset. That is, the tectorial membrane is attached to a structure called the spiral limbus, which is located nearer to the modiolus than the comparable point of attachment for the basilar membrane (a bony structure called the spiral lamina). Figure 3.8 illustrates one of the consequences of these staggered points of attachment. When the basilar membrane is displaced in an upward direction (toward the scala vestibuli), the cilia of the outer hair cells embedded in the tectorial membrane undergo a shearing force in a radial direction (a horizontal direction in the figure). Displacement in a downward direction develops a radial shearing force in the opposite direction. This shearing force is believed to be the trigger that initiates a series of electrical and chemical processes within the

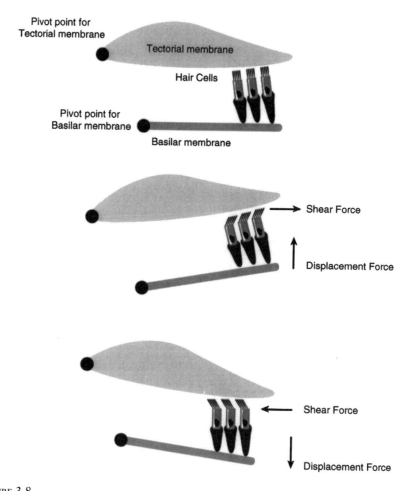

FIGURE 3.8.

Illustration of the mechanism responsible for the generation of shearing forces on the cilia of the outer hair cells. Because the pivot points for the tectorial membrane and basilar membrane, represented in each drawing by the *small black circles,* are offset horizontally, vertical displacement of the basilar membrane creates shearing forces across the cilia in a radial direction (i.e., a push or pull of the cilia in a horizontal, left-to-right direction in the drawings). (Adapted from Zemlin WR: *Speech and Hearing Science: Anatomy and Physiology,* ed 2. Englewood Cliffs, NJ, Prentice-Hall, p 484).

hair cells. This, in turn, leads to the activation of the auditory nerve fibers that are in contact with the base of the hair cell.

A critical element in the conversion of mechanical movements of the basilar membrane to electrical impulses in the auditory nerve is the transduction function served by the inner and outer hair cells in the organ of Corti. The shearing forces applied to the cilia on the tops of these hair cells in response to acoustic stimulation give rise to electrical potentials known generally as receptor potentials. Receptor potentials are common in sensory cells and are only produced in response to a stimulus, unlike resting potentials, which are present in cells at all times in the living organism. Two types of receptor potentials are found in the cochlea: the cochlear microphonic potential and the summating potential. These potentials are generally referred to as gross electrical potentials in that they are measured with electrodes inserted in the cochlea (and sometimes can be recorded from the ear canal) and represent the collective response of hundreds or even thousands of hair cells.

Scientists have been able to record electrical potentials generated by individual hair cells. Again, both resting potentials and receptor potentials have been recorded from individual hair cells. Receptor potentials of single hair cells, referred to as the ac and dc receptor potentials, are somewhat analogous to the grossly recorded cochlear microphonic and summating potentials, respectively. The exact role of the hair cells, their receptor potentials, and the interaction between the two types of hair cells (inner and outer) is unclear. It is clear, however, that damage to the hair cells and the elimination of the receptor potentials produced by the cells greatly diminishes the cochlea's ability to perform a frequency analysis on incoming sounds and reduces the sensory response for sounds of low and moderate intensity.

Some research conducted since the mid-1980s has indicated that the receptor potentials generated by the hair cell trigger mechanical changes in the length of the bodies of the hair cells. When the cilia on the top of the hair cell are sheared in one direction, the receptor potential produced makes the cell body of the hair cell contract. Deflection of the cilia in the opposite direction changes the receptor potential, which causes the cell body of the hair cell to expand or stretch. This expansion and contraction of the hair cells along the length of their cell bodies has been likened to similar events in muscle fibers. Actin, a protein found in muscle fibers that is critical to the fiber's ability to expand and contract, has also been found in hair cells. The net effect of these mechanical changes in the length of the hair cell is to amplify or boost the displacement of the basilar membrane and to create a more vigorous electrical response to the stimulus. The ultimate effect of this elaborate micromechanical system is a much more precise analysis of frequency and a stronger mechanical and electrical response to sounds of low and moderate intensity. Researchers frequently refer to this facilitatory effect of the hair-cell movement as the "cochlear amplifier" because of its enhancement of low- and moderate-intensity sounds.

To understand how changes in the length of the hair cell bodies in response to sound can enhance the basilar membrane's response, consider the following analogy. Imagine that you are bouncing up and down on a large trampoline. You adjust your bounce so that the trampoline is vibrated in an up and down motion with a vertical displacement of 1 foot in each direction. A partner is now positioned beneath the trampoline and is wearing a special helmet, the top of which is attached to the underside of the trampoline's surface at the location corresponding to your point of contact with the trampoline. When your partner squats, the trampoline is pulled down, and when he or she stands, it is returned to a horizontal position. By synchronizing your partner's active vertical movements (using the muscles in his or her legs to alternately squat and stand) with the passive vertical displacement of the trampoline produced by your bouncing, the height of your jump (and the displacement of the trampoline) can be increased or amplified considerably. The trampoline surface is like the basilar membrane, and your partner represents the contracting and expanding hair cell body sandwiched between the basilar membrane and the tectorial membrane. The electrical potentials that perfectly mimic the displacement pattern of the basilar membrane (and the waveform of the sound) keep the two partners synchronized to enhance the vertical displacement. Otherwise, without synchronization, your partner could be pushing upward while you were moving downward on the trampoline and effectively cancel the vertical displacement. Working together, however, the combined efforts of you and your partner produce more activity than you could accomplish by yourself.

If such an active, cochlear amplifier exists, one would expect to be able to measure vibrations coming out of the inner ear when the hair cells have been pushing and pulling on the basilar membrane. Further, if they vibrate the basilar membrane, the oval window and stapes footplate should also vibrate, which should vibrate the rest of the middle-ear ossicles and the eardrum, which, in turn, should produce a measurable sound in the ear canal. In fact, such sounds, known as otoacoustic emissions ("oto" = of the ear, and "acoustic" = sound), have been the focus of an incredible amount of research since their discovery in 1978. They have been measured by placing a tiny microphone deep inside the ear canal.

Otoacoustic emissions, or OAEs, are reviewed in greater detail in the Advanced Material at the end of the chapter. Briefly, there are two general classes of OAEs, spontaneous and evoked. Evoked emissions require a stimulus of some sort to produce them whereas spontaneous emissions simply occur, as the name implies, "spontaneously" (without a stimulus required). Using the preceding trampoline analogy, spontaneous emissions can be thought of as being produced by your partner's continued up and down movement, even when you are no longer on the trampoline. Spontaneous OAEs occur in at least 50% of the normal-hearing young adult population, are more prevalent in females, and are not of much clinical value at present. Evoked OAEs, however, have been demonstrated to be sensitive to damage to the hair cells in the cochlea and are continuing to be explored for clinical uses.

The two primary functions of the auditory portion of the inner ear can be summarized as follows. First, the inner ear performs a frequency analysis on incoming sounds so that different frequencies stimulate different regions of the inner ear. Second, mechanical vibration is amplified and converted into electrical energy by the hair cells. The hair cells are frequently referred to as mechanoelectrical transducers. That is, cells that convert mechanical energy (vibration) into electrical energy (receptor potentials).

Auditory Nerve

The action potentials generated by auditory nerve fibers are called all-or-none potentials. That is, they do not vary in amplitude when activated. If the nerve fibers fire, they always fire to the same degree, reaching 100% amplitude. The action potentials, moreover, are very short-lived events, typically requiring less than 1–2 ms to rise in amplitude to maximum potential and return to resting state. For

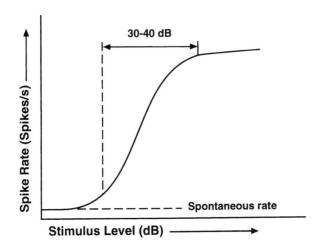

FIGURE 3.9.
An input-output function for a single auditory nerve fiber. As stimulus intensity increases, the firing rate of the nerve fiber increases, but only over a narrow range of 30–40 dB.

this reason, they are frequently referred to as spikes. They can be recorded by inserting a tiny microelectrode into a nerve fiber. When this is done, spikes can be observed even without the presentation of an acoustic stimulus. That is, the nerve fiber has spontaneous activity that consists of random firings of the nerve fiber. The lowest sound intensity that gives rise to a criterion percentage increase (e.g., 20% increase) in the rate at which the fiber is firing is called the threshold for that particular stimulus frequency. As stimulus intensity is raised above threshold, the amplitude of the spikes does not change. They always fire at maximum response. The rate at which the nerve fiber responds, however, does increase with stimulus level. This is illustrated in Figure 3.9, in which an input-output function for a single auditory nerve fiber is displayed. Note that the discharge rate, or *spike rate*, increases steadily with input level above the spontaneous rate until a maximum discharge rate is reached approximately 30–40 dB above threshold. Consequently, a single nerve fiber can code intensity via the discharge rate over only a limited range of intensities. Again, an increase in intensity is encoded by an increase in the firing rate (more spikes per second), not by an increase in the amplitude of the response.

The *solid line* in Figure 3.10 depicts the frequency-threshold curve (FTC) of a single auditory nerve fiber. Combinations of stimulus intensity and frequency lying within the *striped area* bordered by the FTC will cause the nerve fiber to increase its firing rate above the spontaneous rate. Frequency/intensity combinations lying outside this region fail to activate the nerve fiber. The *striped region*, therefore, is frequently referred to as the nerve fiber's response area. (See Vignette 3.2.)

Note that the FTC for the nerve fiber in Figure 3.10 indicates that the nerve fiber responds best to a frequency of 2000 Hz. That is, 2000 Hz is the frequency requiring the least amount of stimulus intensity to evoke a response from the nerve fiber. This frequency is often referred to as the best frequency or characteristic frequency of the nerve fiber. Some nerve fibers have a low characteristic frequency and some have a high characteristic frequency. This is illustrated in the other panels of Figure 3.10.

Figure 3.10.
Frequency-threshold curves (FTCs) for six auditory nerve fibers (*a–f*). The FTC illustrates the intensity required at each frequency to just produce a measurable response in the nerve fiber. The frequency requiring the lowest intensity for a response is known as the "best frequency" or "characteristic frequency." The best frequency for each of the six nerve fibers increases from top (*a*) to the bottom (*f*). The area within each curve, illustrated in *c* by the striped region, represents the response area of the nerve fiber. Any combination of frequency and intensity represented in that area will yield a response from the nerve fiber.

Fibers with high characteristic frequencies come from hair cells in the base of the cochlea, whereas those with low characteristic frequencies supply the apex. As the nerve fibers exit through the bony core of the cochlea, or modiolus, on their way to the brainstem, they maintain an orderly arrangement. The bundle of nerve fibers composing the cochlear branch of the auditory nerve is organized so that fibers with high characteristic frequencies are located around the perimeter, whereas fibers with low characteristic frequencies make up the core of the cochlear nerve. Thus, the auditory nerve is organized, as is the basilar membrane, so that each characteristic frequency corresponds to a place within the nerve bundle. This mapping of frequency of the sound wave to place of maximum activity within an anatomic structure is referred to as *tonotopic organization*. It is a fundamental anatomic property of the auditory system from the cochlea through the auditory cortex.

Vignette 3.2.

Illustration of response area and FTC of nerve fiber.

The frequency-threshold curve, or FTC, of an auditory nerve fiber maps out the response area of the fiber. Combinations of stimulus frequency and intensity falling within the response area produce a response from the nerve fiber, whereas those lying outside this area fail to do so.

The figure illustrates how this area can be mapped out. A series of response histories from an auditory nerve are displayed. The vertical location of these response tracings from the nerve fiber correspond to the level of the sound presented to the ear, as noted along the *y* axis. The lowest tracing, for example, shows the spikes or action potentials (short vertical lines) recorded from this nerve fiber for a sound that had a level of 0 dB SPL as it was increased gradually in frequency from 100 Hz (left-hand portion) to 10,000 Hz (right-hand portion). Notice that only a few spikes occurred during the several seconds required to progress from a sound of 100 Hz to one of 10,000 Hz. This tracing essentially represents the spontaneous activity of the nerve fiber in that the sound was not intense enough to produce a response in the nerve fiber.

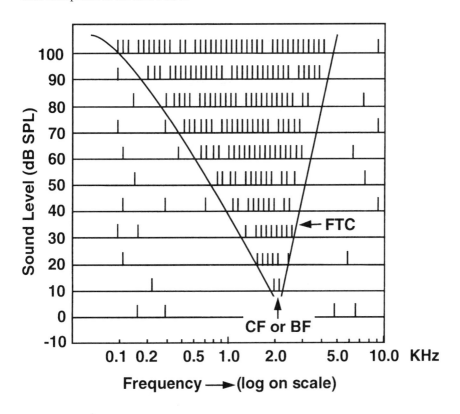

VIGNETTE 3.2.—*continued*

Next, the sound stimulus is increased to 10 dB SPL (second tracing from bottom) and again gradually increased in frequency from 100 to 10,000 Hz. Note now that there is an increase in rate of firing (more vertical lines) near the frequency of 2000 Hz. Thus, this particular nerve fiber appears to respond best (i.e., at the lowest sound intensity) at a frequency of 2000 Hz. This frequency corresponds to this nerve fiber's "best" or "characteristic" frequency (BF or CF).

As the pure tone is increased by another 10 dB to a level of 20 dB SPL, the nerve fiber reveals a broader range of frequencies to which it responds at a rate greater than its spontaneous firing rate. This range now extends from approximately 1500 Hz to 2200 Hz. As we continue to increase the level of the tone in 10-dB steps and sweep the frequency upward from 100 to 10,000 Hz, the frequency range over which the nerve fiber responds continues to broaden. If we were now to draw a line connecting the border between spontaneous activity and increased firing rate at each level to those at adjacent levels, the response area would be defined. This border is essentially the FTC for the nerve fiber. The FTC is sometimes referred to as the "tuning curve" of the nerve fiber because it indicates the frequency to which the nerve fiber is "tuned" (in this case, 2000 Hz). The FTC indicates the response area of the fiber as well as its best frequency. With a best frequency of 2000 Hz, this auditory nerve fiber originated from somewhere in the middle of the cochlea between the high-frequency basal portion and the low-frequency apex.

Temporal or time-domain information is also coded by fibers of the auditory nerve. Consider, for example, the discharge pattern that occurs within a nerve fiber when that stimulus is a sinusoid that lies within the response area of the nerve fiber. The pattern of spikes that occurs under such conditions is illustrated in Figure 3.11. Note that when the single nerve fiber discharges, it always does so at essentially the same location on the stimulus waveform. In Figure 3.11 this happens to be the positive peak of the waveform. Notice also that it may not fire during every cycle of the stimulus waveform. Nonetheless, if one were to record the interval between successive spikes and examine the number of times each interval occurred, a histogram of the results would look like that shown in Figure 3.11. This histogram, known simply as an interval histogram, indicates that the most frequent interspike interval corresponds to the period of the waveform. All other peaks in the histogram occur at integer multiples of the period. Thus, the nerve fiber is able to encode the period of the waveform. This holds true for nerve fibers with characteristic frequencies less than approximately 5000 Hz. As discussed in Chapter 2, if we know the period of a sinusoidal waveform, we know its frequency ($f = 1/T$). Hence, the nerve fibers responding in the manner depicted in Figure 3.11 could code the frequency of the acoustic stimulus according to the timing of discharges. For frequencies up to 5000 Hz, the neural firing is synchronized to the sound stimulus, as in Figure 3.11*A*. By combining synchronized firings for several nerve fibers, it is possible to encode the period of sounds up to 5000 Hz in frequency.

The electrical activity of the auditory nerve can also be recorded from more remote locations. In this case, however, the action potentials are not being measured from single nerve fibers. Recorded electrical activity under these circumstances represents the composite response from a large number of nerve fibers. For this reason, this composite electrical response is referred to frequently as the whole-nerve action poten-

FIGURE 3.11.

A, Illustration of the synchronization of nerve fiber firings to the stimulus waveform. Note that the nerve fiber always fires at the same point of the waveform, although it may not fire every cycle. The intervals between successive firings of the nerve fiber can be measured and stored for later analysis. *B*, A histogram of the intervals measured in *A*, referred to as interspike intervals. An interval of 1 ms was the most frequently occurring interval, having occurred about 180 times. This corresponds to the period of the waveform in *A*.

tial. The whole-nerve action potential can be recorded in human subjects from the ear canal or from the medial wall of the middle ear cavity by placing a needle electrode through the eardrum (with local anesthesia applied, of course!). Because the whole-nerve action potential represents the summed activity of several nerve fibers, the more fibers can be made to fire simultaneously, the greater the amplitude of the response. For this reason, brief abrupt acoustic signals, such as clicks or short-duration pure tones, are used as stimuli. Recall, however, that the traveling wave begins in the base and travels toward the apex. It takes roughly 2–4 ms for the traveling wave to travel the full length of the cochlea from the base to apex. Even for abrupt stimuli, such as clicks, the nerve fibers are not triggered simultaneously throughout the cochlea. Fibers associated with the basal high-frequency region respond synchronously to the stimulus presentation. Those fibers originating further up the cochlea will fire later (up to 2–4 ms later). Those firing in synchrony will provide the largest contribution to the whole-nerve action potential. Consequently, the whole-nerve action potential does not represent the activity of the entire nerve but reflects primarily the response of the synchronous high-frequency fibers associated with the base of the cochlea.

The input-output function for the whole-nerve action potential differs considerably from that described previously for single nerve fibers. For the whole-nerve action potential, the response is measured in terms of its amplitude or latency, not its spike rate. The input-output function of the whole-nerve action potential shows a steady increase in amplitude with increase in stimulus level. This is illustrated in Figure 3.12. Also shown is a plot of the latency of the response as a function of stimulus intensity. Latency refers to the interval between stimulus onset and the onset of the neural response. Note that, as stimulus intensity is increased, the latency of the response decreases. Thus, as response amplitude increases with intensity, response latency decreases. The plot of response latency as a function of stimulus intensity is called a latency-intensity function. The latency-intensity function is of primary importance in clinical electrophysiologic assessment of auditory function.

FIGURE 3.12.
Amplitude-intensity (left ordinate) and latency-intensity (right ordinate) functions for the whole-nerve action potential. As intensity increases, the amplitude (Amp) of the action potential increases and the latency (Lat) of the response decreases.

AUDITORY CENTRAL NERVOUS SYSTEM

Once the action potentials have been generated in the cochlear branch of the auditory nerve, the electrical activity progresses up toward the cortex. This network of nerve fibers is frequently referred to as the auditory central nervous system (auditory CNS). The nerve fibers that carry information in the form of action potentials up the auditory CNS toward the cortex form part of the ascending or afferent pathways. Nerve impulses can also be sent toward the periphery from the cortex or brainstem centers. The fibers carrying such information compose the descending or efferent pathways.

Figure 3.13 is a simplified schematic diagram of the ascending auditory CNS. All nerve fibers from the cochlea terminate at the cochlear nucleus on the same side. From here, however, several possible paths are available. The majority of nerve fibers cross over or decussate at some point along the auditory CNS, so that the activity of the right ear is represented most strongly on the left side of the cortex and vice versa. The crossover, however, is not complete. From the superior olives through the cortex, activity from both ears is represented on each side. All ascending fibers terminate in the medial geniculate body before ascending to the cortex. Thus, all ascending fibers within the brainstem portion of the auditory CNS synapse at the cochlear nucleus and at the medial geniculate body, taking one of several paths between these two points, with many paths having additional inter-

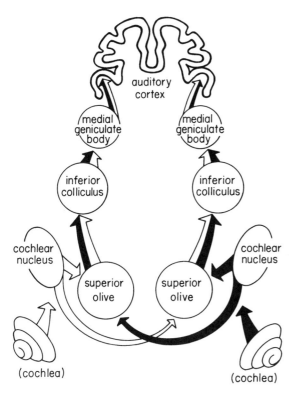

FIGURE 3.13.
The ascending pathways of the auditory central nervous system. The *black arrows* represent input from the right ear; the *white arrows* represent input from the left ear. (Adapted from Yost WA, Nielsen DW: *Fundamentals of Hearing: An Introduction*, ed 2. New York, Holt, Rinehart, & Winston, 1985, p 98.)

vening nerve fibers. Vignette 3.3 describes measurement of the auditory brainstem response and its correlation with anatomic structure.

We have already reviewed the simple coding of information available in the responses of the auditory nerve fibers. The mapping of frequency to place within the cochlea, for example, was seen to be preserved in the responses of the nerve fibers in that fibers having high characteristic frequencies originated from the high-frequency base of the cochlea. The period of the waveform could also be coded for stimulus frequencies less than 5000 Hz. In addition, the intensity of the stimulus was coded over a limited range (30–40 dB) by the discharge rate of the fiber. At the level of the cochlear nucleus, it is already apparent that the ascending auditory pathway begins processing information by converting this fairly simple code into more complex codes. The coding of timing information, for example, is much more

---

Vignette 3.3.
Auditory brainstem response measurements.

It was mentioned earlier that the whole-nerve action potential represented the summed response of many single nerve fibers firing synchronously in response to an abrupt acoustic signal. It was also mentioned that this potential can be recorded remotely from the ear canal. The left-hand portion of the drawing that accompanies this vignette shows a patient with electrodes pasted to the skin of the forehead, the top of the head (vertex), and the area behind the pinna (the mastoid prominence). The tracing in the right-hand portion of this illustration shows the electrical activity recorded from the patient. The acoustic stimulus is a brief click that produces synchronized responses from nerve fibers in the cochlea and the brainstem portion of the auditory CNS. The tracing represents the average of 2000 stimulus presentations presented at a moderate intensity at a rate of 11 clicks per second. Approximately 3 min is required to present all 2000 stimuli and to obtain the average response shown above. Note that the time scale for the x axis of the tracing spans from 0 to 10 ms. This represents a 10-ms interval beginning with the onset of the click stimulus. The tracing shows several distinct bumps or waves, with the first appearing at about 1.5 ms after stimulus onset. This first wave, labeled *I*, is believed to be a remote recording of the whole-nerve action potential from the closest portion of the auditory nerve. Approximately 1 ms later, 2.5 ms after stimulus onset, wave *II* is observed. This wave is believed to be the response of the more distant portion of the auditory nerve. One millisecond later the electrical activity has traveled to the next center in the brainstem, the cochlear nucleus, and produces the response recorded as wave *III*. Wave *IV* represents the activity of the superior olivary complex. Wave *V* represents the response of the lateral lemniscus, a structure lying between the superior olives and the inferior colliculus. Waves *VI* and *VII* (the two unlabeled bumps after wave *V*) represent the response of the latter brainstem structure.

VIGNETTE 3.3.—*continued*

The response shown in the right-hand tracing is known as an auditory brainstem response (ABR). It has proven very useful in a wide variety of clinical applications, from assessment of the functional integrity of the peripheral and brainstem portions of the ascending auditory CNS to assessment of hearing in infants or difficult-to-test patients. Additional related information may be found in the Advanced Material at the end of this chapter.

complex in the cochlear nucleus. In addition, some nerve fibers within the cochlear nucleus have a much broader range of intensities (up to 100 dB) over which the discharge rate increases steadily with sound intensity. As one probes nerve fibers at various centers within the auditory CNS, a tremendous diversity of responses is evident.

Despite this increasing anatomic and physiologic complexity, one thing that appears to be preserved throughout the auditory CNS is tonotopic organization. At each brainstem center and within the auditory portions of the cortex, there is an orderly mapping of frequency to place. This can be demonstrated by measuring the characteristic frequency of nerve fibers encountered at various locations within a given brainstem center or within the cortex.

Another principle underlying the auditory CNS is that of redundancy. That is, information represented in the neural code from one ear has multiple representations at various locations within the auditory system. Every auditory nerve fiber, for example, splits into two fibers before entering the cochlear nucleus, with each branch supplying a different region of the cochlear nucleus. In addition, from the superior olives through the auditory areas of the cortex, information from both ears is represented at each location in the auditory CNS.

Our knowledge of the ascending pathway of the auditory CNS is far from complete. We know even less, however, about the descending pathways. This is due, in part, to the small number of efferent nerve fibers involved in this pathway. There are about two descending efferent fibers for every 100 ascending afferent nerve fibers. Essentially the same brainstem centers are involved in the descending pathway as were involved in the ascending path, although an entirely separate set of nerve fibers is used. The last fiber in this descending pathway runs from the superior olivary complex to enter the cochlea on the same side or the cochlea on the opposite side. These fibers are referred to as either the crossed or the uncrossed olivocochlear bundles. The vast majority (60–80%) of these fibers cross over from the superior olivary complex on one side to the cochlea on the other side and innervate the outer hair cells. The remaining fibers make up the uncrossed bundle and appear to innervate the inner hair cells.

All descending fibers do not terminate at the cochlear nerve fibers. Descending fibers may modify incoming neurally coded sensory information at any of the centers along the auditory CNS. In addition, they may either facilitate or inhibit responses along the ascending auditory pathway. That is, electrical stimulation of some descending fibers increases the discharges recorded from fibers at lower centers, whereas stimulation of other descending fibers results in decreased activity at lower centers. Thus, the descending efferent system regulates, modifies, and shapes the incoming sensory information.

Reflexive contractions of the middle ear muscles due to the presentation of a sound stimulus may also be considered a regulating mechanism for the incoming sensory information. The reflex pathway is illustrated schematically in Figure 3.14. Incoming sensory information enters through the peripheral auditory system and ascends to the superior olive. If the sound is sufficiently intense, descending infor-

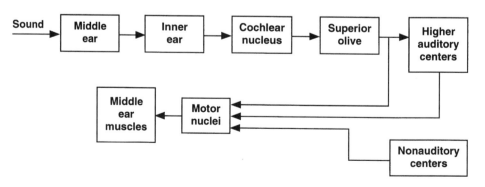

FIGURE 3.14.
The reflex arc for the middle-ear muscle reflex.

mation is routed to motor nuclei that control the contraction of the middle ear muscles. This explains why the reflexive contraction of middle ear muscles due to sound stimuli is a consensual phenomenon, as mentioned previously. Information from the cochlear nucleus goes to both superior olives, so that sound stimulation on one side yields middle ear muscle contraction on both sides.

PERCEPTION OF SOUND

The basic structure and some key aspects of the physiologic function of the auditory system have been reviewed; the remainder of this chapter reviews some fundamental aspects of the perception of sound by humans. We have examined the acoustics involved in the generation and propagation of a sound wave and have reviewed its conversion into a complex neural code. This code of incoming sensory information can influence the behavior of a human subject, whether the sound is the loud whistle of an oncoming train or the cry of a hungry infant. The study of behavioral responses to acoustic stimulation is referred to as psychoacoustics.

Psychoacoustics

Psychoacoustics is the study of the relationship between the sound stimulus and the behavioral response it produces in the subject. We have already discussed how the important parameters of the acoustic stimulus can be measured. Much of psychoacoustics concerns itself with the more challenging task of appropriately measuring the listener's response. Two primary means have evolved through which the psychoacoustician measures responses from the listener. The first, known generally as the discrimination procedure, is used to assess the smallest difference that would allow a listener to discriminate between two stimulus conditions. The end result is an estimate of a threshold of a certain type. A tone of specified amplitude, frequency, and starting phase, for example, can be discriminated from the absence of such a signal. In this particular case, one is measuring the absolute threshold for hearing. That is, the absolute threshold is a statistical concept that represents the lowest sound pressure level at which the tone can be heard a certain percentage of the time. This threshold is often referred to as a detection threshold, because one is determining the stimulus parameters required to just detect the presence of a signal.

Discrimination procedures have also been used to measure difference thresholds. A difference threshold is a statistical concept that indicates the smallest change in a stimulus that can be just detected by the listener. A standard sound that is fixed in intensity, frequency, starting phase, and duration is employed. A comparison stimulus that differs typically in one of these stimulus parameters is then presented. The difference threshold indicates how much the comparison stimulus must differ from the standard signal to permit detection of the difference by the listener a certain percentage of the time.

Many of the discrimination procedures used to measure absolute and difference thresholds were developed over a century ago. Three such procedures, referred to as the classic psychophysical methods, are (*a*) the method of limits, (*b*) the method of adjustment, and (*c*) the method of constant stimuli. Research conducted in more recent years has resulted in two important developments regarding the use of these procedures. First, it was recognized that thresholds measured with these procedures were not uncontaminated estimates of sensory function. Rather, thresholds measured with these procedures could be altered considerably by biasing the subject through various means, such as the use of different sets of instructions or different schedules of reinforcement for correct and incorrect responses. The threshold for the detection of a low-intensity pure tone, for example, can be changed by instructing the listener to be very certain that a tone was heard before responding accordingly, or by encouraging the listener to guess when uncertain. The magnitude of sensation evoked within the sensory system during stimulus presentation should remain unchanged under these manipulations. Yet the threshold was noticeably affected. Threshold as measured with any of these classic procedures is affected by factors other than the magnitude of sensation evoked by the signal. For the audiologist, however, the classic psychophysical procedures have proved to be valid and reliable tools with which to measure various aspects of hearing in clinical settings as long as care is used in instructing the listeners and administering the procedures.

The second recent development that led to a modification of the classic psychophysical procedures was the creation of adaptive test procedures. The current procedure advocated for the measurement of absolute threshold of hearing (discussed in Chapter 4) uses an adaptive modification of the method of limits. Adaptive procedures increase the efficiency of the paradigm without sacrificing the accuracy or reliability of the procedure.

In addition to discrimination procedures, a second class of techniques has been developed to quantify a subject's responses to acoustic signals. These procedures, known generally as scaling techniques, attempt to measure sensation directly. In the study of hearing, they are used most frequently to measure the sensation of loudness, though they have also been used to quantify other sensations, such as pitch. The results from one of these procedures, magnitude estimation, are shown in Figure 3.15. In the magnitude estimation technique, subjects simply assign numbers to the perceived loudness of a series of stimuli. In the case shown in Figure 3.15, the stimuli differed only in intensity. The average results fall along a straight line when plotted on log-log coordinates. Both the *x* axis and the *y* axis in Figure 3.15 are logarithmic. Recall that the decibel scale, the *x* axis in this figure, involved the logarithm of a pressure ratio—that is, SPL in dB = 20 log (p_1/p_2). Comparable results have been obtained for other sensations, such as brightness, vibration on the fingertip, and electric shock. In all cases, a straight line fits the average data very well when plotted on log-log coordinates. From these extensive data, a law was developed that relates the perceived magnitude of sensation (S) to the physical intensity of the stimulus (I) in the following manner: $S = kI^x$, where k is an arbitrary constant and x is an exponent that varies with the sensation under investigation. This law is

FIGURE 3.15.
Hypothetical results from a magnitude estimation experiment in which the perceived loudness was measured for various sound levels. Note that the results fall along a straight line when both axes are logarithmic (recall that the decibel scale incorporates logarithms in the calculation of decibels).

known as Stevens' power law in honor of the scientist S. S. Stevens, who discovered and developed it. A convenient feature of a power function plotted on log-log coordinates is that the slope of the line fit to the data is the exponent, x.

Finally, a procedure that has been used extensively in psychoacoustics to measure auditory sensations via the subject's response is the matching procedure. The matching procedure is a cross between discrimination procedures and scaling procedures in that the technique is similar to that of the method of adjustment (one of the classic psychophysical methods) but its goal is to quantify a subjective attribute of sound, such as loudness or pitch. The matching procedures enable the experimenter to determine a set of stimulus parameters that all yield the same subjective sensation. A pure tone fixed at 1000 Hz and 70 dB SPL, for example, may be presented to one ear of a listener and a second pure tone of 8000 Hz presented to the other ear in an alternating fashion. The subject controls the intensity of the 8000-Hz tone until it is judged to be equal in loudness to the 1000-Hz, 70-dB SPL reference tone. Data in the literature indicate that the 8000-Hz tone would have to be set to 80–85 dB SPL to achieve a loudness match in the case presented above.

Hearing Threshold

Let us now examine how these procedures have been applied to the study of the perception of sound. The results obtained from the measurement of hearing thresholds at various frequencies are depicted in Figure 3.16. Note that the sound pressure level that is just detectable varies with frequency, especially below 500 Hz and above 8000 Hz. The slope of the function in the low frequencies is due to the attenuation of lower frequencies by the middle ear. It is apparent that the frequency contour of the hearing threshold has a minimum in the 2000- to 4000-Hz range. This is attributable, in large part, to the amplification of signals in this frequency range by the outer ear, as discussed earlier in this chapter. The range of audibility of the normal-hearing human ear is described frequently as 20–20,000 Hz. That is,

Figure 3.16.
Average normal threshold sound pressure level plotted as a function of frequency for binaural (two-ear) listening in a free field. (Adapted from Sivian LJ, White SD: Minimum audible pressure and minimum audible field. *Journal of the Acoustical Society of America* 4:288–321, 1933.)

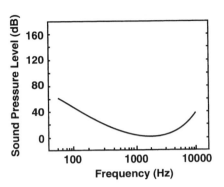

acoustic signals at frequencies above or below this range typically cannot be heard by the normal human ear.

Masking

The phenomenon of masking has also been studied in detail. Masking refers to the ability of one acoustic signal to obscure the presence of another acoustic signal so that it cannot be detected. A whisper might be audible, for example, in a quiet environment. In a noisy industrial environment, however, such a weak acoustic signal would be masked by the more intense factory noise.

The masking of pure tone signals by noise has been studied extensively. To consider the results that have been obtained, however, we must first examine some important acoustic characteristics of the masking noise. Briefly, there are two measures of intensity that can be used to describe the level of a noise. These two measures are the total power (TP) and the noise power per unit (1-Hz) bandwidth, or spectral density (N_o). The TP in dB SPL is the quantity measured by most measuring devices, such as sound level meters. The N_o of the noise, on the other hand, is not measured directly. Rather, it is calculated from the following equation: $10 \log_{10} N_o = 10 \log_{10} TP - 10 \log_{10} BW$, where BW is the bandwidth of the noise in Hertz. The quantity $10 \log_{10} N_o$ is the spectrum level in units of dB SPL/Hz and represents the average noise power in a 1-Hz band. For broad-band noises, the spectrum level determines the masking produced at various frequencies.

Figure 3.17 illustrates data obtained from one of the early studies of masking produced by broad-band noise. These data have been replicated several times since. The lowest curve in this figure depicts the threshold in a quiet environment; all other curves represent masked thresholds obtained for various levels of the noise masker. These levels are expressed as the spectrum level of the masker. Note that the lowest noise levels are not effective maskers at low frequencies. That is, hearing thresholds measured for low-frequency pure tones in the presence of a broad-band noise having $N_o = 0$ dB SPL/Hz are the same as thresholds in quiet. At all frequencies, however, once the noise begins to produce some masking, a 10-dB increase in noise intensity produces a 10-dB increase in masked threshold for the pure tone. Once the noise

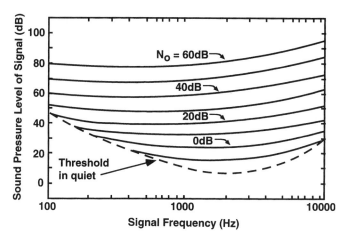

FIGURE 3.17.
Threshold in quiet and masked threshold for various noise spectrum levels (*No*). Threshold was measured at several frequencies in the presence of a broad-band noise. (Adapted from Hawkins JE Jr, Stevens SS: The masking of pure tones and of speech by white noise. *Journal of the Acoustical Society of America* 22:6–13, 1950.)

level that just begins to produce masking is determined, the desired amount of masking can be produced by simply increasing the noise level by a corresponding amount.

How might the masking produced by a noise be affected by decreasing the bandwidth of the noise? Figure 3.18 illustrates data obtained several decades ago from a now classic masking experiment. The results of this experiment, referred to frequently as the "band-narrowing" experiment, have also been replicated several

FIGURE 3.18.
Results from a band-narrowing experiment. Data for two frequencies, 1000 and 4000 Hz, are shown. The critical bandwidths at each frequency are illustrated by *dashed vertical lines*. Note that for bandwidths greater than the critical bandwidth (*CBW*), masking remained unchanged. (Data from Fletcher H: Auditory patterns. *Reviews of Modern Physics* 12:47–65, 1940.)

times since. Masked threshold in dB SPL is plotted as a function of the bandwidth of the masker in Hertz. Results for two different pure-tone frequencies are shown. The *unfilled circles* represent data for a 1000-Hz pure tone, and the *filled circles* depict data for a 4000-Hz pure tone. When the band of masking noise was narrowed, the tone was kept in the center of the noise, and the spectrum level of the noise was held constant. For both frequencies, the masked threshold remains the same as the bandwidth decreases, down to a bandwidth called the critical bandwidth. Continued decreases in bandwidth beyond the critical bandwidth reduce the masking produced by the noise, as reflected in the decrease in masked threshold.

The critical bandwidth, first derived from the band-narrowing masking experiment, has proven to be a concept that applies to a wide variety of psychoacoustic phenomena. For the audiologist, however, one of the most important implications drawn from the band-narrowing experiment just described is that a band of noise having a bandwidth just exceeding the critical bandwidth is as effective a masker for a pure tone centered in the noise as a broad-band noise of the same spectrum level. As we will see in the next chapter, the audiologist frequently needs to introduce masking into a patient's ear. A broad-band masking noise can be uncomfortably loud to a patient. The loudness of the noise, however, can be reduced by decreasing the bandwidth of the noise while maintaining the same spectrum level. A masking noise having a bandwidth only slightly greater than the critical bandwidth will be just as effective as broad-band noise in terms of its masking, but much less loud. The narrower band of noise would be more appropriate for use as a masking sound with patients because of its reduced loudness but equal masking capability.

Loudness

Loudness is another psychoacoustic phenomenon that has been studied extensively. The effects of signal bandwidth on loudness, alluded to in the discussion of masking, for instance, have been investigated in detail. Basically, as the bandwidth of the stimulus increases beyond the critical bandwidth, an increasing number of adjacent critical bands are stimulated, resulting in an increase in loudness. Thus, broad-band signals are louder than narrow-band signals at the same spectrum level.

For pure tones, loudness also varies with frequency. This has been established using the matching procedure described previously. Figure 3.19 depicts so-called equal-loudness contours that have been derived with this technique. A given contour displays the sound pressure levels at various frequencies that are required so as to match the loudness of a 1000-Hz pure tone at the level indicated by the contour. For example, note that on the curve labeled *20*, the function coincides with a sound pressure level of 20 dB SPL at 1000 Hz, whereas on the curve labeled *60*, the function corresponds to 60 dB SPL at 1000 Hz. The contour labeled *60* indicates those combinations of frequencies and intensities that were matched in loudness to a 60-dB SPL, 1000-Hz pure tone. All combinations of stimulus intensity and frequency lying along that contour are said to have a loudness level of 60 phons (correctly pronounced "phones" as in "telephones"). Thus, a 125-Hz pure tone at 70 dB SPL

FIGURE 3.19.

Equal-loudness contours. Each curve displays the combinations of frequency and intensity judged to be equal in loudness to a 1000-Hz tone having a sound pressure level as indicated above each contour. Point *A*, for example, indicates that a 125-Hz tone at 75 dB SPL is as loud as a 1000-Hz tone at 60 dB. (Note that frequency scale is logarithmic.) *MAF*, minimum audible field, or the threshold contour for free-field testing. (Adapted from Fletcher H, Munson WN: Loudness, its definition, measurement, and calculation. *Journal of the Acoustical Society of America* 5:82–108, 1933.)

(point labeled *A* in Fig. 3.19) and an 8000-Hz tone at 58 dB SPL (point labeled *B*) are equivalent in loudness to a 60-dB SPL, 1000-Hz pure tone. All three of those stimuli have a loudness level of 60 phons.

Notice in Figure 3.19 that stimulus intensity must be increased by 110 dB in order to go from a loudness level of 10 phons (threshold) to 120 phons at 1000 Hz. At 100 Hz, only an 80-dB increase is required to span that same change in loudness. From this we can conclude that loudness increases more rapidly at low frequencies than at intermediate frequencies. It took only an 80-dB increase in sound level to go from a sound that was just audible (10 phons) to one that was uncomfortably loud (120 phons) at 100 Hz, whereas an increase of 110 dB was needed to cover this same range of loudness at 1000 Hz.

Another scale of loudness that has been developed is the sone scale. The sone scale is derived by first defining the loudness of a 1000-Hz, 40-dB SPL pure tone as 1 sone. Next, the listener is asked to set the intensity of a second, comparison stimulus so that it produces a loudness sensation either one-half or twice that of the 1-sone standard stimulus. These intensities define the sound levels associated with $^1/_2$

FIGURE 3.20.

The growth of loudness with intensity in quiet (A) and in the presence of a background noise that produced 40 dB of masking (B). (Note that loudness scale is logarithmic.) Functions comparable to B are also obtained in hearing-impaired listeners who have sensorineural hearing loss.

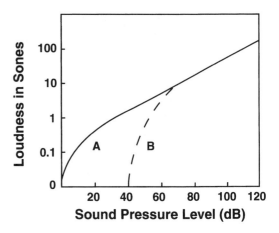

and 2 sones, respectively. This procedure is then repeated, with the sound having a loudness of either $\frac{1}{2}$ or 2 sones serving as the new standard signal. Figure 3.20 illustrates the relationship between the increase of loudness in sones and the increase in sound intensity. Consistent with Stevens' law, described previously, we find that the loudness-growth function is a straight line, with the exception of intensities near threshold, when plotted on log-log coordinates. The slope of this line is 0.6, indicating that Stevens' law for loudness is: $L = kP^{0.6}$, where L is loudness, k is a constant, and P is sound pressure. Note that over the linear range of the function in Figure 3.20, a 10-dB increase in sound pressure level yields a doubling of loudness. That is, at 1000 Hz, an increase in sound pressure level from 40 to 50 dB SPL or from 80 to 90 dB SPL corresponds to a doubling of loudness.

The *dashed line* in Figure 3.20 illustrates a loudness-growth function obtained at 1000 Hz in the presence of a broad-band masking noise. The intersection of the *x* axis by the *dashed line* at 40 dB SPL indicates that the threshold has been elevated 40 dB (from 0 to 40 dB SPL) because of the masking noise. As intensity is increased slightly above threshold, comparison of the two functions indicates that the loudness of a 50-dB SPL tone is greater in the quiet condition (2 sones) than in the masked condition (0.2 sones). At higher intensities, however, the two functions merge, so that an 80-dB SPL tone has a loudness of 16 sones in both cases. Thus, in the masked condition, loudness grows very rapidly to "catch up" with the loudness perceived in the unmasked condition. This rapid growth of loudness is also a characteristic of ears that have a type of hearing loss known as sensorineural hearing loss, which affects the hair cells within the cochlea. The rapid growth of loudness in ears with sensorineural hearing loss is known as loudness recruitment. Its presence helps signify that the hearing loss is caused by pathology within the cochlea. Unfortunately, loudness recruitment presents the audiologist with considerable difficulties in attempting to fit affected patients with amplification devices, such as hearing aids. Low-level sounds must be amplified a specified amount to make them audible to the hearing-impaired listener. If high-level sounds are amplified by the same amount, however, they are uncomfortably loud, just as they would be in a normal ear.

Binaural Hearing

The final section of this chapter deals with the manner in which the information encoded by one ear interacts with that encoded by the other ear. The processing of sound by two ears is referred to as binaural hearing.

The localization of sound in space, for instance, is largely a binaural phenomenon. A sound originating on the right side of a listener, for example, will arrive first at the right ear because it is closer to the sound source. A short time later, the sound will reach the more distant left ear. This produces an interaural (between-ear) difference in the time of arrival of the sound at the two ears. The ear being stimulated first will signal the direction from which the sound arose. As might be expected, the magnitude of this interaural time difference will increase as the location of the sound source changes from straight ahead (called 0° azimuth) to straight out to the side (90° or 270° azimuth). As shown in Figure 3.21A, when the sound originates directly in front of the listener, the length of the path to both ears is the same, and there is no interaural difference in time of arrival of the sound. At the extreme right or left, however, the difference between the length of the path to the near ear and the length of the path to the far ear is greatest (and corresponds to the width of the head). This then will produce the maximum interaural time difference. Figure 3.21B illustrates the dependence of the interaural time difference on the azimuth of the sound source.

For frequencies below approximately 1500 Hz, the interaural time difference could also be encoded meaningfully into an interaural phase difference. From Figure 3.21B, for example, we see that a 60° azimuth results in an interaural time difference of approximately 0.5 ms. This would occur for all frequencies. For a pure tone that completes 1 cycle in 1 ms (frequency = 1000 Hz), this means that the signal to the far ear would be starting 0.5 cycles after the signal to the near ear. The two signals, therefore, would have a 180° phase difference between the two ears. A pure tone of 500 Hz having a 2-ms period and originating from 60° azimuth, however, would only be delayed one-fourth of the period (0.5 ms/2.0 ms), corresponding to a 90° interaural phase difference. We see that, although interaural time differences are the same for all frequencies, the interaural phase differences resulting from these time differences vary with frequency.

Interaural intensity differences are also produced when a sound originates from a location in space. These differences result from a sound shadow being cast by the head. Recall from Chapter 2 that, when the wavelength of the sound is small relative to the dimensions of the object, a sound shadow is produced. The magnitude of the sound shadow created by the head increases with frequency above 500 Hz. It produces interaural intensity differences of 20 dB at 6000 Hz for 90° or 270° azimuth. That is, the intensity of a 6000-Hz pure tone at the near ear is 20 dB greater than that measured at the far ear when the sound originates straight to the side of the listener (90° or 270° azimuth). At 500 Hz, the maximum interaural intensity difference is less than 4 dB. The interaural intensity difference decreases to 0 dB at all frequencies for 0° azimuth (straight ahead).

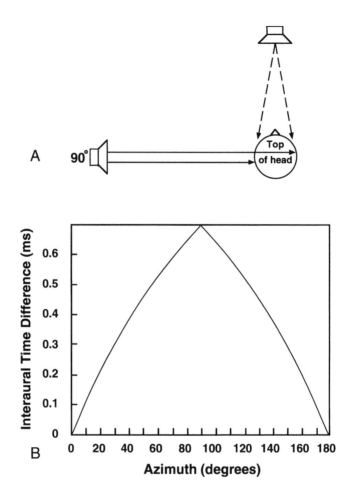

FIGURE 3.21.
A, Path lengths from sound source to the left and right ears for 0° azimuth (*dashed lines*) and 90° azimuth (*solid lines*). B, The interaural (between-ear) time differences as a function of azimuth for the spherical head assumed in A. At 0° and 180°, the sound arrives at the left and right ears simultaneously, resulting in no interaural time difference. The maximum interaural time difference occurs at 90°.

    Thus, there are two primary acoustic cues for the localization of sound in space (specifically, the horizontal plane): interaural time differences and interaural intensity differences. The duplex theory of sound localization in the horizontal plane (left to right) maintains that both cues may be used over a wide range of frequencies by the listener in identifying the location of a sound source, but that interaural time differences predominate at low frequencies and interaural intensity differences predominate at high frequencies. In contemporary theories of sound localization, several additional monaural and binaural cues are included, but interaural time and intensity differences are considered the strongest cues.

Masking is a topic that has also been explored in considerable detail in the bin-aural system. Experiments conducted in the late 1940s and the 1950s indicated that certain combinations of binaural signals and maskers could make the signal more detectable than others. Consider the following example. A noise masker and a pure-tone signal are presented equally and identically to both ears. The signal threshold is then determined—that is, we determine the sound level of the signal required to make it just heard in the presence of the noise. Then the pure-tone sig-nal is removed from one ear, and the signal becomes easier to detect! This release from masking has been named the masking level difference (MLD) and corresponds to the change in threshold between two test conditions. The initial or reference threshold is usually determined for identical maskers and signals delivered to both ears. This is referred to as a diotic condition. Diotic stimulus presentations are those that deliver identical stimuli to both ears. Sometimes the reference threshold involves a masker and signal delivered to only one ear. This is called a monotic condition. After establishing the masked threshold in one of these reference condi-tions, the signal threshold is measured again under any one of several dichotic con-ditions. A dichotic test condition is one in which different stimuli are presented to the two ears. In the example described above, in which the signal was removed from one ear, the removal of the signal made that condition a dichotic one. That is, one ear received the masker and the pure-tone signal, while the other received only the masker. In general, a signal is more readily detected under dichotic masking conditions than under diotic or monotic masking conditions. For a given dichotic condition, the MLD is greatest at low frequencies (100–500 Hz), increases with the intensity of the masker, and is typically 12–15 dB under optimal stimulus condi-tions.

SUMMARY

In this chapter, we have reviewed the structure and function of the auditory system. The anatomy and physiology of the auditory system were discussed in the first portion. The amplification and impedance-matching functions of the outer and middle ear were reviewed. The importance of both a temporal or timing code and a place code (tonotopic organization) within the auditory system was emphasized. Perceptual phenomena, such as loudness and masking, were also reviewed, with an emphasis on those features of clinical relevance.

ADVANCED MATERIAL

More on Anatomy

Earlier in this chapter, the anatomy of the auditory system was overviewed from the outer ear through the auditory cortex. In this section, the anatomy is reviewed in more detail, beginning with the most peripheral structure, the outer ear.

Figure 3.22 is a detailed drawing of the right pinna of a normal adult. This cartilaginous structure has several noteworthy anatomic landmarks. First, the bowl-shaped depression in the middle is the concha, which terminates at its medial end at the entrance to the ear canal (the external auditory meatus). Along the anterior-inferior (front-lower) portion of the concha are two cartilaginous protuberances known as the tragus and antitragus, which are separated, as shown in the figure, by the intertragal notch. The posterior and superior (rear and upper) borders of the concha are formed by a cartilaginous ridge known as the antihelix, which is closely paralleled along the posterior edge of the pinna by the helix. Notice that the helix and antihelix diverge in the superior portion of the pinna and then converge again as they progress anteriorly and inferiorly. The slight depression formed between the helix and antihelix in the anterior superior portion of the pinna is referred to as the triangular fossa.

Medial to the external auditory meatus is the ear canal. The lateral two-thirds of the ear canal are cartilaginous with the medial one-third composed of bone (osseous portion). An epithelium (skin) covering over the cartilaginous and osseous portions of the ear canal is contiguous with the tympanic membrane or eardrum. That is, the lateral-most portion of the tympanic membrane is a layer of epithelium that is a part of the same skin lining the ear canal.

The tympanic membrane itself is a multi-layered structure. Approximately 85% of the tympanic membrane is composed of three types of layers: a lateral epithelial layer, a medial membranous layer that is contiguous with the lining of the middle-ear cavity, and a fibrous layer sandwiched in between the epithelial and membranous layers. The fibrous layer actually contains two sets of fibers: one that is oriented like a series of concentric circles (as in a bullseye target) and another that is oriented in a radial fashion (like spokes on a bicycle wheel with the bullseye as the hub of the wheel). These fibrous layers give the tympanic membrane considerable strength while maintaining elasticity.

FIGURE 3.22.
Several anatomic landmarks of the outer ear.

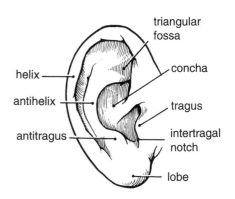

A small portion of the tympanic membrane, an area in the superior-anterior portion that represents about 15% of the total eardrum area, does not contain the two sets of fibers between the epithelial and membranous layers of the eardrum. This portion of the eardrum is known as the *pars flaccida* ("pars" = part and "flaccida" = flaccid or loose). The portion of the tympanic membrane that contains all three types of layers and represents the majority of the eardrum is referred to as the *pars tensa*.

As mentioned, the medial-most layer of the eardrum is a membranous layer that is contiguous with the membranous lining of the middle-ear cavity. Although our focus earlier in the chapter was on the bones and muscles within the middle ear, the middle-ear cavity itself has several noteworthy anatomic landmarks. To review these landmarks and orient you to their location within this tiny cavity, imagine that we've surgically removed the three ossicles while leaving everything else intact and that you've been struck by a "shrink ray" that has reduced you in size so that you can stand on the floor of the middle-ear cavity after being inserted through a tiny surgical slit in the right eardrum. ("Honey, I've shrunk the reader!") You would find yourself standing on a mucous, membranous lining not unlike that which lines the inside of your nose and throat. A bulge running through the floor underneath your feet represents the tunnel or fossa for the jugular vein, one of the main blood vessels carrying blood to the brain.

As you gaze straight ahead in an anterior direction you would notice a small opening in the lower portion of the front wall and some ligaments and a tendon dangling loosely from the upper right portion of the wall. The opening is the entrance or orifice for the eustachian tube; the ligaments represent those previously attached to the anterior process of the malleus, the lateral-most of the three middle-ear ossicles; and the tendon is protruding from a bony structure that houses one of the two middle-ear muscles, the tensor tympani. This muscle would normally be connected via the tendon to the neck of the malleus.

As you look above you, you would notice a partial ceiling that appears to be constructed of bone, although covered, like all the cavity surfaces, with a mucous membrane. This is the tegmen tympany. The unfinished portion of the ceiling or hole in the ceiling above you is the aditus. It opens up into an "attic" known as the epitympanic recess, and leads to a series of air-filled caverns that penetrate the surrounding bone of the skull. The air-filled caverns and pockets are the mastoid air cells.

Directing your gaze to the rear or posterior wall, you would observe two primary landmarks. One is the pyramidal eminence, which is a bony pyramid-shaped structure located in the medial-superior portion of this wall. It houses the other muscle of the middle-ear, the stapedius, which connects via tendon to the stapes. The other landmark, located on the lateral-superior portion of the wall, is the posterior portion of the axial ligaments that attaches to the incus. The axial ligaments, one attaching to the malleus from the anterior wall and the other attaching to the incus from the posterior wall, hold the ossicles in place and help to form the primary axis of rotation for the ossicular chain when it is vibrated by a sound wave striking the eardrum.

Now, as you return to your original position, facing the anterior wall, to your right along the lateral wall of the middle-ear cavity you would observe the membranous layer of the eardrum; to your left, along the medial wall, you would find the oval window and round window. (Remember, you are in the *right* middle-ear cavity, not the left.) A bulge running most of the way across the lateral wall would also be apparent. This bulge is the promontory and is formed by the large basal turn of the adjacent cochlea.

These are some of the highlights of the many anatomic landmarks found in this tiny middle-ear cavity. There are certainly others, such as various nerve fibers and blood vessels, that could be pointed out, but the effects of the shrink ray are starting to wear off and we don't want to leave you trapped in here! ("PPhheeww! Honey, it's okay. I've unshrunk the reader!") The computer diskette accompanying this book provides additional review of the anatomy of the auditory system.

More on Otoacoustic Emissions (OAEs)

As noted previously in the chapter, our knowledge of OAEs has exploded since the early 1980s. Although much remains uncertain about OAEs, an incredible amount has been learned since their discovery in 1978.

It was also noted earlier in the chapter that there are two basic classes of OAE: spontaneous and evoked. The primary distinction between these two classes of OAEs has to do simply with whether or not a sound stimulus is required to elicit the OAE. Spontaneous emissions occur without stimulation, whereas evoked emissions require an acoustic stimulus to be generated. In the remainder of this section we will describe the evoked OAEs in greater detail. More is known about the mechanisms of generation for the evoked emissions, and they have the greatest promise for clinical application.

There are basically three types of evoked OAE: (*a*) transient-evoked OAE (TEOAE), (*b*) distortion-product OAE (DPOAE), and (*c*) stimulus-frequency OAE (SFOAE). The SFOAEs are the most difficult to measure and have been studied the least. They are produced by presenting the ear with a pure tone and examining the sound recorded in the ear canal. The frequency of the emission sound, however, is the same as that of the stimulus tone, and its level is much lower than that of the stimulus. This makes it more difficult to measure and study.

TEOAEs were the first OAEs measured in humans. They are recorded by stimulating the ear with a brief click while recording the sound level in the ear canal with a tiny microphone. A click is a brief sound that has energy spread over a wide range of frequencies. Thus, a wide range of the basilar membrane can be stimulated in an instant. Because of the nature of the traveling wave mechanism in the cochlea, the basilar membrane initially responds to a click with maximum displacement in the high-frequency basal region. The peak displacement of the basilar membrane then travels toward the apex, where maximum displacement occurs in response to low-frequency sounds. Thus, even though the click stimulus instantly presents the ear with sounds of low, mid, and high frequency, it takes longer for the low-frequency sounds to travel to the apex and stimulate the basilar membrane. Assuming that it takes 3 ms for the peak displacement to travel from the basal to the apical portion of the basilar membrane, the low frequencies would maximally stimulate the basilar membrane at the appropriate place about 3 ms after the high frequencies present in the click. Further, the vibrations producing the emissions travel back out of the cochlea at the same rate so that low-frequency sounds would come back out of the cochlea and be measurable by a microphone in the ear canal about 6 ms after the high frequencies appeared.

Figure 3.23 illustrates a representative TEOAE from a normal-hearing young adult. The plot is essentially the acoustic waveform that is recorded in the ear canal by the tiny microphone. The first, large, abrupt portion of the waveform is the click stimulus presented by the earphone. After a brief period of silence, another waveform emerges: a low-level echo! In fact, TEOAEs have frequently been referred to as "cochlear echoes." Careful scrutiny of the echo reveals that the first portion has

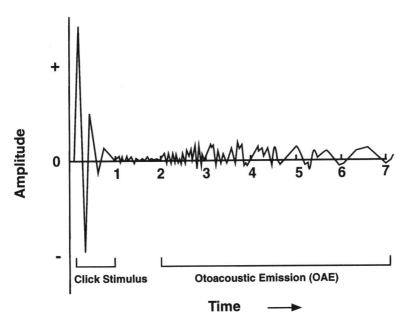

FIGURE 3.23.
An example of a transient-evoked otoacoustic emission (TEOAE). The plot is a waveform showing the sound levels recorded by a tiny microphone placed in the ear canal as a function of time. The large initial portion of the waveform is a recording of the click stimulus presented in the ear canal by the earphone, whereas the lower level and later-appearing portion of the waveform is the "echo" coming back out into the ear canal from the inner ear.

shorter periods or higher frequencies than the later parts of the echo. This is entirely consistent with the scenario described above based on the delays introduced by the traveling wave along the basilar membrane.

TEOAEs are only observed in response to clicks of low and moderate sound level. Animal research has demonstrated that TEOAEs are sensitive to damage, and even reversible injury, to the hair cells. If the measurements described previously in Figure 3.23 were repeated on an individual with hair-cell damage in the high-frequency basal portion of the cochlea, the early parts of the echo would be missing, and only the later-emerging low-frequency emissions originating from the healthy apical region would be observed.

DPOAEs are also being explored for clinical applications. Although DPOAEs can be generated in a variety of ways, the most commonly employed method has made use of two stimulus tones simultaneously introduced into the ear canal. The frequencies of these two pure tones are denoted f_1, f_2, with f_2 being higher in frequency than f_1. Distortion is a characteristic of many systems, including mechanical systems, and can be measured in a variety of ways. One manifestation of distortion in a system is the emergence of tones in the response or output of the system that were not part of the sound stimulus presented to the system. These additional tones are referred to as distortion products. When two tones are presented to the auditory system, the most prominent distortion product that emerges is one that has a frequency corresponding to $2f_1 - f_2$. For reasons beyond the scope of this book, this distortion product is often referred to as the cubic difference tone, or CDT. The CDT is always at a frequency lower than the two input tones. For example, for $f_1 =$ 1000 Hz and $f_2 = 1200$ Hz, the frequency of the CDT is 800 Hz ([2 × 1000 Hz] − 1200 Hz). Although other distortion products have been explored for measurement of DPOAEs, the CDT has been the most thoroughly studied and is the one receiving the most emphasis clinically. Hereafter, unless noted otherwise, the term DPOAE implies measurement of the CDT distortion product.

Because the DPOAE occurs at a frequency close to, but separate from, the input frequencies, it is possible to use sounds of longer duration to evoke the emission. The distortion product is separated from the input frequencies by doing a fast frequency analysis of the sound recorded in the ear canal. Unlike the TEOAE, the DPOAE can be measured over a wide range of sound levels from moderately low to very high. Although there is considerable uncertainty as to whether the same distortion processes are involved over this entire range of sound levels, it appears that the DPOAEs evoked by low-intensity stimuli are sensitive to hair-cell damage in the cochlea much as TEOAEs are. They continue to be explored for possible clinical applications.

More on Auditory Electrophysiology

We briefly highlighted some auditory electrophysiology earlier in this chapter. Here, we seek to expand that coverage somewhat. The focus previously had been placed on peripheral electrophysiology, primarily the cochlear receptor potentials and the action potentials from the auditory nerve. Much of the information reviewed was of receptor potentials from individual hair cells and action potentials from individual nerve fibers.

Although this is the most fundamental form of electrophysiologic information, clinical electrophysiology never makes use of electrical potentials from individual cells. Rather, clinical auditory electrophysiology involves the recording of gross electrical potentials representing the activity of hundreds or thousands of individual hair cells or nerve fibers. These tiny electrical potentials are usually recorded from remote locations on the surface of the head and require amplification and computer averaging of at least several hundred stimulus presentations to be visible.

To give you some perspective on the size and temporal sequence of many of the more common electric potentials used in audiology, consider the hypothetical electrical waveform in Figure 3.24. We have assumed that a special recording electrode has been placed in each ear canal and that a third electrode has been applied to the top of the scalp (vertex). The stimulus is a 2-ms burst of a 2000-Hz pure tone, as shown in the top waveform. This stimulus is presented 1000 times at a rate of 11 tone bursts per second, and the electrical potentials recorded have been averaged together to produce the electrical waveform in the lower portion of the figure. The first electrical potentials to be recorded are the gross cochlear microphonic (CM), which looks like a miniature version of the sound stimulus, and the summating potential (SP), which appears as a vertical shifting of the cochlear microphonic

FIGURE 3.24.
A hypothetical electrical waveform showing the sequence of electrical potentials generated in the auditory system (*bottom portion*) in response to a brief (2-ms) 2000-Hz pure tone (*top portion*). CM, cochlear microphonic; SP, summating potential.

away from the zero line. Next, is the whole-nerve action potential (WNAP), which also corresponds to waves I and II of the auditory brainstem response (ABR). The ABR consists of a series of 5–7 bumps or waves in the electrical waveform that appear in the first 10 ms after the stimulus has been presented. Next, we have a larger and later electrical response known as the middle latency response (MLR), followed by a still larger and later potential referred to as late evoked potential. The MLR is believed to originate from the upper portions of the auditory brainstem, and the late potential comes from the auditory cortex. Thus, the hypothetical electrical waveform shows the progression of electrical activity from the cochlea to the auditory cortex. It should be noted that this waveform is hypothetical in that the recording procedures and stimulus characteristics that are ideal for one type of electrical potential are often not the same ones used to record one of the other potentials. Nonetheless, it suffices to introduce the reader to the various electrical potentials that can be recorded easily from surface electrodes by the audiologist.

Of the electrical potentials available to the audiologist, the one that has received the most investigation and most frequent use clinically is the ABR. The ABR is of value because it is very robust and can be recorded reliably and easily, yet is sensitive to dysfunction occurring from the auditory periphery to the upper brainstem portions of the auditory central nervous system. Thus, it is useful in assisting with detection of neurologic problems along a large portion of the auditory CNS; also, it can be used to estimate the hearing loss in a patient. Although a normal ABR waveform does not indicate normal auditory function (i.e., a problem could lie further up the auditory pathway), an abnormal or absent ABR waveform in response to acoustic stimulation does indicate the presence of a significant hearing loss or neurologic dysfunction in about 95% of such cases. ABR has been used to screen the hearing of newborns and to estimate hearing thresholds in difficult-to-test patients. It is an extremely valuable clinical tool for the audiologist.

REFERENCES AND SUGGESTED READINGS

Durrant JD, Lovrinic JH: *Bases of Hearing Science*, ed 2. Baltimore, Williams & Wilkins, 1984.

Gelfand SA: *Hearing: An Introduction to Psychological and Physiological Acoustics*. New York, Marcel Dekker, 1981.

Hall JW: *Handbook of Auditory Evoked Responses*. Needham, MA, Allyn & Bacon, 1992.

Humes LE: Psychoacoustic foundations of clinical audiology. *In* Katz J (ed): *Handbook of Clinical Audiology*, ed 3. Baltimore, Williams & Wilkins, 1985.

Möller AR: *Auditory Physiology*. New York, Academic Press, 1983.

Moore BCJ: *An Introduction to the Psychology of Hearing*, ed 3. London, Academic Press, 1989.

Pickles JO: *An Introduction to the Physiology of Hearing*, ed 2. London, Academic Press, 1988.

Probst R, Lonsbury-Martin BL, Martin G: A review of otoacoustic emissions. *Journal of the Acoustical Society of America*, 89:2027–2067, 1991.

Shaw EAG: The external ear. *In* Keidel WD, Neff WD, (eds): *Handbook of Sensory Physiology*, vol V(1). New York, Springer Verlag, 1974, pp 455–490.

von Bekesy G: *Experiments in Hearing*. New York, McGraw-Hill, 1960.

Wever EG, Lawrence M: *Physiological Acoustics*. Princeton, NJ, Princeton University Press, 1954.

Yost WA: *Fundamentals of Hearing: An Introduction*, ed 3. New York, Academic Press, 1993.

Zemlin WR: *Speech and Hearing Science: Anatomy and Physiology*, ed 2. Englewood Cliffs, NJ, Prentice-Hall, 1988.

PART II

ASSESSMENT
OF
AUDITORY
FUNCTION

CHAPTER FOUR

AUDIOLOGIC MEASUREMENT

Following completion of this chapter, the reader should be able to:

- Understand the procedures for measuring pure-tone threshold by air conduction and by bone conduction.
- Understand the procedures for measuring hearing sensitivity for speech (speech recognition threshold) and speech recognition.
- Identify situations requiring the use of contralateral masking and understand the concept of masking.
- Recognize the special modifications of these basic measurements needed for application to pediatric populations.
- Understand acoustic immittance measurements.
- Appreciate the way in which each test result represents just one aspect of the complete basic audiologic test battery.

The nature of auditory impairment depends on such factors as the severity of the hearing loss, the age at onset, the cause of the loss, and the location of the lesion within the auditory system. The hearing evaluation plays an important role in determining some of these factors. Audiometric measurement of auditory function can (*a*) determine the degree of hearing loss, (*b*) estimate the location of the lesion within the auditory system that is producing the problem, (*c*) help establish the cause of the hearing problem, (*d*) estimate the extent of the handicap produced by the hearing loss, and (*e*) help to determine the client's habilitative or rehabilitative needs and the appropriate means of filling those needs. This chapter will focus on those tests used most commonly in the evaluation of auditory function. This battery of tests includes pure-tone audiometry, speech audiometry, and acoustic immittance measures.

CASE HISTORY

Before the audiologic evaluation begins, the audiologist obtains a history from the client. For adults, this history may be supplied by completing a printed form prior to the evaluation. The form contains pertinent identifying information for the client, such as home address, social security number, and referral source. Questions regarding the nature of past and present hearing problems, other medical problems, and prior use of amplification are also usually included. The written responses are then followed up during an interview between the audiologist and the client prior to any testing.

For children, the case history form is usually more comprehensive than the adult version. In addition to questions such as the ones mentioned for adults, detailed questions about the mother's pregnancy and the child's birth are included. The development of gross and fine motor skills and the development of speech and language are also probed. The medical history of the child is also reviewed in detail, with special emphasis on childhood diseases (e.g., measles, mumps) capable of producing a hearing loss. (See Chapter 5.)

PURE-TONE AUDIOMETRY

Pure-tone audiometry is the basis of a hearing evaluation. With pure-tone audiometry, hearing thresholds are measured for pure tones at different test frequencies. Hearing threshold is typically defined as the lowest (softest) sound level needed for a person to detect the presence of a signal approximately 50% of the time. Threshold information at each frequency is then plotted on a graph known as an audiogram. Before examining the audiogram, however, we shall describe the equipment used to measure hearing.

Audiometer

An audiometer is the primary instrument used by the audiologist to measure hearing threshold. Audiometers vary from the simple, inexpensive screening devices used in schools and public health programs to the more elaborate and expensive diagnostic audiometers found in hospitals and clinics. Certain basic components, however, are common to all audiometers. Figure 4.1 shows an example of one of these basic units. A frequency selector dial permits selection of different pure-tone frequencies. Ordinarily these frequencies are available at octave intervals ranging from 125 to 8000 Hz. An interrupter switch or presentation button allows presentation of the tone to the listener. A hearing level dial controls the intensity of the signal. Most audiometers can deliver signals spanning a 100-dB range in 5-dB steps. An output selector determines whether the pure tone will be presented to the earphones for air conduction testing (for either the right or the left ear), or whether the tone is to be sent to a bone vibrator for bone conduction testing. Many audiometers also have a masking level dial, which controls the intensity of the masking noise presented to the nontest ear when masking is necessary. The more elaborate diagnostic audiometers not only can generate masking noise and pure-tone signals but also provide a means for measuring the understanding of speech signals.

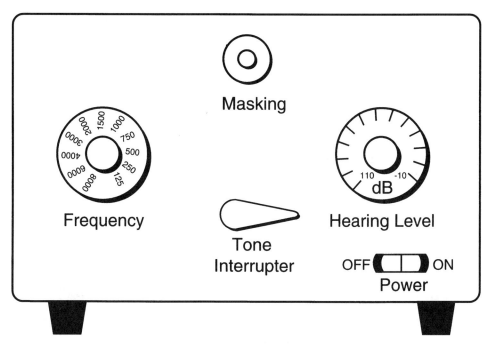

FIGURE 4.1.
The basic components seen on the control panel of a pure-tone audiometer.

Audiogram

The audiogram is a chart used to graphically record the hearing thresholds and other test results. Figure 4.2 shows an example of an audiogram and the associated symbol system recommended by the American Speech-Language-Hearing Association. The audiogram is shown in graphic form, with the signal frequencies (in Hertz) displayed on the *x* axis and the hearing level (in decibels) represented on the *y* axis. The graph is designed in such a manner that 1 octave on the frequency scale is equal in size to 20 dB on the hearing level scale.

The horizontal line at 0 dB hearing level (HL) represents normal hearing sensitivity for the average young adult. However, as described in the previous chapter, the human ear does not perceive sound equally well at all frequencies. Recall that the ear is most sensitive to sound in the intermediate-frequency region from 1000 to 4000 Hz and is less sensitive at both the higher and lower frequencies. Greater sound pressure is needed to elicit a threshold response at 250 Hz than at 2000 Hz in normal ears. The audiometer is calibrated to correct for these differences in threshold sensitivity at various frequencies. Consequently, when the hearing level dial is set at zero for a given frequency, the signal is automatically presented at the normal threshold sound pressure level required for the average young adult to hear that particular frequency (Vignette 4.1).

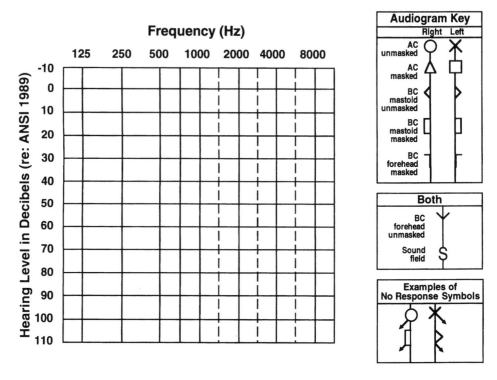

FIGURE 4.2.

Left, Audiogram used for plotting pure-tone air and bone conduction thresholds. *Right*, The *Audiogram Key* displays the symbols commonly used in audiograms. *AC*, air conduction; *BC*, bone conduction.

VIGNETTE 4.1.

Illustration of the relationship between decibels SPL (dB SPL) and decibels HL (dB HL).

The accompanying figure depicts the relationship between the dB HL scale and the dB SPL scale of sound intensity. The circles in the *upper panel* are the data for hearing thresholds of normal-hearing young adults. The triangles in the *upper panel* are hearing thresholds obtained from an individual with a high-frequency hearing loss. Note that increasing hearing loss is indicated by higher sound pressure levels at threshold. At 4000 Hz, for example, the average threshold for normal-hearing young adults is 10 dB SPL; the patient's threshold is 80 dB SPL, indicating a hearing loss of 70 dB. These same data have been replotted on the dB HL scale in the *lower panel*. Note now that the normal hearing threshold has been set to 0 dB HL on this scale at all frequencies. Increasing intensity is shown in a downward direction on the audiogram. Note also that the threshold for the hearing-

Vignette 4.1.—*continued*

impaired subject at 4000 Hz is 70 dB HL. This threshold value itself then directly indicates the magnitude of hearing loss relative to normal hearing. There is no need to subtract the normal-hearing threshold value from the value observed in the impaired ear, as was the case for the dB SPL scale.

FIGURE 4.3.
Classification of hearing impairment in relation to handicap for speech recognition.

Results plotted on the audiogram can be used to classify the extent of a hearing handicap. This information plays a valuable role in determining the habilitative or rehabilitative needs of a hearing-handicapped individual. Classification schemes using the pure-tone audiogram are based on the fact that there is a strong relationship between the threshold for those frequencies known to be important for hearing speech (500, 1000, and 2000 Hz) and the lowest level at which speech can be recognized accurately 50% of the time. The latter measure is generally referred to as the speech recognition threshold, or SRT. Given the pure-tone thresholds at 500, 1000, and 2000 Hz, one can estimate the hearing loss for speech and the potential handicapping effects of the impairment. This is done by simply calculating the average (mean) loss of hearing for these three frequencies. This average is referred to as the three-frequency pure-tone average. Figure 4.3 shows an example of a typical classification system based on the pure-tone average. This scheme, adapted from several other systems, reflects the different classifications of hearing loss as well as the likely effects of the hearing loss on an individual's ability to hear speech. The hearing loss classes, ranging from mild to profound, are based on the pure-tone average at 500, 1000, and 2000 Hz. The classification of normal limits extends to 25 dB HL, and hearing levels within this range have typically been thought to produce essentially no problems with even faint speech. Some evidence indicates that losses from 15 to 25 dB HL, however, can have negative effects educationally on children.

Measurement of Hearing

In pure-tone audiometry, thresholds are obtained by both air conduction and bone conduction. In air conduction measurement, the different pure-tone stimuli are transmitted through earphones. The signal travels through the ear canal, across the middle ear cavity via the three ossicles to the cochlea, and on to the auditory central nervous system, as reviewed in the previous chapter. Air conduction thresholds reflect the integrity of the total peripheral auditory mechanism. When a person exhibits a hearing loss by air conduction, it is not possible to determine the location of the pathology along the auditory pathway. The hearing loss could be the result of (a) a problem in the outer or middle ear, (b) a difficulty at the level of the cochlea, (c) damage along the neural pathways to the brain, or (d) some combination of these. When air conduction measurements are combined with bone conduction measurements, however, it is possible to differentiate outer and middle ear problems (conductive hearing loss) from inner ear problems (sensorineural hearing loss).

In bone conduction measurement, signals are transmitted via a bone vibrator that is usually placed on the mastoid prominence of the skull (a bony prominence located behind the pinna, slightly above the level of the concha). The forehead is another common position for placement of the bone vibrator. A signal transduced through the vibrator causes the skull to vibrate. The pure tone directly stimulates the cochlea, which is embedded in the skull, effectively bypassing the outer ear and middle ear systems. If an individual exhibits a reduction in hearing sensitivity when tested by air conduction yet shows normal sensitivity by bone conduction, the impairment is probably due to an obstruction or blockage of the outer or middle ear. This condition is referred to as a conductive hearing loss. Figure 4.4 gives an audiometric example of a young child with a conductive hearing loss due to middle ear disease. The bone conduction thresholds ([, right-ear thresholds;], left-ear thresholds) appear close to 0 dB HL for all test frequencies. Such a finding implies that the inner ear responds to sound at normal threshold levels. The air conduction thresholds (O-O, right ear; X-X, left ear), on the other hand, are much greater than 0 dB HL. Greater sound intensity is needed for this child to hear the air-conducted pure-tone signals than is required by the average normal hearer. Since the bone conduction thresholds suggest that the inner ear is normal, the loss displayed by air conduction must result from a conductive lesion affecting the outer or middle ear.

The difference between the air conduction threshold and the bone conduction threshold at a given frequency is generally referred to as the air-bone gap. In Figure 4.4, for example, at 250 Hz there is a 30-dB air-bone gap in the right ear and a 40-dB gap in the left ear. Conductive hearing loss is especially prevalent among preschool and young school-age children who experience repeated episodes of otitis media (middle-ear infection). Other examples of pathologic conditions known to produce conductive hearing loss include congenital atresia (absence of ear canals),

FIGURE 4.4.

Pure-tone audiogram demonstrating the relation between air and bone conduction thresholds typifying mild conductive hearing impairment.

blockage or occlusion of the ear canal (possibly by cerumen or earwax), perforation or scarring of the tympanic membrane, ossicular chain disruption, and otosclerosis. These pathologies are described in detail in Chapter 5.

As we noted, hearing thresholds better than a hearing level of 25 dB HL are considered normal. Air-bone gaps of 10 dB or more, however, represent a significant conductive hearing loss and may require medical referral, even if the air conduction thresholds are less than 25 dB at all frequencies.

A sensorineural hearing loss is suggested when the air conduction thresholds *and* bone conduction thresholds are approximately the same (± 5 dB) at all test frequencies. Sensorineural hearing impairment may be either congenital or acquired. Some of the congenital causes include heredity, complications of maternal viral and bacterial infections, and birth trauma. Factors producing acquired sensorineural hearing loss include noise, aging, inflammatory diseases (e.g., measles, mumps), and ototoxic drugs (e.g., aminoglycoside antibiotics). Many of these disorders are also described in Chapter 5. Figure 4.5 gives three different examples of sensorineural hearing impairment. Figure 4.5A shows the audiogram of an adult with a hearing loss resulting from the use of ototoxic antibiotics. This audiogram displays a moderate bilateral sensorineural impairment with a greater hearing loss in the high-frequency region. Figure 4.5B illustrates the audiogram of a child whose hearing impairment resulted from maternal rubella (measles). It can be seen that the magni-

FIGURE 4.5.
Three pure-tone air and bone conduction audiograms. *A*, Moderate bilateral sensorineural hearing loss. *B*, Profound bilateral sensorineural hearing loss. *C*, Low-frequency bilateral sensorineural hearing loss.

tude of this hearing loss falls in the profound category in the region of the most critical frequencies for hearing speech (500–2000 Hz). In fact, the loss is so severe that bone conduction responses could not be obtained at the maximum output of the audiometer at all test frequencies. This is indicated by the downward-pointing arrows attached to the audiometric symbols. Air conduction thresholds also could not be obtained at frequencies above 1000 Hz because the hearing loss was so great.

The majority of sensorineural hearing losses are characterized by audiometric configurations that are flat, trough-shaped, or slightly to steeply sloping in the high frequencies. The latter is probably the most common configuration associated with acquired sensorineural hearing loss. Occasionally, however, patients display a sensorineural hearing loss in which the greatest hearing loss occurs at low and interme-

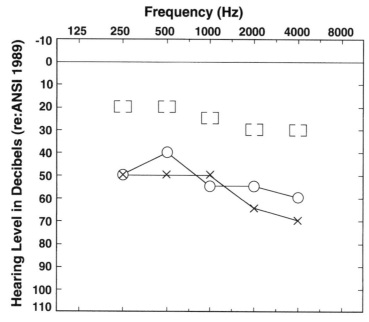

FIGURE 4.6.

Pure-tone audiogram demonstrating the relation between air and bone conduction thresholds indicating a mixed (conductive and sensorineural) type of hearing loss.

diate frequencies, with normal or near-normal hearing sensitivity at the high frequencies. Figure 4.5C shows an example of a typical low-frequency hearing loss. Low-tone hearing loss most commonly results from either some types of hereditary deafness or Ménière's disease. (See Chapter 5.) Young children whose audiograms display low-frequency hearing impairment are difficult to identify and are sometimes the unfortunate victims of misdiagnosis. Because of their near-normal hearing sensitivity in the high frequencies, these children may respond to whispered speech and broad-band stimuli at low intensity levels. In addition, unlike children with a high-frequency hearing loss, their articulation of speech is usually good. These manifestations are not typical of sensorineural hearing loss in children, which makes them more prone to misdiagnosis.

When both air conduction thresholds and bone conduction thresholds are reduced in sensitivity, but bone conduction yields better results than air conduction, the term "mixed hearing loss" is used. That is, the patient's hearing loss is partially conductive and partially sensorineural. Figure 4.6 shows an audiogram depicting mixed hearing loss. Even though hearing loss is evident for both bone and air conduction thresholds, bone conduction sensitivity is consistently better across all test frequencies. This suggests that there has been some damage to the hair cells or nerve endings in the inner ear, causing a reduction in bone conduction thresholds, which is added to the reduction in air conduction thresholds resulting from malfunction of the outer ear or middle ear.

Procedures for Obtaining Threshold

The hearing examination is generally conducted in a sound-treated room where noise levels are kept at a minimum and do not interfere with or influence the hearing test results. Pure-tone audiometry begins with air conduction measurements at octave intervals ranging from 125 or 250 Hz to 8000 Hz; these are followed by bone conduction measurements at octave intervals ranging from 250 to 4000 Hz. (Air conduction measurements at 125 Hz are optional. Some audiometers do not include this frequency.) The initial step in measuring threshold involves instructing the patient as to the listening and responding procedures. The listener is instructed to respond to the pure-tone signals no matter how soft they might be, to respond as soon as the tone is heard, and to stop responding when the sound becomes inaudible. The most common form of response is merely raising or lowering the forefinger. Earphones should be placed carefully and snugly on the patient's head so that the signal source is directed toward the opening of the ear canal.

Because 1000 Hz is considered the frequency most easily heard under headphones, and the threshold at this frequency is the most reliable, it is used as the initial test frequency and is administered first to the better ear. The right ear is tested first if the patient indicates that hearing sensitivity is the same in both ears. The most common procedure for establishing threshold is known as the ascending technique. Figure 4.7 shows an example of this pure-tone procedure. An interrupted signal is presented at a hearing level of approximately 30 dB. If the listener is unable to perceive the tone at this level, the signal is then increased by 20 dB and presented again. This procedure is continued until the listener indicates that a signal has been perceived. For the case shown in Figure 4.7, the initial presentation level

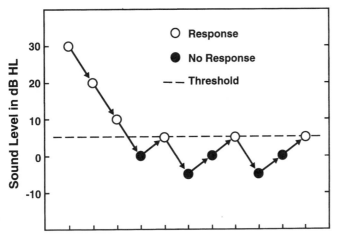

FIGURE 4.7.
Alternating descending and ascending sound level presentations commonly used in obtaining pure-tone thresholds. The x axis simply shows the temporal sequence of tone presentations from beginning (left) to end (right).

of 30 dB HL produced a response in the listener. After each positive response, the intensity dial setting is decreased in 10-dB steps until a hearing level is reached at which there is no response on the part of the listener. Once the patient fails to respond to the signal, the actual ascending technique begins. Following a failure to obtain a response, the signal is increased in 5-dB increments until a response is obtained. Every time a positive response is obtained, the signal is decreased by 10 dB. As soon as the listener's response changes to no response, an ascending series of 5-dB steps is begun again. This process is continued until an intensity level used in an ascending series is found to which the listener responded positively at least 50% of the time. This level is then recorded as the threshold. In practice, if the listener responds at the same *ascending* level for two of two, two of three, two of four, or three of five presentations, this level is considered the threshold. Once this procedure has been completed at 1000 Hz, the examiner goes on to the higher test frequencies (2000, 4000, and 8000 Hz) and then returns to 1000 Hz for a reliability check. The lower frequencies, 500 and 250 Hz, are presented last. After testing all of the frequencies in one ear, the examiner then switches the signal to the opposite ear and repeats the procedures.

Essentially the same procedures are used for obtaining the bone conduction thresholds except that only frequencies from 250 through 4000 Hz are used. A bone vibrator is attached by a tension band to the mastoid prominence of the test ear or to the forehead so that the signal is transmitted via the bone pathways of the skull, bypassing the outer and middle ear. Once pure-tone thresholds have been completed using the same procedures as those described for air conduction, the bone vibrator, if placed on the mastoid prominence, may then be removed and placed on the opposite mastoid prominence for completion of the bone conduction threshold measurements, depending on the agreement observed between the air-conduction and bone-conduction measurements and the need for masking (see below). If the bone vibrator is placed on the forehead, both inner ears can be evaluated from this location and there is no need to move the bone vibrator.

Factors That Can Influence Threshold

To ensure accurate threshold measurement, it is important to take every precaution to eliminate extraneous variables that can influence the threshold test. The following factors are known to be significant.

Proper Maintenance and Calibration of the Audiometer. Like all pieces of electronic equipment, the audiometer is subject to malfunction, especially with extensive use. It is critical that the audiometer be handled carefully to ensure reliable results, and that it be checked electroacoustically and biologically (listening checks) on a periodic basis. Such services can usually be obtained at a university hearing clinic or at the manufacturer's distributorship.

Test Environment. Threshold measurement may also be affected if ambient noise levels are high at the time of the test. The evaluation should be conducted in a sound-treated environment designed specifically for hearing threshold measurement. If such facilities are not available, every precaution should be taken to perform the evaluation in the quietest room possible.

Earphone Placement. Inadequate positioning of the earphones can produce threshold errors as great as 10–15 dB. The audiologist should be sure that the tension band holding the earphones offers a snug yet comfortable fit and that the phones are placed carefully over the ear canal openings. The problems of earphone placement may be especially difficult with hyperactive children, very young children (under 2 years of age), or elderly adults. A popular alternative to conventional earphones is described in Vignette 4.2.

Placement of the Bone Vibrator. In testing for bone conduction, the vibrator is usually positioned on the prominence of the mastoid bone. Thresholds can vary, however, depending on the placement. To ensure the most accurate placement, it is advisable to introduce a comfortably loud pure tone at 1000 Hz and vary the position of the vibrator on the mastoid while asking the subject to report where the signal is loudest. With younger children, such a practice may not be feasible, and special care must be taken to position the vibrator on a prominent portion of the mastoid bone.

The tension of the headband should also be checked on a periodic basis. After extensive use, the headbands for bone vibrators begin to lose tension and reduce the force that holds the vibrator against the mastoid process. Bone conduction thresholds are known to vary depending on the force applied to the vibrator. Again, because most tension bands were designed for adult-sized heads, special care must be taken when positioning the bone vibrator on the head of a child.

Procedures for Young Children

The procedures for pure-tone audiometry previously described are those recommended for older children and adults. Considerable modification of these techniques is required for testing the hearing of younger children. This section will focus on behavioral procedures used with infants and children between the ages of 2 months and 5 years. As noted in the Advanced Material from Chapter 3, however, clinical electrophysiologic measurements, such as the auditory brainstem response, can also be used to provide indirect estimates of hearing threshold in many difficult-to-test populations, including infants and young children. These methods are considered indirect estimators of "hearing" threshold because, unlike the behavioral procedures described below, the presence of an electrophysiologic response measured with electrodes does not always reflect perception of the sound or the sensation of hearing. Behavioral methods are generally required to verify the perception of sound by the listener.

Testing the Younger Infant, Aged 2 Months to 2 Years. A child between the ages of 2 months and 2 years is somewhat easier to evaluate than a newborn because the child's increased maturity results in more sophisticated and reliable responses. By

VIGNETTE 4.2.

Insert earphones—an alternative to conventional headphones.

The drawing that accompanies this vignette illustrates a popular alternative to conventional headphones for testing hearing, known as insert earphones. As shown in the drawing, a long tube (292 mm in length) is used to conduct the sound from a pocket-sized electronic device to a soft foam cylindrical ear insert. The ear insert is a soft foam material that can be compressed temporarily by rolling it between the fingers. While it is compressed, it is inserted deeply into the ear canal and held in place for about 1 min. This allows the foam material to expand and fit snugly in the ear canal. The pocket-sized electronic device is connected to the audiometer just like typical headphones.

Insert earphones have become increasingly popular among audiologists for several reasons. When they are calibrated appropriately, the thresholds measured with them will be the same as those measured with conventional headphones. The insert earphones also reduce the environmental noise levels more than conventional headphones. This enables them to be used in somewhat noisier test areas without the ambient noise affecting test results. The insert phones are also more comfortable to wear and fit children as well as they do adults. Finally, masking (discussed later in this chapter) is needed less frequently when testing by air conduction. They also have some advantages when used to deliver sounds used in clinical electrophysiology, such as the measurement of gross cochlear receptor potentials and the auditory brainstem response.

approximately 3 months of age, attending responses are elicited easily, and the infant is able to determine the location of the sound source in the horizontal plane. The audiologist's assessment of hearing in this age category is generally centered around behavioral observation conducted in a sound-field setting, with the sound delivered by loudspeakers rather than by headphones. Figure 4.8 shows a typical test arrangement for sound-field audiometry. The infant is placed in a high chair or on the mother's lap between two loudspeakers located at a 45° angle from both sides of the child. A controlled auditory signal is then presented at a level well above threshold (usually 50–85 dB HL), and behavioral responses are observed. The signal is decreased systematically in 10- to 20-dB steps for each positive response and increased 10 dB for each negative response. The nature of a positive response varies with the infant's age. Age-appropriate responses are discussed below. Threshold is usually defined as the lowest presentation level at which an infant responds 50% of the time. Some type of visual reinforcement is used to train the infant in the task and to reward the infant for responding appropriately.

The nature of the signal varies. Some clinicians favor the use of various noise-makers, such as a squeeze toy, bell, rattle, or spoon in a cup. Although these signals are considered favorable in that they maintain a certain amount of interest on the part of the child and appear to be effective for eliciting arousal responses in young children or infants, they have inappropriate frequency characteristics. Most noise-makers contain energy at several frequencies. This makes it difficult to define the way in which the hearing loss varies with frequency and, in many cases, to deter-

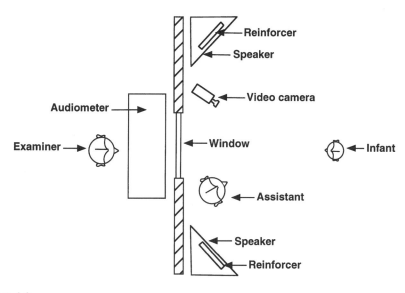

FIGURE 4.8.
Typical sound-field test arrangement for infants and young children. The infant is typically in the mother's lap or seated in a high chair.

mine if a hearing loss is present. If, for example, the infant has normal or near-normal hearing for low frequencies, the use of noisemakers that have energy at low and high frequencies will always produce a normal response in this infant even though a severe or profound high-frequency hearing loss might be present. If noisemakers are chosen as the test signal, the importance of a careful acoustic analysis cannot be overemphasized. The clinician should be familiar with both the frequency and the intensity characteristics of any noisemaker being used for hearing measurement. Most clinicians, however, favor the use of electronically generated signals such as narrow-band and complex noise, warble tones (tones that change slightly in frequency over time), and speech. With these types of test signals, the relevant stimulus parameters, such as intensity and frequency, can be carefully controlled and specified. Our clinical experience suggests that a combination of noisemakers, warble tones (frequency-modulated) or noise, and filtered speech is valuable in the hearing assessment of very young infants.

As mentioned, the kind of behavioral response produced by the young infant will vary with the child's age and the types of stimuli used. Table 4.1 shows an index of the expected auditory response to various sounds for normal-hearing infants. The responses during the early months are typically arousal- or startle-oriented, whereas more sophisticated sound localization responses, such as head turns or eye movements in the direction of the loudspeaker producing the sound, occur with the older infants.

The use of a visual reinforcer in the measurement of hearing for very young infants is extremely important. Delivery of a visual stimulus following the appropriate sound-localization response serves to enhance the response behavior and leads to a more accurate threshold measurement. This technique is sometimes referred to as the conditioned orientation reflex or visual reinforcement audiometry. Visual reinforcers range from a simple blinking light to a more complex animated toy animal.

The scoring of a child's responses is also an important variable in the assessment of very young children. In order to assess sound localization behavior accurately, more than one person should observe the responses of the child. The clinician controlling the audiometer is very involved with the appropriate presentation of the auditory signals and can easily miss a behavioral response. It is desirable to have an assistant in the examination room with the child to help in the scoring of responses.

There are limitations to sound-field audiometry performed with young infants. The most obvious limitations are (*a*) the inability to obtain thresholds from each ear separately, (*b*) the inability to obtain bone conduction thresholds, and (*c*) failure to obtain responses from young children who have severe or profound hearing losses. The latter drawback results simply from the output limitations of typical audiometers when the sound is presented over loudspeakers. Sound-field testing has been considered the test of choice primarily because these children have been considered too young to yield valid earphone data.

TABLE 4.1.
Index of Expected Auditory Responses to Various Sounds of Normal-Hearing Infants

Age	Stimulus			Expected Response
	Noisemakers (dB SPL)	Warbled Pure Tone[a,b] (dB HL)	Speech[a] (dB HL)	
Birth–6 weeks	50–70	78 (SD = 6)	40–60	Eye widening, eye blink, stirring or arousal from sleep, startle
6 weeks–4 months	50–60	70 (SD = 10)	47 (SD = 2)	Eye widening, eye shift, eye blink, quieting; beginning rudimentary head turn by 4 months
4–7 months	40–50	51 (SD = 9)	21 (SD = 8)	Head turn on lateral plane toward sound; listening attitude
7–9 months	30–40	45 (SD = 15)	15 (SD = 7)	Direct localization of sounds to side, indirectly below ear level
9–13 months	25–35	38 (SD = 8)	8 (SD = 7)	Direct localization of sounds to side, directly below ear level, indirectly above ear level
13–16 months	25–30	32 (SD = 10)	5 (SD = 5)	Direct localization of sound on side, above, and below
16–21 months	25	25 (SD = 10)	5 (SD = 1)	Direct localization of sound on side, above, and below
21–24 months	25	26 (SD = 10)	3 (SD = 2)	Direct localization of sound on side, above, and below

[a]Adapted from Northern J, Downs M: *Hearing in Children,* ed. 3. Baltimore, Williams & Wilkins, 1984.

[b]SD, standard deviation.

Testing Children 2 to 5 Years Old. When the child reaches 2–5 years of age, he or she has matured sufficiently to permit the use of more structured procedures in the hearing evaluation. The techniques used most frequently are conditioned play audiometry, tangible reinforcement operant conditioning audiometry (TROCA) or visual reinforcement operant conditioning audiometry (VROCA), and conventional (hand-raising) audiometry.

Conditioned play audiometry is the most well-accepted procedure for measuring the hearing thresholds of children in this age group. The child participates in some form of play activity (e.g., placing a ring on a cone, putting blocks in a box, placing pegs in a hole) each time the signal is heard. The play activity serves as both the visible response for the clinician and the reinforcement for the child. Usually, social reinforcement also accompanies an appropriate response. The child is prevented from playing the game if an inappropriate response is made. The evaluation consists of a conditioning period in which the child is trained to perform the play activity in response to the delivery of a sound stimulus that is clearly audible. This is then followed by a threshold-seeking period. The technique may be employed in a sound-field condition or with earphone and bone conduction measurements. The application of play audiometry is limited to youngsters above the age of 2 years and to children who are not multiply handicapped.

TROCA is a highly structured test procedure that was introduced originally as a means of assessing the hearing sensitivity of mentally retarded children. Although TROCA test procedures vary somewhat from clinic to clinic, the basic principle is that a tangible material, such as candy or trinkets (reinforcer), is automatically dispensed if the child depresses a button when a tone is perceived. If an inappropriate response is made, the child does not receive the reinforcement. TROCA incorporates specialized instrumentation that electromechanically controls the stimulus presentation, monitors the responses, and dispenses the tangible reinforcers. Like conditioned play audiometry, this technique may be employed either in a sound field or with earphone and bone conduction measurements. The use of TROCA has been extended from the mentally retarded population to young children, particularly those classified as difficult-to-test, such as distractible and hyperactive children. It is also considered useful when frequent retesting is required, because reconditioning is seldom needed once the child is trained. The TROCA approach is not considered very successful with children below the age of $2^1/_2$ years.

VROCA differs from TROCA only in that a visual reinforcement is used in place of a tangible reinforcer. Those who desire more detail on the audiometric procedures used with children should consult one of the relevant readings suggested at the end of this chapter.

Masking

When hearing is assessed under earphones or with a bone vibrator, it is not always the case that the ear that the clinician desires to test is the one that is stimulated. Sometimes the other ear, referred to simply as the nontest ear, will be the ear

stimulated by the sound. This situation results because the two ears are not completely isolated from one another. Air-conducted sound delivered to the test ear
through conventional earphones mounted in typical ear cushions is decreased or
attenuated approximately 40 dB before stimulating the other ear via skull vibration. The value of 40 dB for interaural ("between-ear") attenuation is actually a
minimum value. The amount of interaural attenuation for air conduction varies
with the frequency of the test signal but is always more than 40 dB. The minimum
interaural attenuation value for bone conduction is 0 dB. Thus, the bone oscillator
placed on the mastoid process behind the left ear vibrates the entire skull such that
the effective stimulation of the right ear is essentially equivalent to that of the left
ear. It is impossible, therefore, when testing by bone conduction, to discern whether
the right ear or the left ear is responding without some way of eliminating the participation of the nontest ear (Vignette 4.3).

VIGNETTE 4.3.
Understanding the need for masking.

In the drawing that accompanies this vignette, two gremlins named "Lefty"
and "Righty" are shown, one in each of the two adjacent rooms. The two rooms
are separated by a wall that decreases sound intensity by 40 dB. The gremlins' job
is to listen for pure tones in their rooms. When they hear a sound, they are to signal by pushing a button to light a neon sign containing the words "I heard that!"
In the illustration, Righty hears a 10-dB SPL sound coming from the loudspeaker
in his room and presses the button. By using softer and louder intensities, we determine the sound intensity that Righty responds to 50% of the time and call this his
threshold. Righty has a threshold of 10 dB SPL. This is the typical or normal
threshold for most gremlins.

Next, we proceed to measure the hearing threshold of Lefty. Unbeknownst to
us, Lefty has decided to cover his ears with earmuffs! (You have to be careful with
gremlins!) The earmuffs reduce the sound reaching his ears by 60 dB! As we try to
measure Lefty's threshold, we gradually increase the intensity of the sound coming
from the loudspeaker in the left room. Finally, we get a response. About 50% of
the time, we see the neon light flash above the rooms when the presentation level of
the sound is 50 dB SPL. We conclude the Lefty's threshold is 50 dB SPL.

Is our conclusion correct? Probably not. We said that the earmuffs decrease
the sound reaching Lefty's ears by 60 dB and that the typical threshold for gremlins
is 10 dB SPL. If the sound level from the speaker in the left room is 50 dB SPL and
the earmuffs decrease it by 60 dB, then the sound level reaching Lefty's ears is −10
dB SPL. This is well below threshold for gremlins! Yet, we clearly saw the neon
light flash 50% of the time when the left speaker presented a sound level of 50 dB
SPL. By now you have probably discovered that it was Righty responding to the
sound from the left speaker, not Lefty. The wall decreases sound by 40 dB. A 50-

VIGNETTE 4.3.—*continued*

dB SPL sound from the left speaker will be 10 dB SPL in the right room. Righty's threshold is 10 dB SPL, and he responds accordingly by pushing the button and lighting the neon sign. Whenever the sound level presented to one room is 40 dB or more above the threshold of the gremlin in the other room, we can't be sure which gremlin is turning on the neon light.

If we used the loudspeaker in Righty's room to present a noise loud enough to make Righty's threshold higher than 10 dB SPL, we could then proceed to increase the sound from the left speaker above levels of 50 dB SPL. By introducing enough masking noise into Righty's room, we could eventually measure Lefty's real threshold of 70 dB SPL (10 dB SPL normal threshold plus 60 dB from earmuffs).

The gremlins in the drawing are like our inner ears, and the loudspeakers are like the headphones. The wall of 40 dB is the separation between the ears provided by the skull, known as the interaural (between-ear) attenuation. Masking noise is often needed to determine which ear is really responding to sound. This is especially true when testing by bone conduction because there is no interaural attenuation between the two inner ears when the skull is vibrated. Essentially, the 40-dB wall shown above has been removed for bone-conduction testing, and the gremlin with the better hearing always responds. The hearing of the better inner ear is always measured via unmasked bone-conduction testing regardless of where the bone vibrator is placed on the skull.

Masking enables the clinician to eliminate the nontest ear from participation in the measurement of hearing thresholds for the test ear. Essentially, the audiologist introduces a sufficient amount of masking noise into the nontest ear so as to make any sound crossing the skull from the test ear inaudible.

There are two simple rules the audiologist follows in deciding whether to mask the nontest ear; one applies to air conduction testing and the other to bone conduction measurements. Regarding air conduction thresholds, masking is required at a given frequency if the air conduction threshold of the test ear exceeds the bone conduction threshold of the nontest ear by more than 35 dB. Recall that the bone conduction threshold may be equivalent to or better than the air conduction threshold, but never poorer. Thus, if one observes a 50-dB difference between the air conduction thresholds of the two ears at a particular frequency, the difference will be *at least* that great when the air conduction threshold of the test ear is compared with the bone conduction threshold of the nontest ear. Consequently, one need not always determine the bone conduction threshold of the nontest ear prior to deciding whether to mask for air conduction. The following example will clarify this.

The patient indicates that hearing is better in the right ear, and air conduction testing is initiated with that ear. A threshold of 10 dB HL is observed at 1000 Hz. Following completion of testing at other frequencies in the right ear, the left ear is tested. An air conduction threshold of 50 dB HL is observed at 1000 Hz. Is this an accurate indication of the hearing loss at 1000 Hz in the left ear? The audiologist can't be sure. The air conduction threshold for the right ear is 10 dB HL and indicates that the bone conduction threshold for that ear at 1000 Hz is not greater than this value. Thus, there is *at least* a 40-dB difference between the air conduction threshold of the test ear at 1000 Hz (50 dB HL) and the bone conduction threshold of the nontest ear (≤ 10 dB HL). If the skull only attenuates the air-conducted sound delivered to the test ear by 40 dB, then a signal level of approximately 10 dB HL reaches the nontest ear. The level of the crossed-over signal approximates the bone conduction threshold of the nontest ear and may, therefore, be detected by that ear. Now assume that a masking noise is introduced into the nontest ear to raise that ear's threshold to 30 dB HL. If the air-conduction threshold of the test ear remains at 50–55 dB HL, we may safely conclude that the observed threshold provides an accurate indication of the hearing loss in that ear. Why? Because if the listener was actually using the nontest ear to hear the sound presented to the test ear, making the hearing threshold 20 dB worse in the nontest ear (from 10 to 30 dB HL) would also shift the threshold in the test ear by 20 dB (from 50 to 70 dB HL).

When testing hearing by bone conduction, masking is needed whenever the difference between the air conduction threshold of the test ear and the bone conduction threshold of the test ear at the same frequency (the air-bone gap) is ≥ 10 dB. Because the interaural attenuation for bone conduction testing is 0 dB, the bone conduction threshold is always determined by the ear having the better bone conduction hearing. Consider the following example. Air conduction thresholds obtained from both ears reveal a hearing loss of 30 dB across all frequencies in the left ear, whereas thresholds of 0 dB HL are obtained at all frequencies in the right ear. Bone conduction testing of each ear indicates thresholds of 0 dB HL at all frequencies. Is the 30-dB air-bone gap observed in the left ear a real indication of a conductive hearing loss in that ear? Without the use of masking in the measurement of the bone conduction thresholds of the left ear, the clinician can't answer that question confidently. We know that the bone conduction thresholds of the nontest (right) ear will be less than or equal to the air conduction threshold of that ear (0 dB HL). Thus, when we observe this same bone conduction threshold when testing the test (left) ear, either of two explanations is possible. First, the bone conduction threshold could be providing a valid indication of the bone conduction hearing in that ear. This means that a conductive hearing loss is present in that ear. Second, the bone conduction threshold of the test ear could actually be poorer than 0 dB HL, but could simply be reflecting the response of the better ear (the nontest ear with a threshold of 0 dB HL). By masking the nontest ear, we can decide between these two explanations for the observed bone conduction threshold of the test ear. If the bone conduction threshold of the test ear remains unchanged when sufficient masking noise is introduced into the nontest ear, we may safely conclude that it provides an accurate indication of bone conduction hearing in that ear.

As we have seen, the need to mask the nontest ear and the rules for when to mask are relatively straightforward. There are a variety of masking procedures that have been developed to determine how much masking is sufficient. A detailed description of these procedures is beyond the scope of this introductory text. One particular approach, the plateau method, is briefly described in the supplement at the end of this chapter and in the accompanying computer diskette. Additional references on masking can be found at the end of this chapter.

SPEECH AUDIOMETRY

Although pure-tone thresholds tell us much about the function of the auditory system, they do not provide the audiologist with a precise measure of a person's ability to understand speech. Speech audiometry, a technique designed to assess a person's ability to hear and understand speech, has become a basic tool in the overall assessment of hearing handicap. In this section, some of the applications of speech audiometry in the basic hearing evaluation are reviewed.

Speech Audiometer

Speech audiometry generally requires a two-room testing suite—a control room, which contains the audiometric equipment as well as the audiologist, and an evaluation room, where the patient is located (Fig. 4.9). Most diagnostic audiometers include the appropriate circuitry for both pure-tone measurement and speech audiometric evaluation. The speech circuitry portion of a diagnostic audiometer consists of a calibrated amplifying system having a variety of options for input and output of speech signals. Most commonly, the speech audiometer accommodates inputs for a microphone, tape recorder, and compact-disc (CD) player. It is possible to conduct speech testing using "live" speech (microphone) or prerecorded materials. The output of the speech signal may be directed to earphones, a bone vibrator, or a loudspeaker situated in the test room. Speech-audiometric testing via air conduction can be conducted in one ear (monaurally), in both ears (binaurally), or in a sound-field environment. Bone conduction testing is also possible. Many diagnostic

Two Room Test Suite

FIGURE 4.9.
Typical two-room test setup for speech audiometry. Two enclosed rooms are needed, including one for the examiner, because speech is often presented using live voice and a microphone. The enclosed room for the audiologist helps to minimize pick-up of unwanted environmental sounds by the microphone during such testing.

audiometers employ a dual-channel system that enables the examiner to incorporate two inputs at the same time and to direct these signals to any of the available outputs.

To ensure valid and reliable measurements, just as with pure-tone audiometry, the circuitry of the speech audiometer must be calibrated on a regular basis. The acoustic output of the speech audiometer is calibrated in decibels relative to normal hearing threshold (dB HL). According to our most recent standards for speech audiometers, 0 dB HL is equivalent to 20 dB SPL when measured through earphones. There is a difference of approximately 7.5 dB between earphone and sound-field threshold measurements for speech signals. Consequently, 0 dB HL in the sound field corresponds to an output from a loudspeaker of approximately 12 dB SPL. This calculated difference in audiometric zero for earphones and loudspeakers allows us to obtain equivalent speech thresholds in decibels HL under these two listening conditions.

Assessment of Speech Recognition Threshold

SRT is the intensity at which an individual can identify simple speech materials approximately 50% of the time. It is included in the basic hearing evaluation for two specific reasons. First, it serves as an excellent check on the validity of pure-tone thresholds. There is a strong correlation between the average of the pure-tone thresholds obtained at the frequencies known to be important for speech (i.e., 500,

1000, and 2000 Hz) and the SRT. Large discrepancies between the SRT and this pure-tone average (PTA) may suggest functional, or nonorganic, hearing loss. A second important reason for including the SRT in the hearing evaluation is that it provides a basis for selecting the sound level at which a patient's speech recognition abilities should be tested. Finally, besides its use in the basic hearing evaluation, the SRT is also useful in the determination of functional gain in the hearing aid evaluation process. (See Chapter 7.)

Speech Threshold Materials

The most popular test materials used by audiologists to measure SRT are spondaic words. Spondaic words are two-syllable words spoken with equal stress on each syllable (e.g., baseball, hotdog, cowboy). A carrier phrase, such as "say the word," may precede each stimulus item. The spondaic words used most widely by audiologists are taken from the Central Institute for the Deaf (CID) Auditory Test W-1.

Speech Threshold Procedures

Several different procedures have been advocated for determining the SRT using spondaic words. The procedure recommended by the Committee on Audiometric Guidelines of the American Speech-Language-Hearing Association (ASHA) uses most of the 36 spondaic words from the CID W-1 word list. The testing begins by first presenting all of the spondaic words to the client at a comfortable level. This familiarizes the patient with the words to be used in the measurement of threshold.

The actual test procedure is a descending threshold technique that consists of two phases: a preliminary phase and a test phase. In the preliminary phase, the first spondaic word is presented at 30–40 dB above the estimated threshold (pure-tone average) or at 50 dB HL, if an estimate can not be obtained. If the client fails to respond at this level or responds incorrectly, the starting level is increased 20 dB. This is continued until a correct response is obtained. A correct response is then followed by a 10-dB decrease in level until the response changes to an incorrect one. At this level, a second spondee is then presented. The level is decreased in 10-dB steps until two consecutive words have been missed at the same level. The level is then increased 10 dB above the level at which two consecutive spondees were missed. This represents the starting level for the next phase, the test phase.

During the test phase, two spondaic words are presented at the starting level and at each successive 2-dB decrement in level. If five of the first six spondees are repeated correctly, this process continues until five of the last six spondees are responded to incorrectly. If five of the first six stimuli were not repeated correctly, then the starting level is increased 4–10 dB, and the descending series of stimulus presentations is initiated.

The descending procedure recommended by the ASHA begins with speech levels above threshold and "descends" toward threshold. At the first few presentation levels, about 80% (five of six) of the items are correct. At the ending level, about 20% (one of six) spondees are repeated correctly. A formula is used to then calculate the SRT. The SRT represents the lowest hearing level at which an individual can recognize 50% of the speech material.

Assessment of Suprathreshold Speech Recognition

Although the speech threshold provides the clinician with the index of the degree of hearing loss for speech, it does not offer any information regarding a person's ability to make distinctions among the various acoustic cues in our spoken language at conversational intensity levels. Unlike the situation with the SRT, attempts to calculate a person's ability to understand speech presented at comfortably loud levels based on data from the pure-tone audiogram have not been successful. Consequently, various suprathreshold speech recognition tests have been developed for the purpose of estimating a person's ability to understand conversational speech. Three of the more common types of speech recognition tests are phonetically balanced word lists, multiple-choice tests, and sentence tests.

Phonetically Balanced Word Lists

The most popular phonetically balanced (PB) word lists are summarized in Table 4.2. These word lists are referred to as "phonetically balanced" in that the phonetic composition of all lists are equivalent and representative of everyday English speech. All of the PB word lists utilize an open-set response format. The listener is not presented with a closed set of several alternatives for each test item, one of which is the monosyllabic word spoken by the examiner. Rather, the set of possible responses to a test item is open and is limited only by the listener's vocabulary.

For comparison purposes, representative performance-intensity functions for many of these lists appear in Figure 4.10. As evidenced by Figure 4.10, a perfor-

Table 4.2.
A Summary of the Features of Several Common Speech-Recognition Tests

Response Format	Test	No. of Items (Alt.)[a]	No. of Lists[b]	Reference
Open	PAL PB-50	50	20	Egan (1)
	CID W-22	50	4	Hirsh et al. (2)
	NU #6	50	4	Tillman and Carhart (3)
Closed	MRHT	50 (6)	6	House et al. (4)
	CCT	100 (4)	2	Owens and Schubert (5)
	CUNY NST	67–102 (7–9)	1[c]	Levitt and Resnick (6)

[a]Alt., number of alternatives in the multiple-choice, closed response-set tests.

[b]Lists refer to sets of unique words.

[c]Although the same nonsense syllables are used, there are 14 randomizations of these materials available, seven with a female talker and seven with a male talker.

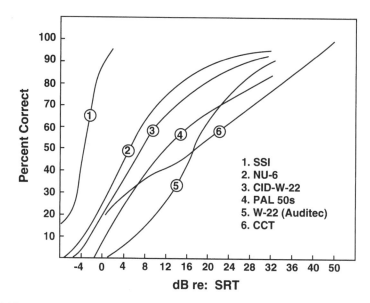

Figure 4.10
Performance-intensity functions of different suprathreshold speech recognition tests. Functions 3 and 5 represent two different recordings of the W-22 material.

mance-intensity function describes performance (for either a group or an individual) in percentage-correct recognition of the test items as a function of the intensity of the speech signal. The intensity of the speech signal is usually specified in decibels above SRT (i.e., decibels sensation level re: SRT, abbreviated dB SL). Because two different recordings of one set of items, the *CID* W-22 lists, are widely used, both of their performance-intensity functions are illustrated in Figure 4.10. This figure readily demonstrates that tests do differ. The most difficult test among these monosyllabic materials is the Psychoacoustic Laboratory (PAL) PB-50s. On the most linear portion of the curve (from 20 to 80% correct), identification performance for this test increases most slowly at a rate of 3.8%/dB. It is of interest to note the differences observed between the functions of the two recorded versions of the CID W-22s (labeled 3 and 5 in Fig. 4.10). Results for the most recent recording (5) are displaced to higher sensation levels than are the results for the original version (3). Such differences illustrate clearly that two different recordings of the same material can yield significantly different performance functions. It is the recorded words that compose the test and not simply the printed list of words.

Multiple-Choice Tests

Some clinicians, unsatisfied with the conventional open-set PB words, directed their attention to alternative test formats for word-recognition testing. The closed-set format inherent with multiple-choice tests was one of the most popular alternatives developed. The closed-set tests provide several advantages over open-set word-recognition tests. The closed-set format eliminates the need to familiarize a

```
VEST  REST
NEST  TEST
BEST  WEST
```

FIGURE 4.11.
Examples of a test ensemble used in the Modified Rhyme Hearing Test (MRHT).

subject with the test vocabulary and reduces the potential for a practice effect. Other advantages of the closed-set format include elimination of examiner bias, ease of administration, and simplified scoring techniques.

Table 4.2 summarizes the features of several popular multiple-choice tests. The most widely recognized multiple-choice test, the Modified Rhyme Hearing Test (MRHT), was introduced in 1968 as a recorded clinical test of speech recognition by a group from the Stanford Research Institute. A sample test ensemble is shown in Figure 4.11. In this and other multiple-choice tests, the choices available to the listener usually differ from one another by only one speech sound.

Another development in multiple-choice tests occurred with the introduction of the California Consonant Test (CCT), a consonant-identification test developed for and standardized on a hearing-impaired population. The CCT is composed of two different scramblings of 100 test items, each of which is arranged within an ensemble of four consonant-vowel-consonant monosyllabic words. For each item, the words are assembled so that either the initial two phonemes are the same, with the final phoneme varying, or, conversely, the final two phonemes are the same, with the initial phoneme varying. Of the 100 test items, 36 consonants are located in the initial position, whereas 64 consonants are found in the final position. Figure 4.12 shows an example consisting of four different test ensembles.

Figure 4.10 shows the performance-intensity function for the CCT (labeled 6). The function for the CCT is distinct from the functions for the other test materials. The slope of the function is only 1.6%/dB. In addition, notice that maximum intelligibility is not reached until signal intensity reaches 50 dB SL (re: SRT).

Another development in speech audiometry is the emergence of closed-set non-sense syllable tests. One such test, the City University of New York (CUNY) Non-sense Syllable Test (NST), is composed of consonant-vowel and vowel-consonant syllables categorized into 11 subtests of 7 to 9 syllables each. The syllables in these

```
BACK   _____   GAVE   _____
BAT    _____   GAME   _____
BATCH  _____   GAZE   _____
BATH   _____   GAGE   _____

THIN   _____   LEASE  _____
TIN    _____   LEASH  _____
SIN    _____   LEAF   _____
SHIN   _____   LEAP   _____
```

FIGURE 4.12.
Examples of four different test ensembles used in the California Consonant Test (CCT).

subtests differ in (*a*) consonant voicing (voiced or voiceless), (*b*) syllable position of the consonant (initial or final position), and (*c*) vowel context (/a, u, i/). With this test, it is possible to obtain a somewhat detailed picture of the *type* of errors made by the listener and not just an indication of the total number of errors made. More detailed knowledge of the types of perceptual errors made by the patient should lead to more effective remediation of their speech understanding difficulties.

Sentence Tests

In an attempt to approximate everyday speech more closely, several speech identification tests have been developed using sentences as the basic test item. An advantage of speech tests using sentence materials over other types of speech tests is that sentences approximate the spectral and contextual characteristics of everyday conversational speech while controlling for sentence length and semantic content. This increases the test's face validity.

The first sentence test designed to clinically assess speech recognition ability was developed and recorded at the CID. At present, however, there are no commercial recordings of these materials. Consequently, the clinical application of the CID sentences is somewhat limited.

One popular sentence test is the Synthetic Sentence Identification (SSI) test. The sentences used in this test were constructed such that each successive group of three words in the sentence was itself meaningful, but the entire sentence was not. The following is an example of a test item from the SSI: "Forward march said the boy had a."

Figure 4.10 shows a sample performance-intensity function for the SSI. Clearly, this test is much easier than other materials represented in this figure. In an effort to increase the difficulty of this test, a competing speech message was mixed with the sentences. For clinical evaluation purposes, it was recommended that the SSI be administered at a message-to-competition ratio of 0 dB; that is, both the speech and the competition are delivered at the same intensity level. This amount of competition yielded performance scores in normal listeners that were comparable to scores obtained with phonetically balanced materials in a quiet environment.

Another sentence identification test, referred to as the Speech Perception in Noise (SPIN) test, has also been developed and evaluated clinically. The eight available lists of the revised SPIN test are each composed of 50 sentences, each being five to eight words in length. The last word of each sentence is the test item. Twenty-five of the sentences contain test items that are classified as having "high predictability," which means that the word is readily predictable given the context of the sentence. Conversely, 25 sentences have test items with "low predictability." An example of a sentence containing a high-predictability test item is: "The boat sailed across the *bay*," whereas an example of a sentence with low predictability using the same test word is: "John was talking about the *bay*." The test's developers also provide a recording of a background of babble-type competition composed of 12 voices reading simultaneously.

Speech Materials for the Pediatric Population

This section reviews some speech materials commonly used to assess the word-recognition skills of children. The major modification required in the evaluation of children is to ensure that the speech material is within the receptive vocabulary of the child under test. The required response, moreover, must be appropriate for the age tested. It would not be appropriate, for example, to ask for written responses from a 4-year-old on a word-recognition task!

The three most popular tests for use with the pediatric population are (*a*) the Phonetically Balanced Kindergarten test (PBK-50s), (*b*) the Word Intelligibility by Picture Identification (WIPI) test, and (*c*) the Northwestern University Auditory Test No. 6 (NU-6). The performance-intensity function for the latter test was described previously in this chapter. The NU-6 materials are appropriate for use with adults and children 8 years of age and older. The PBK-50s, an open-response test, appear to be most suitable for children between the ages of 5 and 7 years.

For many younger children, the open-response design of the PBK-50s and NU-6 provides a complicated task, which causes difficulty in the administration and scoring of the test. For example, a child with a speech problem is difficult to evaluate because oral responses may not represent what the child actually perceived. In addition, children sometimes lose interest in the task because of the tedium associated with this format. Many children's lists have incorporated a closed-set response format to minimize some of these problems.

Probably the most popular multiple-choice test for use with hearing-impaired children is the WIPI test. This test consists of four 25-word lists of monosyllabic words within the vocabulary of preschool-age children. For a given test item, the child is presented with a page containing six pictures, one of which is a picture of the test item. The appropriate response of the child is to point to or touch the picture corresponding to the word perceived. The WIPI test is most appropriate for children between the ages of 2¹⁄₂ and 6 years.

Clinical Decisions in the Assessment of Speech Recognition

The speech recognition score can be influenced (sometimes to a large extent) by several variables, most of which are related to the procedures used in test administration. Because of their important implications for the audiologist, several of these variables are considered below.

Mode of Test Presentation. The audiologist needs to think about the details of test presentation. Speech recognition scores can be affected dramatically by speaker differences, methods used in recording the test materials, and characteristics of the test equipment. When considering the protocol for presenting the test materials, there seem to be three issues of special concern to the clinician: (*a*) whether to use recorded materials or a monitored live-voice presentation, (*b*) whether to use a carrier phrase, and (*c*) how to determine the appropriate intensity level at which to administer the test materials.

Generally, recorded materials offer greater test reliability than monitored live-voice presentations. The score on retest is more similar to results obtained just prior to retest when recorded materials are used. With many clinical populations, however, greater flexibility is needed than is offered by a tape-recorded test. This is frequently the case, for example, when testing young children. Under these circumstances, monitored live-voice presentation is preferred.

A common practice in the assessment of speech recognition is to preface each test item with a carrier phrase such as "Say the word," "You will say," or "Write the word." Carrier phrases are used for two basic purposes. First, they prepare the listener for the upcoming stimulus item, and second, they help the clinician monitor the intensity of the speech signal during monitored live-voice presentation.

Another important consideration for the audiologist is determining the intensity level that is most appropriate for administering a speech recognition test. The objective is usually to estimate the listener's maximum ability to understand speech, often referred to as the "PB-max" when phonetically balanced monosyllabic materials are used. The only true means of obtaining the best speech recognition score is to obtain a complete performance-intensity function. That is, several lists should be presented at successively higher intensity levels. Such a procedure, however, is clinically impractical because of the time required. Instead, clinicians attempt to estimate maximum speech recognition ability from just one intensity level, usually 40 dB above the SRT. The intensity needed to yield a maximum recognition score will vary with the test material used. Figure 4.10 shows the variation in scores that may occur as a function of material. It is noted, for example, that when using the CCT, an intensity of 50 dB SL is required to achieve a maximum score, whereas with the original recordings of the W-22 materials, only 25 dB SL is needed to reach a best score.

Ideally, it is recommended that the clinician administer the speech recognition test at two or three successively higher intensity levels, if time permits. Understandably, however, such a practice is simply not always practical in the clinical milieu. Sometimes the clinician will have to select one intensity level for estimating the PB-max.

Mode of Response. In scoring the responses to a speech recognition test, the most common practice is for the clinician to judge whether the listener's oral response was correct or in error. However, if the patient is able, and if time permits, a written response should be employed in an effort to minimize any biases of the clinician. The patient's written responses are much easier to implement for multiple-choice tests.

Listening Conditions. There are limitations associated with the assessment of speech recognition ability in a quiet environment. First, it is known that many of the available speech recognition tests fail to differentiate among hearing-impaired listeners when administered in a quiet test condition. That is, the tests simply do not appear difficult enough to identify the problems experienced by many listeners with hearing loss. A second disadvantage with performing speech audiometry in quiet is that such a testing condition does not reflect the typical environment encountered in everyday listening situations.

In an attempt to increase the difficulty of the identification task and simulate a more realistic listening environment, audiologists have turned to the use of various background noises and competing messages in the assessment of speech recognition. In 1968, Carhart emphasized the need for clinicians to assess speech recognition ability under conditions that more closely approximated typical listening situations. Carhart's impressions on this subject can best be summarized by his statement, ". . . once we have developed good methods for measuring a patient's capacity to understand speech under adverse listening conditions we will possess the audiological tools for dealing much more insightfully with his everyday listening problems" (7). Unfortunately, there are no standardized procedures, to date, for assessing recognition under adverse listening conditions, even though there is an abundance of literature in this area.

Several types of background noises or competition have been used in speech recognition tests, including white noise, filtered and shaped noise, modulated white noise, cafeteria noise, and spoken messages (from one to several talkers). All such background signals are known to degrade the perception of the speech signal to various degrees. Unfortunately, the addition of background noise also increases the variability of test results and reduces the reliability of the data. Nonetheless, by measuring recognition under adverse listening conditions, the clinician is able to assess more adequately the communicative handicap imposed by the patient's hearing impairment.

Masking. In speech audiometry, just as in pure-tone measurements, cross-over can occur from the test ear to the nontest ear. Consequently, when the level of the speech signal presented to the test ear exceeds the bone conduction threshold of the nontest ear by more than 35 dB, masking may be necessary.

ACOUSTIC IMMITTANCE MEASUREMENT

Impedance, as mentioned in Chapter 2, is defined as the opposition to the flow of energy through a system. When an acoustic wave strikes the eardrum of the normal ear, a portion of the signal is transmitted through the middle ear to the cochlea, while the remaining part of the wave is reflected back out the external canal. The reflected energy forms a sound wave traveling in an outward direction with an amplitude and phase that depend on the opposition encountered at the tympanic membrane. The energy of the reflected wave is greatest when the middle ear system is stiff or immobile, as in such pathologic conditions as otitis media with effusion and otosclerosis. On the other hand, an ear with ossicular-chain interruption will reflect considerably less sound back into the canal because of the reduced stiffness. A greater portion of the acoustic wave will be transmitted to the middle ear under these circumstances. The reflected sound wave, therefore, carries information about the status of the middle ear system.

The reciprocal of impedance is admittance. An ear with a high impedance has a low admittance, and vice versa. Admittance describes the relative ease with which energy flows through a system. Some commercially available devices used by the clinician measure quantities related to acoustic impedance of the middle ear, whereas others measure quantities related to acoustic admittance. In an effort to provide a common vocabulary for results obtained with either device, professionals have decided to use the term "immittance." Immittance itself is not a physical quantity but simply a term that can be used to refer to either impedance data or admittance data.

The measurement of acoustic immittance at the tympanic membrane is an important component of the basic hearing evaluation. This sensitive and objective diagnostic tool has been used to identify the presence of fluid in the middle ear, to evaluate eustachian tube and facial nerve function, to predict audiometric findings, to determine the nature of hearing loss, and to assist in diagnosing the site of auditory lesion. This technique is considered particularly useful in the assessment of difficult-to-test persons, including very young children.

Figure 4.13 shows how this concept may be applied to actual practice. A pliable probe tip is inserted carefully into the ear canal and an airtight seal is obtained so that varying amounts of air pressure can be applied to the ear cavity by pumping air into the ear canal or suctioning it out. A positive amount of air pressure (usually

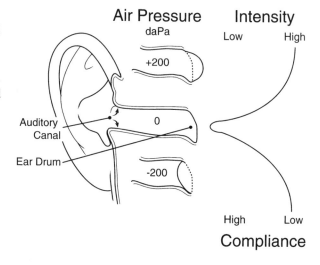

FIGURE 4.13.
Concepts of immittance applied in practice. The *middle column* shows three different air pressures developed in the ear canal (+200, 0, and −200 daPa), and the *dotted line* in the drawings at the top and bottom of this column represent the resting position of the eardrum (at 0 daPa). The *right column* shows both the sound intensity of the probe tone recorded in the ear canal as the air pressure is changed from +200 daPa (*top*) to −200 daPa (*bottom*) and the corresponding changes in the compliance of the middle ear.

FIGURE 4.14.
Components of an immittance instrument.

+200 daPa)[a] is then introduced into the airtight ear canal, forcing the tympanic membrane inward. The eardrum is now stiffer than it is in its natural state because of the positive pressure created in the ear canal. A low-frequency pure tone is then introduced, and a tiny microphone measures the level of the sound reflected from the stiffened eardrum. A low-frequency tone is used because this is the frequency region most affected by changes in stiffness. (See Chapter 2.) Keeping the intensity of the probe tone introduced into the ear canal constant, the pressure is then reduced slowly, causing the tympanic membrane to become more compliant (less stiff). As the tympanic membrane becomes increasingly compliant, more of the acoustic signal will be passed through the middle ear, and the level of the reflected sound in the ear canal will decrease. When the air pressure in the ear canal equals the air pressure in the middle ear, the tympanic membrane will move with the greatest ease. As the pressure is reduced further, the tympanic membrane is pulled outward, and the eardrum again becomes less mobile. As before, when the eardrum becomes stiffer or less compliant, more low-frequency energy is reflected off the tympanic membrane, and the sound level within the ear canal increases.

Figure 4.14 illustrates the basic components of most immittance instruments. The probe tip is sealed in the ear canal, providing a closed cavity. The probe con-

---

[a] daPa is a measure of air pressure in units of dekaPascals. 1 daPa = 10 Pa = 1.02 mm H_2O. Millimeters (mm) H_2O refers to the amount of pressure needed to push a column of water in a special tube to a given height in millimeters. For measurements of immittance, air pressure is generally expressed relative to ambient air pressure. That is, ambient air pressure is represented as 0 daPa, and a pressure 100 daPa above ambient pressure is represented as +100 daPa.

tains three small ports that are connected to (*a*) a sound source that generates a low-frequency (usually 220- or 660-Hz) pure tone, (*b*) a microphone to measure the reflected sound wave, and (*c*) an air pump and manometer for varying the air pressure within the ear canal.

Immittance Test Battery

Three basic measurements—tympanometry, static acoustic immittance, and threshold of the acoustic reflex—commonly make up the basic acoustic immittance test battery.

Tympanometry

Acoustic immittance at the tympanic membrane of a normal ear changes systematically as air pressure in the external canal is varied above and below ambient air pressure (see Fig. 4.13). The normal relationship between air pressure changes and changes in immittance is frequently altered in the presence of middle ear disease. Tympanometry is the measurement of the mobility of the middle ear when air pressure in the external canal is varied from +200 to −400 daPa. Results from tympanometry are then plotted on a graph, with air pressure along the *x* axis and immittance, or *compliance*, along the *y* axis.[b] Figure 4.15 illustrates some of the tympanograms commonly seen in normal and pathologic ears.

Various estimates have been made of the air pressure in the ear canal that results in the least amount of reflected sound energy from normal middle ears. This air pressure is routinely referred to as the peak pressure point. A normal tympanogram for an adult (Fig. 4.15*a*) has a peak pressure point between −100 and +40 daPa, which suggests that the middle ear functions optimally at or near ambient pressure (0 daPa). Tympanograms that peak at a point below the accepted range of normal pressures (Fig. 4.15*b*) suggest malfunction of the middle ear pressure-equalizing system. This malfunction might be due to eustachian tube malfunction, early or resolving serous otitis media, or acute otitis media. (These and other disorders are described in detail in Chapter 5.) Ears that contain fluid behind the eardrum are characterized by a flat tympanogram at a high impedance or low admittance value without a peak pressure point (Fig. 4.15*c*). This implies an excessively stiff system that does not allow for an increase in sound transmission through the middle ear under any pressure state.

The amplitude (height) of the tympanogram also provides information about the compliance or elasticity of the system. A stiff middle ear (as in, for example,

---

[b] Throughout this text, we have assumed that immittance measurements are made with an impedance meter. With such a device, immittance values are described in arbitrary units, frequently labeled "compliance." These devices do not actually measure compliance.

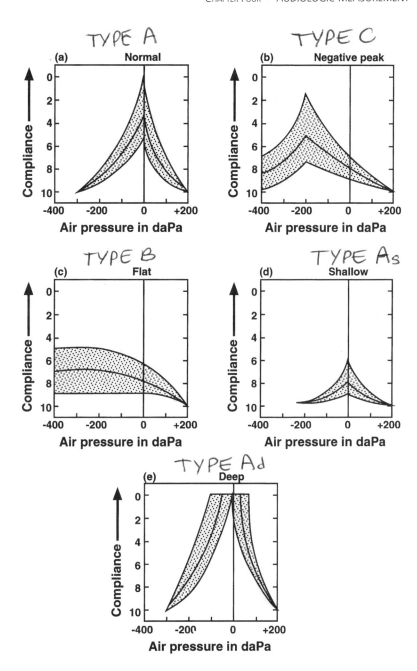

FIGURE 4.15.

Tympanometric configurations seen in normal and pathologic ears. Measured tymp-manograms falling in the *dotted regions* would be classified using the label at the top of each tympanogram (normal, negative peak, flat, etc.).

ossicular-chain fixation) is represented by a shallow amplitude, suggesting high acoustic impedance or low admittance (Fig. 4.15*d*). Conversely, an ear with abnormally low acoustic impedance or high admittance (as in an interrupted ossicular chain or a hypermobile tympanic membrane) is revealed by a tympanogram with a very high amplitude (Fig. 4.15*e*).

As noted, most tympanograms are measured using low-frequency probe tones introduced into the ear canal; frequencies of 220 and 660 Hz are the most commonly used frequencies. In recent years, however, there has been increased interest in the use of multiple probe-tone frequencies in which a family of tympanograms are obtained for a wide range of probe frequencies. This has usually been accomplished by sweeping the probe tone frequency from a low to a high value at each of several air-pressure values or by sweeping the air pressure from positive to negative (or vice versa) air pressures at each of several probe-tone frequencies. Use of multiple probe-tone frequencies allows measurement and specification of the resonant frequency of the middle ear. Although it has been suggested that changes in the resonant frequency observed with multiple-frequency tympanograms can improve the diagnostic capabilities of tympanometric measurements, the clinical usefulness of this additional information remains to be firmly established. It does appear, however, that multiple-frequency tympanograms may be more useful than those obtained using only a 220-Hz or 660-Hz probe tone in detecting the presence of fluid in the middle ears of young infants (under 4 months of age).

Static Acoustic Immittance

Static acoustic immittance measures the ease of flow of acoustic energy through the middle ear and is usually expressed in "equivalent volume" in cubic centimeters. To obtain this measurement, immittance is first determined under a positive pressure (+200 daPa) artificially induced in the canal. Very little sound is admitted through the middle ear under this extreme positive pressure, with much of the acoustic energy reflected back into the ear canal. Next, a similar determination is made with the eardrum in its most compliant position, thus maximizing transmission through the middle ear cavity. The arithmetic difference between these two immittance values, usually recorded in cubic centimeters (cm^3) of equivalent volume, provides an estimate of immittance at the tympanic membrane. Compliance values less than or equal to 0.25 cm^3 of equivalent volume suggest low acoustic immittance (indicative of stiffening pathologies), and values greater than or equal to 2.0 cm^3 generally indicate abnormally high immittance (suggestive of ossicular discontinuity or healed tympanic membrane perforations).

Acoustic Reflex Threshold

The acoustic reflex threshold is defined as the lowest possible intensity needed to elicit a middle ear muscle contraction. Contraction of the middle ear muscles evoked by intense sound results in a temporary increase in the middle ear impedance. As noted in Chapter 3, the acoustic reflex is a consensual phenomenon; acoustic stimulation to one ear will elicit a muscle contraction and subsequent impedance change in both ears. Usually, the acoustic reflex is monitored in the ear canal contralateral to the ear receiving the sound stimulus. Figure 4.16 shows how it is measured. A headphone is placed on one ear, and the probe assembly is inserted into the contralateral ear. When the signal transduced from the earphone reaches an intensity sufficient to evoke an acoustic reflex, the stiffness of the middle ear is increased in both ears. This results in more sound being reflected from the eardrum, and a subsequent increase in sound pressure is observed on the immittance instrument. In recording the data, it is standard procedure to consider the ear stimulated with the intense sound as the ear under test. Because the ear stimulated is contralateral to the ear in which the reflex is measured, these reflex thresholds are referred to as contralateral reflex thresholds. It is also frequently possible to present the loud reflex-activating stimulus through the probe assembly itself. In this case, the reflex is both activated and measured in the same ear. This is referred to as an ipsilateral acoustic reflex.

In the normal ear, contraction of middle ear muscles occurs with pure tones ranging from 65 to 95 dB HL. A conductive hearing loss, however, tends to either elevate or eliminate the reflex response. When acoustic reflex information is used in conjunction with tympanometry and static acoustic immittance measurements, it serves to substantiate further the existence of a middle ear disorder. With unilateral conductive hearing loss, failure to elicit the reflex depends on the size of the air-bone gap and on the ear in which the probe tip is inserted. If the stimulus is pre-

FIGURE 4.16.
Example of how an acoustic reflex is obtained for contralateral stimulus presentation. Essentially, for ipsilateral measurements, the functions of the probe tip and the earphone are combined so that the reflex-eliciting stimulus and the immittance change that results from the muscle contraction can be measured in the same ear.

sented to the good ear and the probe tip is placed on the affected side, an air-bone gap of only 10 dB will usually abolish the reflex response. If, however, the stimulus is presented to the pathologic ear and the probe is in the normal ear, a gap of 25 dB is needed to abolish or significantly elevate the reflex threshold.

Acoustic reflex thresholds can also be useful in differentiating whether a sensorineural hearing loss is due to a lesion in the inner ear or to one in the auditory nerve. For hearing losses ranging from mild to severe, the acoustic reflex threshold is more likely to be elevated or absent in ears with neural pathology than in those with cochlear damage. The pattern of acoustic reflex thresholds for ipsilateral and contralateral stimulation across both ears, moreover, can aid in diagnosing brainstem lesions affecting the reflex pathways in the auditory brainstem. (See Chapter 3 for a brief overview of these pathways.)

Special Considerations in the Use of Immittance with Young Children

Immittance can be most valuable in the assessment of young children, although it does have some diagnostic limitations. Further, although electroacoustic immittance measures are ordinarily simple and quick to obtain, special consideration and skills are required to obtain these measures successfully from young infants.

Although immittance tests may be administered to neonates and young infants with a reasonable amount of success, tympanometry may have limited value with children younger than 7 months of age. Below this age, there is a poor correlation between tympanometry and the actual condition of the middle ear. In very young infants, a normal tympanogram does not necessarily imply that there is a normal middle ear system. However, a flat tympanogram obtained in an infant strongly suggests a diseased ear. Consequently, it is still worthwhile to administer immittance tests to this population.

Another limitation of immittance measurements is the difficulty of obtaining measurements from a hyperactive child or a child who is crying, yawning, or continually talking. A young child who exhibits excessive body movement or head turning will make it almost impossible to maintain an airtight seal with the probe tip. Vocalization produces middle ear muscle activity that in turn causes continual alterations in the compliance of the tympanic membrane, making immittance measurements impossible. With difficult-to-test and younger children, specialized techniques are needed to keep the child relatively calm and quiet. For young children, it is always recommended that a second person be involved in the evaluation. While the child is sitting on the parent's lap, one person can place the earphone and insert the probe tip while a second person manipulates the controls of the equipment. With infants below 2 years of age, placing the earphones and headband on the child's head is often distracting. It may be helpful to remove the earphone from the headband, rest the band over the mother's shoulder, and insert the probe tip into the child's ear. It is also helpful to use some distractive techniques that will occupy the child's attention during the test (Vignette 4.4).

VIGNETTE 4.4.

Distractive techniques used in evaluating young children with immittance.[a]

Flashlight

Direct the light toward the child or shine it on objects or people well within the child's visual field. Constantly change the rate of movement from slow to fast. If habituation occurs, take the child's hand and repeatedly place it over the light source.

Animated Toys

Introduce animated toys only as required at critical times necessary to complete the test. Avoid movement artifacts by keeping the toy well out of the reach of the child.

Cotton Swab

Gently brush the back of the child's hand, arm, or leg in a slow, even motion. Make the distraction visual as well as tactile by making oscillatory or exaggerated movements of the swab.

Pendulum

Using a bright and unusually shaped object, make a pendulum with about an 18-inch string. This technique is highly effective if the examiner swings the pendulum about in various motions within various areas of the infant's vision. Swing the pendulum rather slowly in short excursions, permitting easy visual following. Frequently stop or alter the swinging motion to provide novelty to the pendular action.

Mirror

To an infant less than 1 year of age who is capable of reacting and attending to faces, a large mirror is sometimes irresistible, at least for a period sufficiently long to place a probe tip and to perform the impedance test battery.

Toys That Produce Sounds

Toys or other devices that emit intense sounds should be avoided since they may evoke an acoustic or other reflexive response from the child. Toys that produce softer sounds in no way interfere with the test and can therefore by used effectively, especially if the sound is novel.

Food

Children, like adults, seem to enjoy sweets, and although swallowing and sucking movements are notorious for producing artifacts in the tympanogram and reflex measures, food can still be used as a distractive technique. Flavored gelatin or soft-drink powder in water, honey, or sweetened lemon juice can be dropped into the child's mouth at intervals during the test. Avoid taking measures until the reflexive sucking action has subsided. Administering small amounts of liquid at well-spaced intervals can keep the child occupied for many minutes.

VIGNETTE **4.4**—*continued*

Watch

In front of the child, simply remove one's wristwatch, manipulate or wind it well out of reach of the child or point to it.

Shoe

A simple yet effective technique is to begin lacing and unlacing a child's shoe, either on or off his foot. This should be carefully timed to coincide with the insertion of the test tip into the ear. Move slowly and methodically and do not appear to have any object in mind except to lace and unlace the shoe.

Action Toys

A variety of toys are available that perform repetitive actions, such as a monkey that climbs down a stick pole. Often these are not the best distractive devices because children 1 year and older often wish to handle or manipulate this type of toy.

Wad of Cotton or Tissue

A cotton ball can facilitate effective passive attention by balancing the cotton on the hand, arm, or knee of the child or on the hand of the assistant. It can be squeezed or otherwise manipulated; it can be blown or allowed to fall repeatedly from the hand. A tissue can also be used as a parachute, torn slowly into shapes, rolled into small balls and placed in the child's hand, waved, punctured, and so forth.

Tape

A roll of adhesive or paper surgical tape has been found to be one of the most effective distractive devices available in the clinic. Bits of tape can be torn off or stuck on various parts of the child's or examiner's anatomy. The child can be allowed to pull the tape off, objects can be picked up with the adhesive side of the tape, fingers can be bound together, links can be made with small strips, rings can be formed, fingernails covered, and innumerable other totally nonmeaningful manipulations can be performed. Tape works wonders for the few seconds necessary for obtaining immittance measures.

Lollipop

A lollipop can be utilized when the child is cradled and partially immobilized in the examiner's or parent's arm. The examiner can stroke the child's lips or tongue with the lollipop. Careful spacing of the lollipop sampling permits completion of the entire immittance test pattern.

Miscellaneous Devices

Tongue blades, cotton swabs, colored yarn, or similar devices are all effective as distractive devices. They are best utilized when manipulated or "played with" by the examiner. If the child insists, he can be allowed to manipulate the device. Care must be taken to permit only passive action so as to reduce movement artifact while the test is proceeding.

From Northern JL: Acoustic impedance in the pediatric population. *In* Bess FH (ed): *Childhood Deafness: Causation, Assessment and Management.* New York, Grune & Stratton, 1977.

BASIC AUDIOLOGIC TEST BATTERY

In the measurement of auditory function, the most meaningful information can be gleaned only when the entire test battery of pure-tone and speech audiometry together with immittance measurements is used. If just one or two of these procedures are employed, valuable clinical information will be lost, since each of these clinical tools offers a unique and informative set of data. In particular, the reader should keep in mind the differences between pure-tone measures and electro-acoustic-immittance measurements. Pure-tone audiometry does not measure the immittance of the middle ear, just as immittance does not measure hearing sensitivity. Although an abnormal audiogram strongly suggests the presence of a hearing loss, abnormal immittance does not. Abnormal immittance findings in the absence of significant hearing loss, on the other hand, can be sufficient grounds for medical referral. A test-battery approach is essential. Vignettes 4.5–4.7 show examples of applications of the test battery.

ADDITIONAL SPECIAL TESTS

The basic audiologic test battery determines whether or not the patient has any hearing loss; what effect the hearing loss, if present, has on speech understanding; and whether the nature of the hearing loss is conductive, sensorineural, or a combination of the two (mixed). The immittance battery can also evaluate middle ear function regardless of whether a measurable hearing loss is present. Thus, the basic audiologic test battery is able to determine where in the peripheral portion of the auditory system a lesion may be.

Additional special auditory tests are needed, however, to determine if lesions are present in more central portions of the ascending nervous system, such as the auditory nerve, brainstem, or cortex. A patient with a life-threatening tumor affecting the auditory nerve, for example, will frequently have pure-tone test results consistent with a high-frequency sensorineural hearing loss. Other components of the basic hearing test battery, however, may provide some "warning signs" suggesting that the lesion responsible for the hearing is affecting the auditory nerve. For example, the hearing loss in such cases usually affects the high frequencies and is different in the two ears, often leaving one ear completely unaffected. In addition, speech recognition scores in the impaired ear are often reduced much more than would be expected on the basis of the pure-tone hearing loss. Finally, acoustic reflex thresholds for the affected ear are typically elevated above the normal range (> 100 dB HL). Although these features are typical for many patients with tumors affecting the auditory nerve, many cases manifest only one or two of these features. Patients with inner ear pathology, moreover, may also manifest one or more of these features.

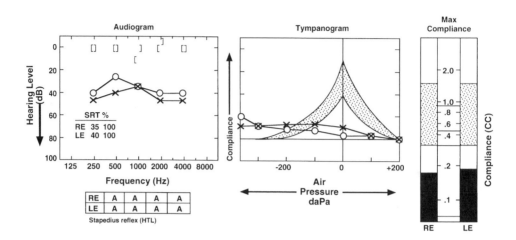

VIGNETTE 4.5.

A 6-year-old child with bilateral otitis media

The accompanying charts show a mild-to-moderate bilateral hearing loss for air conduction; bone conduction thresholds are normal in both ears. Such a discrepancy between air conduction and bone conduction thresholds suggests a conductive loss. The SRTs are compatible with the pure-tone data; when the signal is made comfortably loud, suprathreshold speech recognition is excellent in both ears. Good speech recognition is consistent with a middle ear disorder. Immittance confirms the impression of a conductive loss. The shaded areas on the tympanogram and static immittance forms represent normative data. The tympanograms are flat, the static immittance is well below normal, and acoustic reflexes are absent in both ears. This general pattern is consistent with a middle ear complication and strongly suggests a fluid-filled middle ear, thus requiring a medical referral. If however, there is no evidence of previous middle ear problems and the child has no complaints, a recheck should be recommended in 3 weeks. If the same results are obtained, the child should be referred to the family physician.

Educationally, such a problem can be relatively serious if medical intervention does not result in a speedy return to completely normal hearing levels. Such children are likely to appear listless and inattentive in the classroom, and their performance soon begins to deteriorate. Both the teacher and the parents should receive an explanation of these probable consequences from the audiologist. In counseling the teacher, emphasis should be placed on establishing favorable classroom seating, supplementing auditory input with visual cues, articulating clearly and forcefully, and frequently reiterating assignments. If the condition does not respond readily to medical treatment, amplification, along with other remedial measures such as speechreading instruction and training in listening skills, should not be ruled out. Above all, the child will need patient understanding while the hearing level is diminished and sometimes fluctuating from one day to the next.

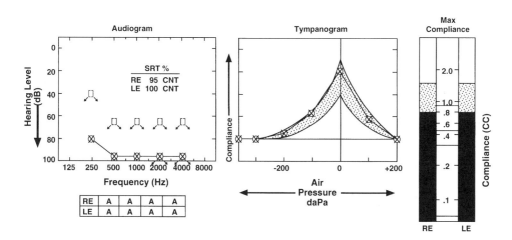

Vignette 4.6.

An 8-year-old child with a bilateral severe-to-profound sensorineural hearing loss

The pure-tone results in the accompanying figure display a severe-to-profound sensorineural hearing loss. Bone conduction responses could not be obtained at the maximum output limits of the audiometer. The SRTs using selected spondees were compatible with the pure-tone data. Suprathreshold speech recognition scores could not be obtained because of the severity of the loss. Immittance results on both ears show tympanograms and static immittance values to be within the normal range. Acoustic reflexes are absent in both ears, but these usually cannot be elicited with a hearing loss in excess of 85 dB HL.

These audiologic results confirm the irreversibility of the hearing impairment, which is so severe that the best possible special education opportunities must be made available. Periodic audiologic evaluations are highly important in the optimal educational management of such children. Frequently they suffer ear infections that further reduce their already greatly depressed level of sensitivity. At such times, the amplification program that has been recommended for them must be modified temporarily while medical treatment is being obtained.

Vignette 4.7.

Adult with a bilateral mild-to-moderate sensorineural hearing loss

The pure-tone results accompanying this vignette show a bilateral sloping sensorineural hearing loss in an elderly adult. The SRTs are compatible with the pure-tone data, and suprathreshold speech recognition is only fair to good, even when the signal is made comfortably loud. Immittance results show normal tympanograms and static immittance for both ears, with acoustic reflexes present, but elevated, bilaterally.

Normally, an adult with this battery of results will be either a successful user of individual amplification, a highly competent speechreader, or both. It may still be necessary to provide special assistance in the form of training in auditory and visual communication (speechreading) skills.

A battery of special auditory tests has been developed to assist in the identification of lesions occurring central to the cochlea or inner ear. These lesions are referred to as retrocochlear lesions. Historically, this test battery was based on a variety of behavioral tests that used pure tones as stimuli. After several years of test development and refinement, most of these tests were still only 60–70% accurate in identifying retrocochlear impairments. Many individuals with cochlear hearing loss were falsely identified as having retrocochlear lesions, and still more retrocochlear lesions were identified as cochlear.

Today's battery of special auditory tests consists of five basic tests, only one of which involves behavioral measurements in response to pure-tone stimulation (threshold tone decay). The five test procedures measure (*a*) threshold tone decay, (*b*) performance-intensity functions for speech materials, (*c*) acoustic reflex threshold, (*d*) acoustic reflex decay, and (*e*) auditory brainstem responses (see Chapter 3). This contemporary test battery is 90–95% accurate in identifying retrocochlear lesions. In addition, as noted in Chapter 3, diagnostic application of evoked otoacoustic emissions is being explored and may become a component of the test battery in the future.

Detailed descriptions of these procedures are beyond the scope of this book. It is important to note only that the basic audiologic test battery is limited in its diagnostic usefulness. Additional special auditory tests can be performed in the event that any of the retrocochlear warning signs described above are found after performing the basic tests. Readers who desire to learn more about the special auditory test battery can consult the Suggested Readings at the end of this chapter.

SUMMARY

We have reviewed the basic components of the test battery used in the measurement of auditory function. This includes the measurement of pure-tone threshold by air and bone conduction, speech audiometry, and immittance measurements. The results from these various approaches, when used as a battery, give the audiologist good insight into the nature and extent of the auditory disorder.

ADVANCED MATERIAL

More on Masking

In terms of masking, this chapter focused on its underlying concepts and on recognizing when it is necessary. In this supplemental material, the focus is on how to mask. As mentioned, several methods are available to mask the nontest ear for measurement of hearing threshold by air and bone conduction. This supplement briefly describes a common clinical method known as the plateau method (8).

This method is very simple and quite popular. Once the audiologist has determined that masking is needed for either air or bone conduction measurements, a low-intensity noise is delivered to the nontest ear. The noise might be a narrow-band noise with frequency content similar to the test tone, or it might be a broad-band noise. Once introduced into the nontest ear, the noise is increased in 5-dB steps. If threshold for the tone in the test ear never changes while increasing the noise level in the nontest ear to high intensities, then this is the true threshold of the test ear.

Frequently, however, this is not the case. At some point, the noise level will be increased in the nontest ear and make the tone in the test ear inaudible. At this point, threshold for the tone in the test ear is then measured again while the noise remains in the nontest ear. The noise level is increased 5 dB again, and the threshold is then re-established. Frequently during this portion of the plateau method, the level of the noise and tone are alternately increased by 5 dB several times. This is because both the tone and the noise are heard in the nontest ear. The tone is heard in that ear because it crosses over through the skull from the test ear while the noise is introduced directly into the nontest ear.

Eventually, the noise level will be raised by 5 dB several times with no change in threshold for the pure tone. At this point, the noise has eliminated the participation of the nontest ear in the detection of the tone, and the tone is producing sensation in the test ear. Increasing the noise level under these circumstances causes no shift in hearing threshold for the pure tone because the noise is in the nontest ear and the tone is now being heard in the test ear. The range of noise levels that fail to shift the threshold for the tone is referred to as the plateau. The level of the tone during the plateau represents the true threshold of the test ear at that frequency. Figure 4.17 illustrates the gradual increase in masking noise level up to the plateau, which occurs at a hearing level corresponding to the true hearing threshold of the test ear. Generally, the plateau should be 20–30 dB in width prior to termination of the masking procedure.

If the noise level in the nontest ear is increased further, beyond the plateau, the threshold of the pure tone will eventually begin to increase again (Fig. 4.17). This is known as overmasking and occurs when the noise in the nontest ear crosses over through the skull to the test ear and begins to mask the pure tone. During over-masking, the tone and noise will again be alternately increased in 5-dB steps, depending on the intensity of the noise during the plateau and the output limits of the audiometer. "Minimum masking" occurs at the noise level that first produces the plateau, and "maximum masking" occurs at the noise level at the end of the plateau, just prior to overmasking.

Additional details about masking methods are beyond the scope of this introductory text. The reader is referred to Hood (8), Studebaker (9), and Martin (10) for additional details about the plateau method, as well as alternative procedures.

FIGURE 4.17.
Plateau method of clinical masking. Masked bone-conduction threshold in the right ear (y axis) is plotted as a function of the masking noise level delivered by a headphone to the non-test (left) ear (x axis). The unmasked air-conduction threshold in the test ear was 30 dB HL, whereas both bone-conduction thresholds and the air-conduction threshold in the left ear were all 10 dB HL. Thus, there is a 20-dB air-bone gap in the right ear, according to the unmasked thresholds. Note, however, that the *masked* bone-conduction threshold of the right ear increases to 30 dB HL at the plateau, indicating that the 30-dB hearing loss in the right ear is sensorineural and not conductive. (The air-bone gap has diminished to 0 dB under masking.)

Practice Diskette

The computer diskette included with this book contains some tutorials for use with this chapter. These diskettes use animated characters to simulate the behavior of the patient and give you some hands-on practice in measurement of hearing threshold, use of masking, and immittance measurements. *Try it! You'll like it!*

REFERENCES

1. Egan J: Articulation testing methods. *Laryngoscope* 58:955–991, 1948.

2. Hirsh IJ, Davis H, Silverman SR, Reynolds FG, Eldert E, Benson RW: Development of materials for speech audiometry. *Journal of Speech and Hearing Disorders* 17:321–337, 1952.

3. Tillman TW, Carhart R: *An Expanded Test for Speech Discrimination Using CNC Mono-syllabic Words.* Northwestern University Auditory Test No. 6. Technical Report No. SAM-TR-66-55, USAF School of Aerospace Medicine, Brooks Air Force Base, Texas, 1966.

4. House AS, Williams CE, Hecker MHL, Kryter KD: Articulation testing methods: conso-nantal differentiation in a closed-response set. *Journal of the Acoustical Society of America* 20:463–474, 1965.

5. Owens E, Schubert ED: Development of the California consonant test. *Journal of Speech and Hearing Research* 20:463–474, 1977.

6. Levitt H, Resnick SB: Speech reception by the hearing impaired: methods of testing and the development of new tests. In Ludvigsen C, Barfod J (eds): Sensorineural Hearing Impaired and Hearing Aids. *Scandinavian Audiology Supplement* 6:107–130, 1978.

7. Carhart R: Future horizons in audiological diagnosis. *Annals of Otology, Rhinology, Laryngology* 77:706–716, 1968.

8. Hood JD: The principles and practice of bone-conduction audiometry: a review of the pres-ent position. *Laryngoscope* 70:1211–1228, 1960.

9. Studebaker GA: Clinical masking in air- and bone-conducted stimuli. *Journal of Speech and Hearing Disorders* 29:23–35, 1964.

10. Martin FN: Minimum effective masking levels in threshold audiometry. *Journal of Speech and Hearing Disorders* 39:280–285, 1974.

SUGGESTED READINGS

American Speech-Language-Hearing Association: Guidelines for audiometric symbols. *ASHA* 32(Suppl 2):25–30, 1990.

American Speech-Language-Hearing Association: Guidelines for determining threshold level for speech. *ASHA* 30(3):85–90, 1988.

Bess FH: Clinical assessment of speech recognition. *In* Konkle DF, Rintelmann WF (eds): Principles of Speech Audiometry. Baltimore, University Park Press, 1982.

Bess FH: The minimally hearing impaired child. *Ear and Hearing* 6:43–47, 1985.

Bluestone CD, Beery QC, Paradise JL: Audiometry and tympanometry in relation to middle ear effusions in children. *Laryngoscope* 83:594–604, 1963.

Carhart R, Jerger JF: Preferred method for clinical determination of pure-tone thresholds. *Journal of Speech and Hearing Disorders* 24:330–345, 1959.

Diefendorf AO: Pediatric audiology. *In* Lass NJ, McReynolds LV, Northern JL, Yoder DE (eds): *Handbook of Speech-Language Pathology and Audiology.* Philadelphia, BC Decker, 1988.

Jerger S: Speech audiometry. *In* Jerger J (ed): *Pediatric Audiology.* San Diego, College Hill Press, 1984.

House AS, Williams CE, Hecker MHL, Kryter KD: Articulation testing methods: consonan-tal differentiation in a closed-response set. *Journal of the Acoustical Society of America* 20:463–474, 1965.

Katz J: *Handbook of Clinical Audiology*, ed 4. Baltimore, Williams & Wilkins, 1993.

Northern JL: Acoustic impedance in the pediatric population. *In* Bess FH (ed): *Childhood Deafness: Causation, Assessment and Management*. New York, Grune & Stratton, 1977.

Northern JL, Downs MP: *Hearing in Children*, ed 4. Baltimore, Williams & Wilkins, 1991.

Olsen WO, Matkin ND: Speech audiometry. *In* Rintelmann WF (ed): *Hearing Assessment*. Baltimore, University Park Press, 1979.

Sanders JW: Masking. *In* Katz J (ed): *Handbook of Clinical Audiology*, ed 2. Baltimore, Williams & Wilkins, 1978, p 124.

Sanders JW: Diagnostic audiology. *In* Lass NJ, McReynolds NJ, Northern JL, Yoder DE (eds): *Handbook of Speech-Language Pathology and Audiology*. Philadelphia, BC Decker, 1988.

Schwartz D, Josey AF, Bess FH (eds): Proceedings of meeting in honor of Professor Jay Sanders. *Ear and Hearing* 8:4, 1987.

Shanks JE, Lilly DJ, Margolis RH, Wiley TL, Wilson RH: Tympanometry. *Journal of Speech and Hearing Disorders* 53:354–377, 1988.

Tillman TW, Olsen WO: Speech audiometry. *In* Jerger J (ed): *Modern Developments in Audiology*. New York, Academic Press, 1973.

CHAPTER FIVE

PATHOLOGIES OF THE AUDITORY SYSTEM

Following completion of this chapter, the reader should be able to:

- Understand the system used to classify auditory disorders.
- Discuss the most common disorders affecting the external ear and middle ear.
- Be familiar with typical disorders affecting the cochlea.
- Identify the most common disorders affecting the auditory central nervous system.
- Develop an appreciation and an understanding of the physical symptoms and audiologic manifestations associated with most of these disorders.

A variety of disorders, both congenital and acquired, directly affect the auditory system. These disorders can occur at the level of the external ear, the external auditory canal, the tympanic membrane, the middle ear space, the cochlea, the auditory central nervous system, or any combination of these sites. The following review offers a discussion of some of the more commonly seen disorders that can impair the auditory system.

CLASSIFICATION OF AUDITORY DISORDERS

All auditory disorders can be divided into two major classifications: exogenous (outside the genes) and endogenous (within the genes). Exogenous hearing disorders are those caused by inflammatory disease, toxicity, noise, accident, or injury that inflicts damage on any part of the auditory system. Endogenous conditions originate in the genetic characteristics of an individual. An endogenous auditory defect is transmitted from the parents to the child as an inherited trait. However, not all congenital (present at birth) hearing disorders are hereditary, nor are all hereditary disorders congenital. For example, the child whose hearing mechanism is damaged in utero by maternal rubella is born with a hearing loss. This hearing loss is congenital but not hereditary. On the other hand, some hereditary defects of

FIGURE 5.1.
Percentage of individuals that exhibit exogenous and endogenous types of hearing loss.

hearing may not manifest themselves until adulthood. A breakdown of the estimated percentage of individuals with exogenous and endogenous types of hearing loss is shown in Figure 5.1.

Genetic Transmission of Hearing Loss

As Figure 5.1 shows, hearing loss due to hereditary factors is thought to make up about 50% of all auditory disorders. It is estimated that there are 150–175 different genetic syndromes that include hearing loss as a primary feature. In addition, there are about 16 types of genetic deafness that are known to occur without any other associated anomalies. Whether occurring as one manifestation of a particular syndrome or with no other abnormalities, hereditary hearing loss is usually governed by the Mendelian laws of inheritance. According to these genetic laws, genetic traits may be dominant, recessive, or X-linked (sex linked). Genes are located on the chromosomes, and, with the exception of those genes that are located on the sex chromosomes of males, they come in pairs. One member of each gene pair (and the corresponding member of a chromosome pair) is inherited from each parent. Humans have 22 pairs of autosomes, or non–sex-determining chromosomes, and one pair of sex-determining chromosomes. The sex chromosome pair for females consists of two X chromosomes, and for males, one X and one Y chromosome. In the process of human reproduction, each egg and each sperm cell carries one-half the number of chromosomes of each parent. When the egg is fertilized, the full complement of chromosomes is restored, so that half of a child's genes are from the mother and half are from the father.

Autosomal Dominant Inheritance

In autosomal dominant inheritance, the trait is carried from one generation to another. The term "autosomal" implies that the abnormal gene is not located on one of the two sex chromosomes. Typically, one parent exhibits the inherited trait, which may be transmitted to 50% of the offspring. This does not mean that half the children in a given family will necessarily be affected. Statistically, there is a 50% chance that any given child, whether male or female, will be affected (Vignette 5.1). Autosomal dominant inheritance is believed to account for about 20% of cases of genetically caused (endogenous) deafness. Because of the interaction of a number of genes, some traits may manifest themselves only partially; for example, only a very mild hearing loss may be observed despite a genetic structure indicating profound hearing loss.

VIGNETTE 5.1.
Illustration of Mendelian Laws

For this demonstration, you will need two paper cups and five poker chips or checkers: three of one color and two of another. For the first illustration, select one chip of one color and three of the other color. We will assume that you have one black chip and three white ones. Divide the four chips into two pairs, each pair representing a parent. The black chip represents a dominant gene for deafness. Whenever it is paired with another black chip or a white chip, it dominates the trait for hearing, resulting in deafness in the person with the gene. In this example, we have one deaf parent (one black chip, one white chip) and one normal-hearing parent (two white chips).

Each parent contributes one gene for hearing status to each offspring. When the deaf parent contributes the gene for deafness (black chip), the offspring will always be deaf. This is because the normal-hearing parent has only recessive genes for normal hearing (white chips) to contribute to the offspring. Separate the black chip from the deaf parent and slide it toward you. Slide each of the white chips from the other parent toward you, one at a time. For both of these possible offspring, the child will be deaf (a black chip paired with a white one). Now return the chips to the parents and slide the white chip from the deaf parent close to you. Slide each of the white chips from the normal parent closer to you, one after the other. Notice that when the deaf parent contributes a gene for normal hearing (white chip), the offspring will have normal hearing. This is true for pairings of each gene from the normal-hearing parent. For these two possible gene pairings, the offspring would have normal hearing.

In toto, there were four possible gene pairings for the offspring. Of these, two were predicted to produce deafness and two were predicted to result in normal hearing. In this illustration of autosomal dominant deafness, the odds are that 50%, or one-half, of the offspring from these two parents will be deaf.

Now, remove one of the white chips and replace it with a black one. Form two pairs of chips in front of you, each having one black and one white chip. In this case, the black chip represents the gene for deafness again, but it is recessive. That is, the gene for normal hearing (white chip) is dominant. There will again be four possible pairings of the chips in the offspring, one from each parent. Examine the various combinations of genes by first sliding one chip closer to you from the parent on the left. Examine two possible pairings for each gene from the parent on the right. Now repeat this process by sliding the other chip from the parent on the left closer to you. When you have finished, you should have observed the following four pairs of chips for the offspring (black-white, black-black, white-black, white-white). In this case of autosomal recessive deafness, only one of the possible combinations would produce a deaf offspring (black-black). The probability of a deaf child is one in four, or 25%. Two of the three normal-hearing offspring, however, will carry a gene for deafness (black-white chip pairs). These offspring are referred to as "carriers" of the trait.

It is sometimes difficult to understand that the Mendelian laws of hearing are only probabilities. In the case of autosomal recessive deafness, for example, one might think that if the parents had four offspring, they would have one deaf child. That is only the probability. They could very well have four normal-hearing children or four deaf children. To see how this occurs, place one black and one white chip in each of the two paper cups. Shake up the left cup and draw a chip. Repeat the process with the right cup. Examine the two chips (genes) selected, one from each cup (parent). Record the outcome (deaf or normal hearing) and replace chips in the cups. Do this 20 times, representing five families of four offspring each. When you're finished, you will likely find some families of four that had two, three, or four deaf offspring. If you did this an *infinite* number of times, however, 25% of the offspring would be deaf, as predicted by Mendelian laws for autosomal recessive deafness.

Autosomal Recessive Inheritance

In contrast to autosomal dominant inheritance, both parents of a child with hearing loss of the autosomal recessive type are clinically normal. Appearance of the trait in the offspring requires that an individual possess two similar abnormal genes, one from each parent. The parents themselves are often heterozygous carriers of a single abnormal recessive gene. This means that each carries two different genes, one normal and one abnormal with respect to a particular gene pair. Offspring carrying two of either the normal or the abnormal type of gene are termed "homozygotes." Offspring may also be heterozygotes like their parents, carrying one of each gene type. If no abnormal gene is transmitted, the offspring is normal for that trait. If there is one abnormal gene, the child becomes a carrier for the trait. Finally, if two abnormal genes, one from each parent, are transmitted, the offspring is affected and becomes a homozygous carrier. The probability that heterozygote parents will bear an affected, homozygous child is 25% in each pregnancy on the basis that each child would inherit the abnormal gene from both the father (50% chance) and the mother (50% chance). Since the laws of probability permit this type of hearing loss to be transmitted without manifestation through several generations, the detection of the true origin is often quite difficult. Recessive genes account for the majority of cases of genetic hearing loss and can account for as much as 80% of childhood deafness.

X-Linked Inheritance

In the X-linked type of deafness, affected males are linked together through carrier females. In this pattern, inherited traits are determined by genes located on the X chromosome. As noted earlier, normal females have two X chromosomes, whereas males possess one X and one Y chromosome. Sons receive their Y chromosomes from their fathers; their X chromosomes are inherited from their mothers. Daughters, on the other hand, receive one X chromosome from their fathers and the other from their mothers. In an X-linked trait, a carrier female has a 50% probability that each of her sons will be affected and a 50% probability that each of her daughters will be carriers. All the daughters of an affected male would be carriers, but there is never a father-to-son transmission of the trait itself. About 2–3% of deafness occurs as a result of X-linked inheritance.

Site of Lesion

Also important in the classification of an auditory disorder is the location of the lesion. We have already learned that lesions occurring in the outer or middle ear cause conductive hearing loss that is frequently amenable to medical treatment. If damage occurs to the nerve endings or to the hair cells in the inner ear, the hearing loss is sensorineural. Hearing losses resulting from damage to the auditory nerve after it leaves the cochlea are sometimes designated neural. When damage occurs to the nerve pathways within the auditory central nervous system (see Chapter 3), the resulting condition is often known as central auditory impairment.

One other variable that can be used in the classification of auditory disorders, but that does not require detailed explanation here, is time of onset. Typically, the hearing loss is described, in part, with consideration of when the impairment was thought to occur (i.e., prior to delivery or after birth). Time of onset will be discussed in more detail later in this chapter.

DISORDERS OF THE OUTER EAR AND MIDDLE EAR

Conductive hearing losses occur when there is a complication somewhere between the outer ear and the middle ear. A person with a conductive hearing loss exhibits normal threshold sensitivity by bone conduction measurements and decreased threshold values via air conduction. In Chapter 4, this was referred to as an air-bone gap.

A variety of disorders can produce a conductive hearing loss. All of them result in the alteration of the mechanics of the external ear or the middle ear system. Some of these mechanical changes might include blockage of the external or middle ear, increasing the stiffness of the tympanic membrane or middle ear system, or increasing the mass of the middle ear. These alterations in the mechanics of the outer and middle ear produce varying degrees and configurations of hearing loss. Recall from Chapter 2 that increasing the stiffness of a mechanical system has its greatest effect at low frequencies. Similarly, changing the mass of a mechanical system primarily affects the high frequencies. The specific configuration of the audiogram will depend on the specific mechanical alterations produced by the disorder. Although the conductive loss might make it difficult to hear conversational speech, the ability to understand spoken messages is usually not impaired when speech is presented at comfortably loud levels.

Outer Ear Disorders

Deformities of the Pinna (Auricle) and External Ear Canal

A wide variety of external ear malformations or anomalies can take place; most are due to an inherited trait. Such anomalies of the external ear can occur in isolation or as part of an anomaly complex that produces a variety of other alterations to the skull and face (called craniofacial defects). Pinna deformity can range from very mild malformations, which are difficult for the layperson to identify, to the more severe forms of the condition, such as total absence of the pinna or complete closure of the ear canal.

The most severe form of pinna deformity is called *microtia*, a term that implies a very small and deformed pinna. Microtia is often associated with *atresia*, a term used to denote the absence or closure of the external auditory meatus. Importantly, atresia can also occur without significant pinna abnormalities or as part of a constellation of other craniofacial defects. Figure 5.2 shows examples of the variations in pinna deformities.

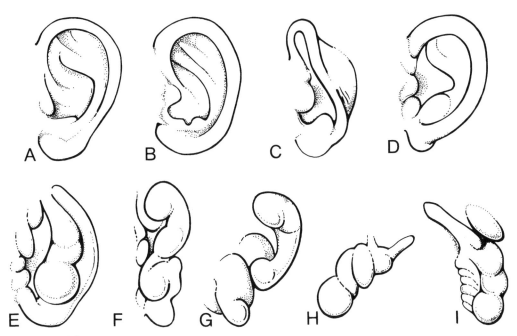

FIGURE 5.2.
Examples of variations in pinna deformities. Examples *A–D* represent mild deformities, whereas examples *E–I* represent severe pinna deformities.

Microtia and atresia are bilateral in 15–20% of cases, are known to affect the right ear more frequently than the left, and are slightly more prevalent in males. The severity of the pinna deformity will sometimes offer an indication of the corresponding status of the middle ear space. A patient with microtia, for example, can also exhibit malformations of the middle ear ranging from minor deformities of the ossicles to a total absence of the middle ear cavity. Generally speaking, the more severe the deformation of the outer ear, the greater the conductive hearing loss. Figure 5.3 shows an example of a conductive hearing loss seen in a severe case of microtia.

External Otitis

A number of diseases can cause acute external otitis, which originates from viruses or bacteria. One of these diseases, referred to as herpes simplex, invades the pinna or ear canal. The disease resembles the herpes seen on the face or other parts of the body. Another inflammatory disease is viral bullous myringitis, a complication that involves the outer layer of the tympanic membrane and then spreads laterally to the external canal. In rare instances, these diseases can produce severe swelling of the canal and subsequent hearing loss.

Collapsed Canal

An occasional clinical finding is the collapse of an ear canal brought about by the pressure that results from earphone placement. The pressure of the earphones

FIGURE 5.3.
Audiometric example of hearing loss seen in a severe case of bilateral microtia with atresia.

against the side of the head moves the pinna forward and thus causes the soft carti-laginous part of the ear canal to close. This condition is thought to occur in about 3% of a clinical caseload and affects both children and adults. There is a tendency, however, for this condition to occur more frequently in adults, especially in the elderly population. Importantly, the collapsed canal has also been reported to occur in neonates. A collapse of the ear canal can produce a conductive hearing impair-ment on the order of 15–30 dB HL, with the greatest loss occurring at 2000 Hz. The use of insert earphones, described in Chapter 4, eliminates the problem of col-lapsing ear canals.

Cerumen and Foreign Bodies

In some individuals, the ear canal generates excessive amounts of cerumen (ear-wax). If not removed on a periodic basis, this can accumulate and block the trans-mission of sound to the middle ear. The ear canal is also sufficiently large to accept foreign objects such as matches, paper clips, and pencil tips. Portions of these objects inserted by either children or adults can be lost in the ear canal and remain there for many years. This can result in mild forms of conductive hearing loss. Audiologists who plan to specialize in the pediatric population should recognize that children have been known to insert seeds or beans into the ear canal. The ear canal is warm and moist and provides an excellent growing environment! When the seed or bean expands, the child experiences pain and loss of hearing.

Finally, sharp objects inserted into the ear canal can pierce or tear the tympanic membrane. Such trauma can also cause disruption of the ossicular chain. Self-induced perforations of the tympanic membrane and/or separation of the ossicles can result in a mild-to-moderate conductive hearing loss. The audiologist should make a practice of inspecting the ear canal with an otoscope prior to conducting an audiologic examination.

Cysts and Tumors

The external ear and ear canal can serve as a site for both cysts and tumors. A cyst is a closed cavity or sac that lies underneath the skin and is often filled with a liquid or semisolid material. A cyst is primarily of cosmetic importance unless it becomes infected. If swollen from infection, a cyst can cause hearing loss.

Tumors, both benign and malignant, can arise from the pinna or ear canal. Benign tumors can have a vascular origin or can simply be an outgrowth of bone. Malignancies more frequently arise from the pinna but can, in rare circumstances, arise in the ear canal. Occasionally, these lesions become quite large and close off the ear canal.

Middle Ear Disorders

The Problem of Otitis Media

An important middle ear disorder frequently seen by the audiologist is otitis media, one of the most common diseases in childhood. Otitis media refers to inflammation of the middle ear cavity. It is considered an important economic and health problem because of its prevalence, the cost of its treatment, the potential for secondary medical complications, and the possibility of long-term nonmedical consequences. The clinical audiologist must be familiar with this middle ear disorder and have a grasp of such important topics as the classification of otitis media, its natural history and epidemiology, its cause, its management, and its potential complications.

Classification of Otitis Media. Otitis media is often classified on the basis of the temporal sequence of the disease. That is, the disease is categorized according to the duration of the disease process. For example, acute otitis media (AOM) typically will run its full course within a 3-week period. The disease begins with a rapid onset, persists for a week to 10 days, and then resolves rapidly. Some of the more common symptoms associated with AOM include a bulging, reddened tympanic membrane, pain, and upper respiratory infection. If the disease has a slow onset and persists for 3 months or more, it is referred to as chronic otitis media (COM). Symptoms associated with COM include a large central perforation in the eardrum and discharge of fluid through the perforation. Subacute otitis media refers to a disease that has persisted beyond the acute stage but has not yet become chronic.

Otitis media is also classified according to the type of fluid that is observed by the physician in the middle ear cavity. If the fluid is purulent or suppurative, like

Table 5.1.
Clinical Classification of Otitis Media and Commonly Used Synonyms

Classification	Synonyms
Otitis media without effusion	Myringitis
Acute otitis media	Suppurative OM, purulent OM, bacterial OM
Otitis media with effusion	Secretory OM, nonsuppurative OM, serous OM, mucoid OM
Chronic otitis media	Suppurative OM, purulent OM

OM, otitis media

the fluid found most often in AOM, it will contain white blood cells, some cellular debris, and many bacteria. AOM is sometimes referred to as acute suppurative otitis media or acute purulent otitis media. A fluid that is free of cellular debris and bacteria is described as *serous*, and the term *serous otitis media* is used to describe this condition. Sometimes the fluid is mucoid because it has been secreted from the mucosal lining of the middle ear. This fluid is thick in substance and contains white blood cells, few bacteria, and some cellular debris. When mucoid fluid is present, the disease may be referred to as mucoid otitis media, or secretory otitis media. Table 5.1 summarizes the most commonly employed descriptions of otitis media and their associated synonyms. In addition, Figure 5.4 illustrates a normal tympanic membrane along with several pathologic conditions including serous otitis media, otitis media with bubbles in the fluid, and acute otitis media.

Natural History and Epidemiology of Otitis Media. To understand fully the nature of otitis media, one must appreciate the natural history and epidemiology of the disease. *Natural history* and *epidemiology* are terms used to denote the study of the relationships of various factors that determine the natural frequency and distribution of a disease. It has already been stated that otitis media with effusion is one of the most prevalent diseases in childhood (Vignette 5.2). Depending on the study reviewed, 76–95% of all children have at least one episode of otitis media by 6 years of age. In addition, it is found that the prevalence of the disease peaks during the early years of life. The prevalence of otitis media is typically greatest during the first 2 years of life and then decreases with increasing age. Importantly, there appears to be a relationship between the age of onset and the probability of repeated episodes. Children who appear to be prone to middle ear disease and experience five to six bouts within the first several years of life have usually experienced their first episode of the disease during the first 18 months of life. Seldom does a child become otitis-prone if the first episode occurred after 18 months of age.

Otitis media varies slightly with gender, with more cases seen in males than in females. There is seasonal variation in otitis media, with higher occurrence during winter and spring. Some groups are more at risk for middle ear disease than others. Some of the groups considered more at risk for otitis media are children with cleft palate and other craniofacial disorders, those with Down syndrome, and those with

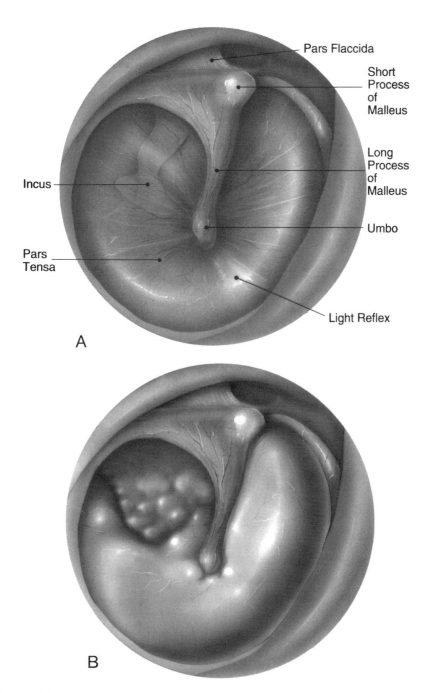

Pars Flaccida

Short
Process
of
Malleus

Long
Process
of
Malleus

Umbo

Incus

Pars
Tensa

Light Reflex

A

B

FIGURE 5.4.
Normal tympanic membrane (*A*) and three pathologic conditions: *B*, serous otitis media; *C*, serous otitis media with air bubbles; and *D*, acute otitis media. (From English GM: *Oto-laryngology*. Hagerstown, MD, Harper & Row, 1976.)

Figure 5.4.
Continued

VIGNETTE 5.2.
Prevalence of Middle Ear Disease in Children

The prevalence of middle ear disease is increasing; in fact, it is reaching epidemic proportions. For children below the age of 6 years, otitis media is the most common reason for a doctor visit. According to the Centers for Disease Control in Atlanta, ear infection diagnoses increased 178% between 1975 and 1990. Moreover, in 1975, there were 10 million doctor visits for ear aches; by 1990, there were 25 million visits, costing more than $1 billion annually. Nine out of every ten children will have at least one ear infection; most will have at least one acute ear infection by age 3, and more than one-third of all children will have three acute infections. Why is the prevalence of ear infections increasing? Most authorities agree that day care is responsible. Children in day care have a much higher prevalence of upper respiratory infections and, subsequently, ear infections.

The extent of the management for ear infections is also substantial. For example, the most common surgery on children is myringotomy with insertion tubes (see Fig. 5.9), a procedure used to drain fluid and restore hearing. In addition, the cost of antibiotics commonly prescribed for ear infections amounts to several billion dollars in annual world-wide sales. Clearly, middle ear disease has become one of the major health care problems among children in the United States.

learning disabilities. Children who reside in the inner city and children who attend day-care centers are also prone to suffer from middle ear disease, as are Native Americans.

Cause of Otitis Media. It is commonly believed that otitis media develops because of eustachian tube obstruction. As mentioned in Chapter 3, the eustachian tube is important to a healthy middle ear because it provides for pressure equalization and fluid drainage. If the pressure-equalization system is obstructed, a negative pressure can develop in the middle ear cavity. The negative pressure literally sucks the fluid from the membranous lining of the middle ear canal. The fluid that has accumulated from the mucosal lining of the middle ear has no place to escape because the eustachian tube is blocked. Vignette 5.3 shows a representation of this general process. A number of factors may produce eustachian tube obstruction,

---

VIGNETTE 5.3.
Development of Acute Otitis Media (AOM)

The drawings that accompany this vignette illustrate the general pattern of events that can occur in AOM. Panel *A* shows the landmarks of a normal middle ear system. Note the translucency and concavity of the tympanic membrane. Note also the appearance of the eustachian tube, especially at the opening in the nasopharyngeal area. Panel *B* shows that the pharyngeal end of the eustachian tube has been closed off by swelling due to pharyngeal infection or possibly an allergy. More specifically, the upper respiratory infection produces a congestion of the mucosa in the nasopharyngeal area, the eustachian tube, and the middle ear. The congestion of the mucosa of the tube produces an obstruction that prevents ventilation of the middle ear space. Also, the tympanic membrane is retracted inward because of negative pressure due to absorption from the middle ear. Finally, bacteria from the oral pharyngeal area are drawn up the eustachian tube to the middle ear space. Panel *C* illustrates a full-blown condition of AOM. Fluid secretions from the goblet cells of the mucosal lining of the middle ear are now trapped and have no way to leave the middle ear cavity. The bacteria drawn from the eustachian tube proliferate in the secretions, forming a viscous pus. Observe also that the tympanic membrane is no longer retracted but is bulging.

Panel *D* shows a condition that may well result following antimicrobial treatment. The bacteria have been killed by the antibiotics, and a thin or mucoid-type fluid remains. Other possible outcomes following medical treatment might be the return to a completely normal middle ear, as in *A*, or a condition like the one shown in *B*.

The onset of otitis media with effusion, although asymptomatic, would follow a similar pattern of events. Recurrent episodes of AOM or middle ear disease with effusion are probably due to abnormal anatomy or physiology of the eustachian tube.

VIGNETTE 5.3—*continued*

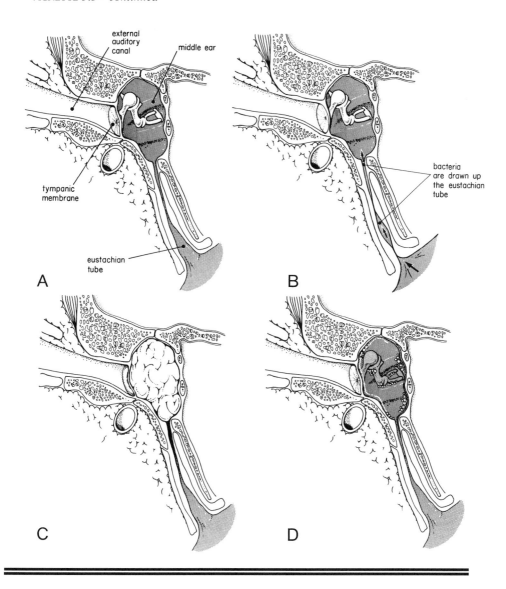

including large adenoid tissue in the nasopharyngeal area and inflammation of the mucous lining of the tube. It is also important to note that the muscular opening function of the eustachian tube is poor in children with otitis media and in children with histories of middle ear disease. In fact, in general, the muscle responsible for opening and closing the tube (tensor veli palatini) is less efficient among young infants and children. Moreover, the position of the eustachian tube in children lies at an angle of only 10° in relation to the horizontal plane, whereas in adults this angle is 45° (Fig. 5.5). Further, the tube is much shorter in young infants. Because

FIGURE 5.5.
Anatomic illustration of the eustachian tube in an infant ear compared with that of the adult ear. Note that the tube of an infant lies more on a horizontal plane.

INFANT EAR

ADULT EAR

of the angle and shortness of the tube in children, fluid is able to reach the middle ear from the nasopharyngeal area with greater ease and has greater difficulty escaping from the middle ear cleft.

Nonmedical Complications Associated with Otitis Media. Hearing loss is considered the most common complication of otitis media. Although the nature of the loss is usually conductive, sensorineural involvement can also occur. In general, the prevalence rate depends on the criteria used to define hearing loss. Unfortunately, prevalence data are difficult to determine because of the lack of well-controlled studies in this area. Too often, there is limited information with regard to testing conditions, calibration of equipment, type of threshold procedure employed, definition of hearing loss, and diagnosis of the disease.

Figure 5.6 shows an audiometric profile typical of individuals with otitis media with effusion. It is seen that the hearing loss for air conduction is fairly flat. The

Figure 5.6.
Audiometric profile of otitis media with effusion. Filled circles represent air conduction thresholds; open triangles represent bone conduction thresholds.

average amount of air conduction loss through the speech frequency range (500–2000 Hz) is 25 dB HL. The bone conduction loss averages 3 dB HL through the speech frequencies, producing a mean air-bone gap of roughly 22 dB.

The degree of hearing loss ranges from normal sensitivity to hearing losses as great as 50 dB HL. Figure 5.7 shows a distribution of the expected hearing loss subsequent to otitis media with effusion. These data illustrate the number of ears falling within various hearing loss categories. Within the speech frequency range, fewer than 50 ears (7.7%) showed an average loss of 10 dB HL or less, and only five ears showed losses of 50 dB HL or more. The vast majority of ears exhibited losses between 16 and 40 dB HL, with 21–30 dB HL being the most common hearing loss category.

Although otitis media is usually manifested as a conductive hearing loss, sensorineural hearing loss may be associated with the more severe forms of COM. It is believed that toxic products from the fluid can pass through the round window and damage the cochlea. The damage to the inner ear produces high-frequency sensorineural hearing loss. The longer the fluid remains in the middle ear, the greater the potential for sensorineural involvement.

Another complication that may result from longstanding middle ear disease with effusion is deficiency in psychoeducational and/or communicative skills. It is widely suspected that otitis-prone children are more susceptible to delays in speech, language, and cognitive development, and in education. The research done in this area, however, has been severely criticized, and a cause-effect relationship cannot be assumed at the present time.

Medical Complications Associated with Otitis Media. A number of medical complications are associated with otitis media. The most common medical complications are COM with associated cholesteatoma, perforations or retraction pockets of the tympanic membrane, tympanosclerosis, adhesive otitis media, and facial paralysis.

FIGURE 5.7.
Distribution of degree of hearing loss in middle ear disease with effusion.

COM and Associated Cholesteatoma. Cholesteatoma refers to the accumulation of cellular debris developed from perforations of the tympanic membrane. Sometimes this pseudotumor becomes infected and causes some erosion of the ossicles. No typical audiometric configuration is associated with cholesteatomas, and the loss may vary from 15 to 55 dB HL.

Perforation of the Tympanic Membrane. Spontaneous perforations usually occur subsequent to acute infections but may also be associated with COM. Perforations of the tympanic membrane produce hearing deficits in the mild-to-moderate category, provided there are no ossicular defects. The hearing loss is a result of reduction in the areal ratio between the tympanic membrane and oval window and the direct coupling of sound waves to the round window. (See Chapter 3 for a discussion of these mechanisms.) Figure 5.8 illustrates several different perforations of the tympanic membrane.

Tympanosclerosis. Tympanosclerosis is characterized by white shale-like plaques on the tympanic membrane and deposits on the ossicles. It occurs most often following COM, which, when resolved, leaves a residual material. The shale-like plaques create a stiffening effect on the tympanic membrane and the ossicular chain, producing conductive hearing loss in the low frequencies.

Adhesive Otitis Media. Adhesive otitis media is a thickening of the mucous membrane lining the middle ear cavity. It can cause fixation of the ossicles and subsequent hearing loss.

Facial Paralysis. Facial paralysis may occur in the course of acute or chronic otitis media. The facial nerve passes through the middle ear area in a bony tube called the fallopian canal. It is possible for the fallopian canal to become eroded and expose the facial nerve to the toxic effects of the infection.

FIGURE 5.8.
Perforations in three different tympanic membranes. *A*, Attic perforation and associated cholesteotoma. *B*, Marginal perforation. *C*, Large central perforation. (From English GM: *Otolaryngology*. Hagerstown, MD, Harper & Row, 1976.)

C

FIGURE 5.8.
Continued.

Management of Otitis Media. The most common means of treating AOM is the routine administration of antimicrobial agents. These antibiotics are designed to combat the various pathogens thought to exist within the middle ear fluid. The drugs ampicillin and amoxicillin are frequently administered in the management of AOM. Importantly, even when appropriate antimicrobial agents have been prescribed and the fluid is sterilized, the effusion may persist for 2 weeks to 3 months. Antihistamines and decongestants have also been used in the treatment of middle ear disease. This form of treatment, however, has recently been shown to be ineffective.

A common surgical approach to the management of both suppurative and non-suppurative otitis media is a myringotomy. Myringotomy is a surgical procedure that involves making an incision in one of the inferior quadrants of the tympanic membrane, as shown in Figure 5.9. In the acute forms of the disease, a myringotomy is performed when there is severe pain or toxicity, high fever, failure to respond to antimicrobial therapy, or some serious secondary medical complication. In secretory otitis media, a myringotomy is more commonly done, usually in order to remove fluid and restore hearing sensitivity. The eardrum incision can heal quickly, however, and the fluid reappears. To avoid this possibility and to ensure sustained middle ear aeration, ventilating tubes or grommets are often inserted into the eardrum (Fig. 5.10).

Tonsillectomy and adenoidectomy are also considered as a management approach to otitis media. Although tonsillectomy does not seem to be an effective

FIGURE 5.9.
Myringotomy. Note the bulging appearance of the tympanic membrane. (From English GM: *Otolaryngology*. Hagerstown, MD, Harper & Row, 1976.)

FIGURE 5.10.
Ventilating tube or grommet.

treatment protocol, adenoidectomy is a common surgical procedure for the management of otitis media. In general, this approach is undertaken when a patient does not respond to medical therapy, large adenoids are present, and there is no evidence of nasal allergy. Under these conditions, it is assumed that the eustachian tube blockage causing the middle ear disease is due to enlarged adenoids. The adenoids are removed to free the eustachian tube from the blockage.

A more radical surgical approach is required if chronic disease permanently impairs basic structures within the middle ear. When alteration of the middle ear structures is required, a surgical technique known as tympanoplasty is performed.

Otosclerosis

Otosclerosis, sometimes referred to as otospongiosis, is a common cause of conductive hearing loss and is reported to affect 5–10% of the Caucasian population. Otosclerosis means "hardening of the ear" and is manifested by a build-up of spongifying bone on the osseous labyrinth, usually in the area of the oval window. The build-up of bone around the oval window immobilizes the footplate of the stapes and interferes with sound transmission to the inner ear. Although the focus of the lesion is usually limited to the region of the oval window, the growth of spongy bone can also invade the walls of the cochlea. When the cochlea becomes involved, sensorineural hearing loss may ensue, producing a condition called cochlear otosclerosis.

The disease is about 2.5 times as common in women as in men and may be exacerbated during pregnancy. The disease occurs less frequently in blacks and Orientals and usually has its onset when the individuals are in their 20s, 30s, or 40s. Finally, bilateral otosclerosis is much more common than unilateral disease, although the latter will be seen in 10–15% of cases.

The cause of otosclerosis is not clearly understood. Most would agree that the disease has a genetic predisposition, since about 50% of affected patients report a similar condition in other family members. The mode of transmission is thought to be autosomal dominant with variable expressivity.

Audiologic Manifestations of Otosclerosis. A progressive conductive hearing loss is the primary result of otosclerosis. The affected patient will typically exhibit an audiometric configuration similar to that shown in Figure 5.11. This figure depicts the air and bone conduction thresholds of a 35-year-old female patient with surgically confirmed otosclerosis. The hearing loss has progressed somewhat gradually for several years, beginning at the age of 25 years. Notice the moderate hearing thresholds for air conduction with greater loss in the low-frequency region, and the relatively normal bone conduction thresholds. An exception to the latter is the slight reduction of bone conduction hearing at 2000 Hz. The bone conduction loss at 2000 Hz is characteristic of otosclerosis and is referred to as the "Carhart notch" because Carhart was the first to report this notching phenomenon. Immittance measurements in otosclerotic cases are also uniquely characteristic and typically manifest absent acoustic reflexes, abnormally low compliance values, and a shallow tympanogram. Figure 5.12 shows an audiometric example of a patient with both stape-

FIGURE 5.11.
Audiometric example of otosclerosis.

FIGURE 5.12.
Audiometric example of combination of stapedial and cochlear otosclerosis.

dial and cochlear involvement from otosclerosis. Note that a mixed hearing loss is present, representing a conductive component due to stapes fixation and a sensorineural component due to the spread of the spongy bone to the cochlea.

Management of Otosclerosis. The most common approach to the management of otosclerosis is surgery of the stapes. The ideal candidates for stapes surgery are those with relatively normal bone conduction thresholds (0–20 dB HL, 500–2000 Hz) and air conduction values in the 35- to 65-dB HL range (500–2000 Hz). Surgical candidates usually exhibit an air-bone gap of at least 15 dB and have speech-recognition scores of 60% or better.

One surgical approach to otosclerosis is stapes mobilization, which is simply a loosening of the stapes with a chisel-like instrument. A limitation of this technique is that in many cases, fixation of the stapes and subsequent conductive hearing loss can recur. An alternative and more accepted approach is stapedectomy. A stapedectomy involves removal of the fixed stapes footplate and all or a portion of the stapedial arch and substitution of a prosthetic device for the stapes. In cases of complete stapedectomy and the incorporation of a prosthetic device, the oval window is sealed with a graft or an absorptive sponge. Surgery usually results in complete or nearly complete restoration of hearing. Figure 5.13 shows examples of two surgical procedures.

Other Ossicular Disorders

The ossicles other than the stapes can also be partially or completely fixed. The ossicles can also be pulled apart, or disarticulated, producing a variety of different conductive hearing losses. For example, the malleus and the incus can become

A   B

FIGURE 5.13.
Two surgical procedures on the stapes. *A*, Stapes mobilization. *B*, stapedectomy. (From Goodhill V [ed]: *Ear Diseases, Deafness and Dizziness.* Hagerstown, MD, Harper & Row, 1979.)

fixated, or there can be fixation of the malleus alone or the incus alone without any involvement of the stapes. These conditions are sometimes referred to as "pseudo-otosclerosis," and the audiologic manifestations often mock what we would expect to find in otosclerosis.

In contrast to fixation, it is possible to have discontinuity, or disarticulation, of the ossicles, again producing a significant conductive hearing loss. A discontinuity of the ossicles can be caused by a degenerative process or by some traumatic experience. For example, the introduction of a sharp object into the ear canal could pierce the tympanic membrane and cause a dislocation of the ossicles. A similar effect can result from a skull fracture, wherein the impact to the head produces a dislodging of the ossicular chain. In addition, degeneration of the ossicles is possible when a disease process (particularly a cholesteatoma) is present. Under these conditions, the individual will exhibit a substantial conductive hearing loss in the neighborhood of 50–60 dB.

COCHLEAR AND RETROCHOCHLEAR PATHOLOGY

Millions of Americans have sensorineural hearing loss as a consequence of cochlear pathology. For children, conductive hearing loss produced by middle ear pathology, as reviewed earlier in this chapter, is probably the most common type of hearing loss. For adults, however, sensorineural hearing loss resulting from underlying cochlear pathology is probably the most common type of hearing impairment. Recall from the previous sections of this chapter that conductive hearing loss was usually medically treatable, either through surgery, medication, or a combination of the two. With sensorineural hearing loss, however, this is usually not the case. The hearing loss is typically permanent. For those individuals with significant sensorineural hearing loss, the usual course of action is to seek assistance from amplification, often a personal wearable hearing aid. Hearing aids and other types of amplification for the hearing impaired are described in detail in Chapter 7.

The description of the hearing loss produced by cochlear pathology as "sensorineural" seems particularly appropriate. Recall that a sensorineural hearing loss is one in which the threshold by bone conduction is the same as that by air conduction (within 5 dB). The threshold when the inner ear is stimulated directly through skull vibration (bone conduction) is the same as when the entire peripheral auditory system is stimulated (air conduction). If thresholds for air conduction and bone conduction are both elevated to the same degree, then all that can be concluded is that there is some pathology in the auditory system at or central to the inner ear. The presence of a sensorineural hearing loss does not tell us where along the auditory pathway the pathology is; it only eliminates the outer and middle ears as possibilities. The pathology could be affecting the sensory receptors within the cochlea, or the neural pathways leading from the cochlea to higher centers of the auditory system, or both the sensory and neural structures. In this context, then, "sensorineural" hearing loss is a very appropriate label.

The term *sensorineural hearing loss* is also an appropriate label for the hearing loss resulting from cochlear pathology for another reason. In cochlear pathology, the sensory receptors within the cochlea are destroyed. Exactly how this occurs depends on the specific etiology. Research conducted during the past 10–15 years suggests that the sensory destruction quickly becomes sensorineural damage. Once the hair cells within the organ of Corti are destroyed, a phenomenon known as retrograde degeneration occurs. Retrograde degeneration refers to the destruction of connecting anatomic structures located more central to the structure that was destroyed. Destruction of the sensory hair cells within the organ of Corti results in the eventual degeneration of the first-order afferent nerve fibers communicating with the damaged hair cells. Most patients with sensorineural hearing loss due to cochlear pathology, therefore, most likely have underlying damage to both the sensory (cochlea) and neural (nerve fibers) portions of the auditory system.

When a sensorineural hearing loss is observed, how do the audiologist and physician determine whether it is due to cochlear pathology or to a problem lying further up the ascending neural pathways (called "retrocochlear" pathology)? As mentioned in Chapter 4, several steps are involved in establishing the diagnosis. The case history taken by the audiologist or physician can provide some important clues as to the location of the problem. The presence of other, frequently nonauditory, complaints, such as dizziness, loss of balance, and ringing in the ears (tinnitus), can aid the physician in establishing the diagnosis. A particular pattern of results from the basic audiology test battery may alert the physician to a probable underlying cause. The presence of a high-frequency sensorineural hearing loss in just one ear, for example, is a common audiometric configuration in some types of retrocochlear pathology. Finally, special tests can be performed on the patient at the physician's request. These tests may be auditory, in which case they are performed by the audiologist, or they may be nonauditory. An example of a nonauditory special test is electronystagmography (ENG), which tests the vestibular system and may also be performed by an audiologist. Another nonauditory test, one not performed by the audiologist, might involve some form of tomography. Tomography provides a visual image of the brain and brainstem structures. The most definitive auditory special test involves the measurement of the auditory brainstem response, or ABR. This test may also be administered by an audiologist. (The ABR was described in Chapters 3 and 4.)

Discussion of the special tests, auditory and nonauditory, that aid the physician in establishing the diagnosis is beyond the scope of this book. Suffice it to say that such tests exist and that the audiologist is frequently asked to perform them. Many types of cochlear and retrocochlear pathology, however, do produce a typical pattern of results on the basic audiologic test battery. The remainder of this chapter describes several of these pathologies and their audiologic profiles.

Cochlear Pathology

Prior to describing some specific causes of cochlear pathology, some general characteristics shared by most patients with cochlear pathology are noteworthy. First, for the most part, studies of human cadavers have revealed a close correspondence between the location of the damage along the length of the cochlea and the resulting audiometric configuration. For example, if postmortem anatomic studies of a patient's ear reveal damage in the basal high-frequency portion of the cochlea, then a recent audiogram obtained prior to death would most likely indicate the presence of a high-frequency sensorineural hearing loss. Although there are exceptions, it is generally the case in cochlear pathology that the audiometric configuration provides at least a gross indication of the regions of the cochlea that were damaged by the pathology (Vignette 5.4). A high-frequency sensorineural hearing loss reflects damage to the basal portion of the cochlea, a low-frequency sensorineural hearing loss suggests damage to the apical region of the cochlea, and a broad hearing loss extending from low to high frequencies reflects an underlying lesion along the entire length of the cochlea.

In sensorineural hearing loss due to cochlear pathology, there is a close correspondence between the frequencies that demonstrate hearing loss and the region along the length of the cochlea that is damaged. There is a less certain correspondence, however, between the degree of hearing loss at a particular frequency and the degree of damage at the corresponding location in the cochlea. One popular conception is that mild or moderate sensorineural hearing loss is due to destruction of the outer hair cells, whereas more severe hearing loss reflects damage to both the outer and inner hair cells.

There are also several perceptual consequences of sensorineural hearing loss due to cochlear pathology. Except for those with profound impairments, patients with cochlear pathology most commonly complain that they can hear speech but can't understand it. This may be especially true when listening against a background of noise. The patient with cochlear pathology also frequently experiences a phenomenon known as loudness recruitment. This phenomenon was discussed earlier, in Chapter 3. The hearing loss makes low-intensity sounds inaudible. Moderate-intensity sounds that are comfortably loud to a normal-hearing person may be barely audible to the person with cochlear pathology. At high intensities, however, the loudness of the sound is the same for both a normal ear and one with cochlear pathology. Let us assume, for example, that a pure tone at 2000 Hz having a level of 110 dB SPL is uncomfortably loud for both a normal listener and a person with cochlear pathology. The person with cochlear pathology, however, has a hearing threshold at 2000 Hz of 60 dB SPL, whereas the normal listener's threshold is 10 dB SPL. Thus, for the normal listener, the intensity of the tone has to be increased 100 dB to increase the loudness of the tone from "just audible" (threshold) to "uncomfortable." For the person with cochlear pathology, however, an increase in intensity of only 50 dB was needed to cover the same range of loudness (from "just audible" to "uncomfortable"). Loudness increases more rapidly in the ear with cochlear pathology than in the normal ear. This is known as loudness recruitment.

The presence of loudness recruitment makes it more difficult to fit a hearing aid on a person with cochlear pathology. Low-level sounds need to be amplified to be made audible to the hearing-impaired person. High-intensity sounds, however, cannot be amplified by the same amount or the hearing aid will produce sounds that are uncomfortably loud to the wearer. Possible solutions to this dilemma when fitting the patient with a hearing aid are described in more detail in Chapter 7.

Finally, the patient with cochlear hearing loss may have accompanying speech abnormalities. Depending on the severity, configuration, and age of onset of the hearing loss, the speech may be misarticulated. In addition, if the cochlear pathology produces sensorineural hearing loss in the low and intermediate frequencies, the patient

VIGNETTE 5.4.

Illustration of the Relationship between Location of Cochlear Damage and Hearing Loss[a]

The three figures accompanying this vignette illustrate the correspondence between the region of the cochlea that is damaged and the resultant hearing loss that is measured. The upper portion of each figure shows a "cochleogram" from three monkeys that were exposed to intense noise. A cochleogram depicts the percentage of hair cells (HCs) within the organ of Corti that remain at various locations along the length of the cochlea after noise exposure. The percentages are determined after careful microscopic examination of the cochlea.

In panel A, the monkey was exposed to a low-frequency noise. This resulted in destruction of outer hair cells (OHCs) in the region roughly 15–25 mm from the base of the cochlea. Prior to sacrificing the animal to examine the type and extent of damage produced by the noise, the audiogram in the lower portion of the panel was obtained. A sensorineural hearing loss in the low and intermediate frequencies was produced.

When another monkey was exposed to a high-frequency noise (panel B), the cochleogram (upper portion) indicated that the damage appeared in the basal portion of the cochlea. Note that the audiogram obtained from the same monkey after the noise exposure and just prior to sacrifice (lower portion) revealed the presence of a high-frequency sensorineural hearing loss. As the damage to the sensory hair cells within the organ of Corti progressed from an apical (panel A) to a basal (panel B) region of the cochlea, the audiogram reflected the change as a shift from a low-frequency to a high-frequency sensorineural hearing loss.

Panel C shows a cochleogram and audiogram from a monkey exposed to a wide-band noise. Note that the damage is much more extensive, affecting both the apical and basal portions of the cochlea. The damage, however, is most severe in the basal region. This is again reflected in the audiogram. The audiogram shows a broad hearing loss extending from low to high frequencies, more severe in the high frequencies.

[a] Adapted from Moody DB, Stebbins WC, Hawkins JE Jr, Johnsson L-G: Hearing loss and cochlear pathology in the monkey [macaca] following exposure to high levels of noise. *Archives of Oto-Rhino-Laryngology* 220:47–72, 1978.

will typically use speech levels that are inappropriately loud, especially while talking without wearing a hearing aid. This is because the feedback that a speaker normally receives by bone conduction is not available to assist in regulating the voice level.

Now that we have reviewed some features shared by most individuals with cochlear pathology, the remainder of this section will examine several types of pathology. The pathologies described here are by no means an exhaustive compilation. In keeping with the general mission of this book, the pathologies described were selected because of their common occurrence either in the general population or among children.

High-Risk Factors

A number of complications can arise prior to birth, during the birth process, or soon after birth that cause hearing loss. Many of these complications are factors included in the so-called high-risk register. The high-risk register is a checklist of conditions known to exhibit a higher-than-normal prevalence of hearing loss. These conditions for newborns include familial history of hearing loss, congenital infections (e.g., rubella), craniofacial anomalies, low birthweight, hyperbilirubinemia, ototoxic medications, bacterial meningitis, severe depression at birth (Apgar scores[a] =0–4 at 1 min; 0–6 at 5 min), prolonged mechanical ventilation, and stigmata or other findings associated with a syndrome known to include a sensorineural and/or conductive hearing loss.

Some of the above risk indicators are self-explanatory (e.g., family history of hearing loss, craniofacial anomalies, bacterial meningitis, low birthweight, congenital infection, and ototoxic medications); others, however, need further explanation. *Hyperbilirubinemia* occurs when the bilirubin concentration in the blood exceeds 6–8 mg/dl. Once this level is reached, the child's skin becomes yellowish, a condition sometimes referred to as jaundice. Hyperbilirubinemia is a very complex metabolic complication that is thought to result from the production of too much bilirubin or the inability of the system to clear the bilirubin from the blood by the liver. *Severe depression at birth*, sometimes referred to as asphyxia, is an interruption of oxygen to the body, including the brain. In newborns, asphyxia results from an interruption of the placenta or maternal bloodflow before birth. Another possible factor is a blockage of the infant's airway during the delivery process. Asphyxia can damage the inner ear and/or auditory regions of the brain. *Prolonged mechanical ventilation* is a fairly recent addition to the high-risk register and is most often associated with infants who have severe pulmonary complications such as persistent pulmonary hypertension in the newborn (PPHN). PPHN occurs typically in near full-term or post-term infants and is characterized by hypoxemia (i.e., subnormal

---

[a] The Apgar score is a common tool for describing the amount of depression exhibited by the infant. Apgar scores consist of five criteria: *(a)* heart rate, *(b)* respiratory rate, *(c)* muscle tone, *(d)* response to stimulation, and *(e)* color. The highest possible score is 10.

oxygenation of blood), which results in increased pulmonary vasoconstriction and, subsequently, a decrease in pulmonary circulation. Such children have a 25 times greater risk for hearing loss than other babies in the neonatal intensive care unit. Finally, *stigmata* or other findings associated with a syndrome are simply landmarks of a syndrome that might be associated with hearing impairment. A complete listing of the 1993 High-Risk Register for both newborns and infants is summarized in Tables 6.1 and 6.2 in Chapter 6.

Viral and Bacterial Diseases

Severe viral and bacterial infections can result in varying degrees and patterns of sensorineural hearing loss. Infectious disease can be transmitted to the child by the mother in utero, a condition referred to as prenatal, congenital, or sometimes perinatal disease. These terms carry slightly different meanings, yet are often used synonymously. The term *prenatal* refers to something that occurs to the fetus before birth. *Congenital* also implies before birth, but usually prior to the 28th week of gestation. Finally, the word *perinatal* pertains to a condition that occurs in the period shortly before or after birth (from 8 weeks prior to birth to 4 weeks after). A disease can also be acquired later in life, and this is usually referred to as a *postnatal* condition. The following discussion reviews some of the more common prenatal and postnatal infectious diseases known to cause hearing loss.

Prenatal Diseases. Many of the prenatal diseases are categorized as part of the TORCH complex, an acronym used to identify the major infections that may be contracted in utero. In the acronym TORCH, *T* stands for toxoplasmosis, *O* is for other, *R* is for rubella, *C* is for cytomegalovirus, and *H* is for herpes simplex. Some have used the mnemonic (S)TORCH, where *S* stands for syphilis. Any disease of the (S)TORCH complex is considered a high-risk factor for hearing loss, and it is therefore important for the audiologist to have some general knowledge of these infectious conditions. Table 5.2 summarizes the (S)TORCH diseases and describes the expected hearing loss with each. In addition, Figure 5.14 illustrates the audiometric patterns known to occur with most of the (S)TORCH agents. Let us now briefly review these conditions.

Syphilis. Syphilis is transmitted to the child by intrauterine infection from the mother. Syphilis may manifest itself anytime from the 1st to the 6th decade of life. When the age of onset is early (before 10 years), the sensorineural hearing loss is profound and bilateral with sudden onset. With adult onset, the hearing loss is fluctuating and asymmetric and may appear either suddenly or gradually. Dizziness is also commonly associated with this condition. Figure 5.14D illustrates just one possible audiometric configuration associated with adult-onset syphilis.

Toxoplasmosis. Toxoplasmosis is a disease caused by an organism (*Toxoplasma gondii*) that is transmitted to the child via the placenta. It is thought that the infection is contracted by eating uncooked meat or making contact with feces of cats. As noted from Table 5.2, about 17% of infected newborns exhibit sensorineural hearing loss. The hearing loss is typically moderate and progressive (Fig. 5.14B).

Rubella. Rubella is perhaps the most well-recognized disease of the (S)TORCH

TABLE 5.2.
Clinical Manifestations of the (S)TORCH Complex

Disease	Primary Symptoms	Prevalence of Hearing Loss (%)	Type and Degree of Hearing Loss
Syphilis	Enlarged liver and spleen, snuffles, rash, hearing loss	35	Severe to profound bilateral SNHL; configuration and degree varies
Toxoplasmosis	Chorioretinitis, hydrocephalus, intracranial calcifications, hearing loss	17	Moderate to severe bilateral SNHL; may be progressive
Rubella	Heart and kidney defects, eye anomalies, mental retardation, hearing loss	20–30	Profound bilateral SNHL— "cookie-bite" audiogram is common; may be progressive
Cytomegalovirus	Mental retardation, visual defects, hearing loss	17	Mild to profound bilateral SNHL; may be progressive
Herpes simplex	Enlarged liver, rash, visual abnormalities, psychomotor retardation, encephalitis, hearing loss	10	Moderate to severe unilateral or bilateral SNHL

SNHL, sensorineural hearing loss.

complex. Rubella, sometimes referred to as German measles, infects the mother via the respiratory route. The virus is carried by the bloodstream to the placenta and to the fetus. If the mother contracts the virus during the 1st month of pregnancy, there is a 50% chance that the fetus will be infected; in the 2nd month, a 22% chance; and in subsequent months, about a 6–10% chance. Table 5.2 lists some of the more frequently encountered symptoms. One of the symptoms is a severe-to-profound bilateral sensorineural hearing loss (Fig. 5.14C). The child will display a trough- or bowl-shaped configuration or a corner-type audiogram. Children with **maternal rubella** have been known to exhibit both conductive and mixed-type hearing losses, although such instances are rare.

Cytomegalovirus (CMV). CMV is easily the most common viral disease known to cause hearing loss. About 33,000 infants are born each year with CMV. Ninety percent of the symptomatic children who survive (about 20% die) will exhibit complications. One of the common complications is sensorineural hearing loss. The

FIGURE 5.14.
Audiometric examples of *A*, cytomegalovirus (CMV); *B*, toxoplasmosis; *C*, rubella; *D*, syphilis.

hearing loss ranges from mild to profound and can be progressive. Figure 5.14A shows an example of a severe-to-profound hearing loss. The virus is passed from the mother to the fetus via the bloodstream.

Herpes Simplex Virus (HSV). HSV is a sexually transmitted disease, and the acquired virus is passed on to the fetus in utero or during the birth process. Only 4% of infected infants survive without complication. Some of the complications of the disease include central nervous system involvement, psychomotor retardation, visual problems, and hearing loss. Sensorineural hearing loss occurs when HSV is contracted in utero.

Postnatal Infections. Several postnatal infections produce sensorineural hearing loss. The cochlear damage produced by these viral or bacterial infections appears to result from the infecting agent entering the inner ear through the blood supply and nerve fibers. Figure 5.15 shows sample audiometric patterns for several postnatal conditions. The following is a brief review of those diseases that would be encountered most frequently by the audiologist.

Bacterial Meningitis. Hearing loss is the most common consequence of acute meningitis (Fig. 5.15*B*). Although the pathways used by the organisms to reach the inner ear are not altogether clear, several routes have been suggested. These include the bloodstream, the auditory nerve, and the fluid supply of the inner ear and the middle ear. The prevalence of severe-to-profound sensorineural hearing loss among patients with this disorder is about 10%. Another 16% will exhibit transient conductive hearing loss. Interestingly, some patients with sensorineural hearing loss will exhibit partial recovery, although such a finding is rare.

Mumps. Mumps is recognized as one of the more common causes of unilateral sensorineural hearing loss. The hearing loss is usually sudden and can vary from a mild high-frequency impairment to profound loss. Figure 5.15*C* illustrates a case of unilateral severe high-frequency hearing loss. Both children and adults are affected.

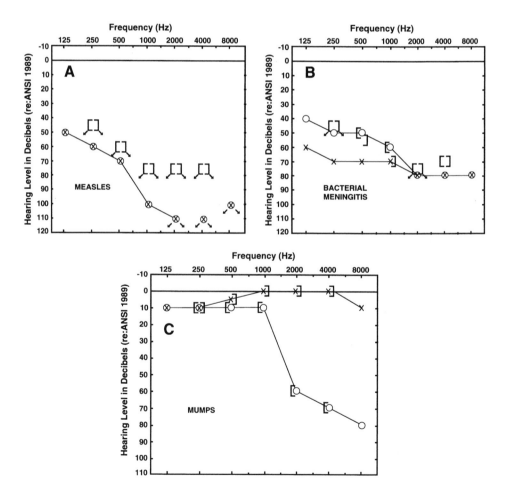

FIGURE 5.15.
Audiometric examples of *A*, measles; *B*, bacterial meningitis; and *C*, mumps.

Since it is uncommon for this disease to be subclinical, children with hearing loss resulting from mumps are not usually identified until they first attend school.

Measles. Measles is another cause of sensorineural hearing loss. Hearing loss affects 6–10% of measles patients. A typical audiometric configuration is a severe-to-profound bilateral high-frequency sensorineural impairment (Fig. 5.15A). Patients with measles also can show conductive hearing impairment.

Herpes Zoster Oticus. The first symptom associated with this disease is a burning pain close to the ear. Shortly thereafter, eruption of vessicles (small sac-like bodies) occurs in the ear canal and sometimes on the face, neck, or trunk. Common symptoms include facial paralysis, hearing loss, and vertigo. The loss is usually a severe bilateral high-frequency hearing impairment.

Ménière's Disease

Ménière's disease is typically defined as a symptom complex affecting the membranous inner ear. It is characterized by progressive or fluctuating sensorineural hearing loss, episodic vertigo, and, frequently, tinnitus (ringing or buzzing in the ear) that varies in both degree and type. Some have added the symptoms of a feeling of fullness and pressure in the ear to the classic signs associated with this disorder. The most commonly reported etiologies of Ménière's disease include allergies, adrenal-pituitary insufficiency, vascular insufficiency, hypothyroidism, and even psychologic disorders.

Vertigo is considered the most characteristic symptom of Ménière's disease. It can occur in attacks that are extremely severe, lasting anywhere from a few minutes to several days. In its more severe forms, the vertigo can be accompanied by extreme nausea and vomiting.

Tinnitus, a ringing sound in the ears, often precedes an episode and subsequently serves as a warning signal for an impending attack. The tinnitus usually increases as the hearing loss associated with the disease increases. Most patients with Ménière's disease describe their tinnitus as a low-pitched narrow band of noise, much like a roaring sound.

The audiologic manifestation associated with this disease is most often characterized by a low-frequency, sometimes fluctuating, sensorineural hearing impairment (Fig. 5.16). Although it has long been assumed that the disease is most often unilateral, estimates of bilateral involvement range from about 5% to 60%. In the later stages of the disease, the fluctuating nature of the hearing loss decreases, and the high frequencies become more involved. Typically, one sees good word-recognition scores and special auditory test results consistent with a cochlear lesion.

Ototoxic Drugs

A negative side effect of some antibiotic drugs is the production of severe high-frequency sensorineural hearing loss. A group of antibiotics known as aminoglycosides are particularly hazardous. This group, also commonly referred to as the "mycin" drugs, includes streptomycin, neomycin, kanamycin, and gentamicin. A

FIGURE 5.16.
Audiometric example of hearing loss due to Ménière's disease.

variety of factors can determine whether hearing loss is produced in a specific patient. These factors include the drug dosage, the susceptibility of the patient, and the simultaneous or previous use of other ototoxic agents.

Ototoxic antibiotics reach the inner ear through the bloodstream. The resulting damage is greater in the base of the cochlea, and outer hair cells are typically the primary targets, with only limited damage appearing in other cochlear structures. As shown in Figure 5.17, this results in an audiometric pattern of moderate-to-severe high-frequency sensorineural hearing loss in both ears.

Some ototoxic drugs cause a temporary or reversible hearing loss. Perhaps the most common such substance is aspirin. When taken in large amounts, aspirin can produce a mild-to-moderate temporary sensorineural hearing loss.

Noise-Induced Hearing Loss

Exposure to intense sounds can result in temporary or permanent hearing loss. Whether or not a hearing loss actually results from exposure to the intense sound again depends on several factors. These factors include the acoustic characteristics of the sound, such as its intensity, duration, and frequency content (amplitude spectrum), the length of the exposure, and the susceptibility of the individual.

When the intense sound is a broad-band noise, such as might be found in industrial settings, a characteristic audiometric pattern emerges following the exposure. This audiometric configuration is shown in Figure 5.18. It is frequently referred to as a "4k notch," which reflects the sharp dip in the audiogram at 4 kHz.

FIGURE 5.17.
Audiometric example of hearing loss due to ototoxicity.

More detailed measurements of the hearing loss produced by exposure to broad-band noise reveal that the notch in the audiogram is as likely to appear at 3 or 6 kHz as at 4 kHz. Because 3 and 6 kHz are not routinely included in audiometric testing, however, the notch is less frequently observed at these two frequencies.

FIGURE 5.18.
Audiometric pattern associated with noise-induced hearing loss.

This same "4k notch" configuration is observed both in temporary hearing loss following brief exposures to broad-band noise and in permanent hearing loss following prolonged exposure to such noise.

Many theories attempt to explain why the region around 4 kHz appears to be more susceptible to the damaging effects of broad-band noise. One theory is that, although the noise itself may be broad-band, with roughly equal amplitude at all frequencies, the outer ear and ear canal resonances (see Chapter 3) have amplified the noise in the 2–4 kHz region by the time the noise reaches the inner ear. Thus, this region shows the greatest hearing loss. Other theories suggest that the region of the cochlea associated with 4 kHz is more vulnerable to damage because of differences in cochlear mechanics, cochlear metabolism, or cochlear blood supply. Whatever the underlying mechanism, damage is greatest in that region of the cochlea associated with 4 kHz. The damage again appears to be more marked in the outer hair cells, although this can vary with the acoustic characteristics of the noise.

Presbycusis

Beyond about age 50 years, hearing sensitivity deteriorates progressively, especially in the high frequencies. The progression is somewhat more rapid for men than for women. Figure 5.19 shows the progression of hearing loss in both men and women as a function of age. The more rapid decline of hearing with age in men may not reflect differences in aging per se, but may reflect their more frequent participation in noisy recreational activities such as hunting, snow-mobiling, or operating power tools (e.g., lawn mowers, chain saws, table saws).

The data in Figure 5.19 suggest that aging results in a sloping high-frequency sensorineural hearing loss that gets progressively more severe with advancing age. It should be noted, however, that audiometric configurations other than sloping ones can be observed in the aged. The sloping high-frequency audiogram described above is typical of the most common types of presbycusis, known as sensory and neural presbycusis. At least two other types of presbycusis have been described. These are referred to as metabolic and mechanical presbycusis and are generally associated with flat and very gradually sloping audiometric configurations, respectively. As mentioned, however, these configurations are much less common.

As shown in Figures 5.17, 5.18, and 5.19, the audiometric configurations associated with ototoxic antibiotics, noise-induced hearing loss, and sensory or neural presbycusis are all very similar. In all three cases, a bilateral high-frequency sensorineural hearing loss is usually observed. The underlying cochlear damage is also very similar: the basal high-frequency region of the cochlea is the main area of destruction and the outer hair cells are primarily affected. Accompanying retrograde destruction of first-order afferent nerve fibers is also typically observed, as is usually the case in cochlear pathology.

Degenerative changes associated with aging have also been observed in the brainstem and cortical areas of the ascending auditory pathway in some cases.

FIGURE 5.19.

Hearing loss progression as a function of age in women (*left*) and men (*right*). (Adapted from Lebo CP, Reddell RC: The presbycusis component in occupational hearing loss. *Laryngoscope* 82:1399–1409, 1972).

These central changes, when present, can seriously compound the communicative impairment experienced by the elderly person with sensorineural hearing loss. Approximately 5–15% of elderly persons may have central auditory deficits affecting their ability to communicate.

Retrocochlear Pathology

Retrocochlear pathology refers to damage to nerve fibers along the ascending auditory pathways from the internal auditory meatus to the cortex. Most often a tumor is involved, although not always, as in the case of multiple sclerosis.

In many cases, the auditory manifestations of the retrocochlear pathology are subtle. Frequently, for example, no hearing loss is measured for pure tones. The possibility that a tumor along the auditory pathway will fail to produce measurable hearing loss for pure tones can be understood when one recalls the multiple paths by which information ascends through the brainstem within the auditory system (Chapter 3). Recall that after the first-order ascending neurons terminated in the cochlear nucleus, a variety of paths were available for the neurally transmitted information to ascend to the cortex. Thus, if the tumor is located central to the cochlear nucleus, the information required for the detection of a pure tone can easily bypass the affected pathway and progress to the cortex.

For the detection of a pure tone, many of the brainstem centers along the ascending auditory pathways probably serve simple relay functions and perform little processing of the signal. For more complex signals, such as speech, however, some preprocessing probably takes place in the brainstem prior to complete processing by the cortex. Still, in many brainstem and cortical disorders, speech recognition appears normal in quiet. This appears to be due to the multiple cues available in the speech signal that assist in its recognition. Some of the cues processed by a brainstem or a cortical center can be eliminated from the total information reaching the cortex by the presence of a tumor without producing a misperception of the speech signal. The patient is simply using several of the remaining cues that are not affected by the presence of the tumor. If, however, the speech signal is degraded by filtering, adding noise, temporal interruption, and so forth, the cues of the speech signal become less redundant. Every cue in the speech signal is now needed for its correct recognition. Individuals with retrocochlear pathology in the brainstem or cortex typically perform poorly on speech-recognition tests involving the recognition of degraded speech signals.

Again, a detailed description of retrocochlear disorders and the tests developed for their detection is beyond the scope of this book. Many special speech-recognition tests making use of degraded speech have been developed for this population. In addition, as mentioned previously, the ABR and other auditory evoked potentials are also of tremendous assistance to the physician in establishing a diagnosis of retrocochlear pathology.

Retrocochlear pathology that occurs at the first-order afferent nerve fibers, unlike that occurring at higher centers along the ascending auditory pathway, typically does result in abnormal performance on the basic audiologic test battery.

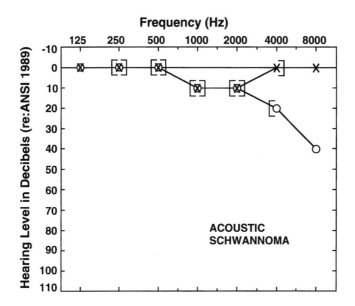

FIGURE 5.20.
Audiometric pattern associated with acoustic schwannoma.

These tumors, referred to as acoustic schwannomas, acoustic neurinomas, acoustic neurilemomas, or acoustic neuromas, typically produce a high-frequency sensorineural hearing loss that is either unilateral or asymmetric between the two ears (Fig. 5.20). Most patients will also complain of tinnitus on the affected side, and slightly more than half of these patients complain of dizziness. Speech-recognition performance may range from normal to extremely poor at moderate intensities, but it typically becomes poorer as speech level is increased to high intensities. Acoustic reflexes are usually absent or present at elevated levels when the affected ear is stimulated. A special test, known as acoustic reflex decay, measures the amplitude of the middle ear muscle contraction over time during stimulation by intense pure tones. Patients with acoustic schwannoma who have a measurable reflex threshold typically show pronounced reflex decay, especially when stimulated with pure tones at or below 1000 Hz. If several of the above-mentioned audiologic results are observed, the patient should be referred for additional testing. This will most likely involve measurement of the ABR and other special auditory and nonauditory tests.

NONORGANIC HEARING LOSS

The audiologist may obtain audiometric evidence of hearing loss when there is no organic basis to explain the impairment. Some of the terms commonly used to describe this phenomenon are nonorganic hearing loss, pseudohypoacusis, functional hearing loss, and psychogenic deafness. The cause for nonorganic hearing loss varies and is not clearly understood. Sometimes a patient purposely feigns a hearing loss to gain a benefit (e.g., monetary compensation), or the patient offers incorrect audiometric information because of a psychological disturbance. Whatever the reason, the audiologist must be able to determine whether a nonorganic hearing loss is present and, if so, the extent of the nonorganic impairment. Sometimes, a nonorganic hearing impairment will coexist with an organic hearing loss.

A number of audiometric signs can alert the audiologist to the possibility of a nonorganic hearing loss. These signs include the source of the referral (e.g., insurance company referring because of a claim), inappropriate behavior during the interview (e.g., exaggerated effort to speechread or to listen), and inconsistent audiologic test results (e.g., poor test-retest reliability). An obvious clue to nonorganic hearing loss is incompatibility between the pure-tone average and the speech recognition threshold (SRT). Recall from Chapter 4 that the pure-tone average and the SRT are related ($\pm$ 10 dB). A person exaggerating a hearing impairment for pure tones cannot always provide equivalent hearing loss data for speech and thus will usually exhibit an SRT that is considerably lower (softer) than the pure-tone average. Such a result should alert the audiologist to the possibility of a functional problem. Numerous other special tests have been developed to detect nonorganic hearing loss. However, detailed discussion of these tests is beyond the scope of this book. Readers who want to learn more about these tests should refer to the Suggested Readings at the end of the chapter.

SUMMARY

The auditory system, marvelously complex and intricate, is nevertheless vulnerable to assault and damage from disease, trauma, genetic imperfection, extreme environmental conditions (i.e., noise), and aging. Many conditions affect both children and adults and can affect all levels of the auditory system, resulting in conductive, sensorineural, or retrocochlear hearing problems.

REFERENCES AND SUGGESTED READINGS

Bess FH (ed): *Hearing Impairment in Children.* Parkton, MD, York Press, 1988.

Carhart R: Clinical application of bone conduction audiometry. *Archives of Otolaryngology* 51:798–807, 1950.

Dahl AJ, McCollister FP: Audiological findings in children with neonatal herpes. *Ear and Hearing* 9:256–258, 1988.

Eichwald J, Mahoney T: Apgar scores in the identification of sensorineural hearing loss. *Journal of the American Academy of Audiology* 4:133–138, 1993.

English GM (ed): *Otolaryngology*. Hagerstown, MD, Harper & Row, 1976.

Fria TJ, Cantekin EI, Eichler JA: Hearing acuity of children with otitis media with effusion. *Archives of Otolaryngology* 111:10–16, 1985.

Gerkin KP: The high risk register for deafness. *ASHA* 26:17–23, 1984.

Goodhill V (ed): *Ear Diseases, Deafness, and Dizziness*. Hagerstown, MD, Harper & Row, 1979.

Jerger J, Jerger S: *Auditory Disorders*. Boston, Little Brown, 1981.

Joint Committee on Infant Hearing 1994 Position Statement, Draft, 1994.

Kavanaugh J (ed): *Otitis Media and Child Development*. Parkton, MD, York Press, 1986.

Lebo CP, Reddell RC: The presbycusis component in occupational hearing loss. *Laryngoscope* 82:1399–1409, 1972.

Moody DB, Stebbins WC, Hawkins JE Jr, Johnsson L-G: Hearing loss and cochlear pathology in the monkey (macaca) following exposure to high levels of noise. *Archives of Oto-Rhino-Laryngology* 220:47–72, 1978.

Northern JL (ed): *Hearing Disorders,* ed 4. Boston, Little Brown, 1991.

Parving A: Congenital hearing disability—epidemiology and identification: a comparison between two health authority districts. *International Journal of Pediatric Otorhinolaryngology* 27:29–46, 1993.

Shambaugh GE, Glasscock ME: *Surgery of the Ear*. Philadelphia, WB Saunders, 1980.

Shuknecht HF: *Pathology of the Ear*. Cambridge, Harvard University Press, 1974.

CHAPTER SIX

SCREENING AUDITORY FUNCTION

OBJECTIVES

Following completion of this chapter, the reader should be able to:

- Understand how screening programs can improve hearing care.
- Evaluate the efficiency of a screening tool and a screening procedure.
- Know the recommended screening procedures used to identify hearing loss or middle ear disease in different age groups.
- Understand the need for and the importance of follow-up programs.

An important component of any comprehensive management strategy for the hearing impaired is an appropriate screening program. Screening is designed to separate persons who have an auditory disorder from those who do not in a simple, safe, rapid, and cost-effective manner. Screening programs are intended to be preventive measures that focus on early identification and subsequent intervention. The objective is to minimize the consequences of hearing loss or middle ear disease as early as possible so that the disorder will not produce a handicapping condition.

The purpose of this chapter is to present information on screening for hearing loss and middle ear disease. The review will cover the general principles of screening, discuss screening procedures for hearing loss and otitis media used with different age groups, and recommend follow-up protocols for those identified as having an auditory disorder.

UNDERSTANDING THE PRINCIPLES OF SCREENING

Factors That Determine Whether to Screen

How does one know whether to screen for the presence of a particular disorder? Several criteria are used in establishing the value of screening for a specific disorder. First, a disorder should be important. If left unidentified, the disorder should significantly damage an individual's functional status. It is also essential that the program be capable of reaching those who could benefit. Another important criterion is the prevalence of the disorder, or how frequently it occurs within a given population. There should be acceptable criteria for diagnosis. Specific symptoms of a disease must occur with sufficient regularity that it can be determined with assurance which persons have the disorder and which do not. Once detected, the disease should be treatable. Diagnostic and treatment resources must also be available so that adequate medical and educational follow-up can be implemented. Finally, the health system must be able to cope with the program, and the program must be cost-effective. It is generally believed by most, but not all, that hearing loss in people of all ages and middle ear disease in children satisfy many of these criteria and that screening for auditory disorders is justifiable, at least for selected populations (e.g., children at risk for hearing loss).

What is an Acceptable Screening Test?

A screening test must be selected that will most effectively detect the conditions to be identified. A good screening tool should be acceptable, reliable, valid, safe, and cost-effective. An acceptable test is simple, easy to administer, readily interpretable, and generally well received by the public. A reliable test should be consistent, providing results that do not differ significantly from one test to the next for the same individual. It does little good, for example, to have a screening test that the same healthy individual passes five times and fails five times when the test is administered 10 times in succession. Furthermore, the test should allow examiners to be consistent in the evaluation of a response. Two different examiners testing the same person should obtain the same results.

Validity may best be defined by asking, "Are we measuring what we think we are measuring?" The emphasis in this question is on what is being measured. For example, a clinician who wants to identify middle ear disease has selected a screening test that involves the measurement of hearing. Such a test would not be valid because, although it might reliably measure a child's hearing loss, it cannot indicate the presence or absence of otitis media. Validity consists of two components: sensitivity and specificity. Sensitivity refers to the ability of a screening test to identify accurately an ear that is abnormal (whether from hearing loss or from otitis media); specificity denotes the ability of a screening tool to identify normal ears. Thus, a valid test is one that identifies a normal condition as normal and an abnormal one as abnormal.

Finally, a good screening test is one that is safe and cost-effective in relation to the expected benefits. Since the instruments designed to screen for hearing loss and middle ear disease are considered safe and reasonable in cost, the greatest direct expense is usually the salary for personnel. Other factors should be taken into consideration when estimating the expense of a screening program. These include the time required to administer the test, the cost of supplies, the number of individuals to be screened and rescreened, and the cost of training and supervising screeners. The following formula has been suggested to estimate the cost of a school screening program:

$$\text{Cost/child} = \frac{S}{R} + \frac{C+(M \times L)}{(N \times L)}$$

where C = cost of equipment in dollars, S = salary of the screening personnel in dollars per hour, L = lifetime of the equipment in years, M = annual maintenance cost in dollars, R = screening rate in children per hour, and N = number screened per year. This formula could also be modified for determining the cost of an adult screening program.

Calculation of the costs of any screening program should also consider indirect costs, such as the cost of the comprehensive audiologic assessment, monitoring, and intervention that would occur as a result of the screening. A special concern is the cost associated with "false-positive" tests, those individuals who fail the screen but who have normal hearing. For children, such costs might include a parent's lost time from work, transportation to health care facilities, administration of unnecessary follow-up tests, and, possibly, unnecessary treatment, as well as the more human cost of the anxiety of parents or caring others, the potential of misunderstanding, and the disturbance of family function. Finally, the possible cost savings resulting from a screening program must be entered into the equation. For example, educational costs might be reduced as a consequence of early identification and subsequent intervention.

Principles of Evaluating a Screening Test

In this section, we will cover some of the basic principles of how to assess the usefulness of a screening test. Figure 6.1 sets the stage for understanding this process. Our primary goal is to distinguish within the population at large those individuals who exhibit an auditory disorder ($A + C$) from those who do not ($B + D$). Within the group with an auditory disorder, subgroup A are those people with the disorder who test positive (true positives); subgroup C are those with the disor-

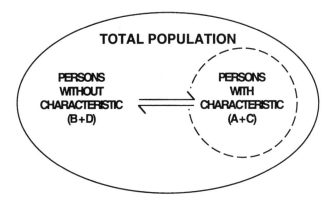

FIGURE 6.1.
The screening process. The purpose is to differentiate those who exhibit an auditory disorder in the population at large from those who do not.

der who test negative (false negatives). Within the group without an auditory disorder, subgroup *B* are those persons without the disorder who test positive (false positives); subgroup *D* are all those persons without the disorder who test negative (true negatives).

Any screening test must be evaluated against an independent standard, often referred to as a "gold standard." The results of the gold standard test are universally accepted as proof that the disease or disorder is either present or absent. In the case of hearing loss, pure-tone audiometry typically serves as the gold standard for any screening tool, whereas for middle ear disease the gold standard is usually pneumatic otoscopy or electroacoustic immittance. Figure 6.2 illustrates how the characteristics of a screening test can be evaluated against the gold standard. Toward this end, several terms and definitions need to be understood. First is sensitivity $[100A/(A + C)]$. (The factor 100 is introduced to convert the result to a percentage.) We have already learned that sensitivity refers to the proportion of individuals with the characteristic correctly identified by the test. If 100 subjects have a hearing loss and the test correctly identifies 75 of them, the sensitivity of the test would be 75%. Sensitivity is typically affected by the severity or duration of the characteristic. This is only logical in that, the milder an impairment is, the closer it is to a normal condition and the more difficult it is to distinguish from normal. However, the measure is not affected by prevalence. Another important measure is specificity, $[100D/(B + D)]$, which refers to the proportion of individuals without the characteristic correctly identified by the test. If, in a group of 100 normal subjects, the test identifies 70 as normal and 30 as abnormal, the specificity would be 70%. Like sensitivity, specificity is not affected by the prevalence of the disorder. The best screening tool will be one that provides the highest degree of both sensitivity and specificity.

It is possible to vary the accuracy of a screening test by altering the pass/fail criteria. A cutoff on a hearing screening test, for example, might be 15 dB HL or 40 dB HL. A 15-dB HL cutoff will provide high sensitivity but lower specificity. This is because the 15-dB HL criterion will result in a larger portion of near-normal subjects being classified as hearing-impaired. If a 40-dB HL cutoff is used, however,

	Gold Standard Test		
	Characteristic		
	Present	**Absent**	**Total**
Positive	A	B	A + B
Negative	C	D	C + D
Totals	A + C	B + D	A + B + C + D

FIGURE 6.2.
A decision matrix for calculating the operating characteristics of a screening test.

sensitivity will decrease but specificity will increase. The 40-dB HL cutoff will miss some of the mildly impaired near-normal subjects but will avoid misclassifying most of the subjects with normal hearing.

An important concept in any screening program is the prevalence of the disorder that is to be screened. Prevalence (derived from the word *prevail*) refers to the proportion of individuals in the population who demonstrate the characteristic $[100(A + C)/(A + B + C + D)]$. An important use of prevalence data is as a pre-test indicator of the probability of the disorder being present. For example, if the prevalence of hearing loss in the elderly is 30%, then when an older person walks into a hearing clinic you know that there is a 30% chance of hearing impairment before you conduct any tests. To illustrate how the prevalence of a disorder may be important to a screening program, consider the following two extremes. If 99% of the population has the disorder, it is easier to simply assume that everyone has it and treat it accordingly. In this case we would only be mistreating 1% of the population. If one in a million people have the disorder (prevalence = 0.0001%), then it may be safer and more efficient to assume that no one has it. Failure to screen for such a disorder would miss 0.0001% of the population.

Additional test characteristics of key importance in screening for a disorder are positive predictive value, the probability of an individual having the disorder when the test is positive, and negative predictive value, the probability of not having the disorder when the test is negative. Unlike sensitivity and specificity, predictive values are very dependent on the prevalence of the disorder in the population being tested. For a disorder of very low prevalence, even a highly specific test is likely to have a low positive predictive value. To illustrate, a test that has a sensitivity of 90% and a specificity of 90% in detecting a disorder will have a positive predictive value of 79.4%, and thus a false-positive rate of 20.6%, if the prevalence of the disorder is 30%. However, the positive predictive value decreases to 50% if the prevalence is only 10% and to 8.3% if the prevalence is only 1%.

In most hearing clinic settings, especially when screening for hearing loss, we need tests that yield maximum accuracy. The ideal test would be one that always gave positive results in anyone with a hearing loss and negative results in anyone without a hearing loss. Unfortunately, no such test exists. As a rule, one attempts to maximize the sensitivity and specificity of a screening test. This is done by evaluating different pass/fail criteria and test protocols in comparison to the gold standard. Vignettes 6.1 and 6.2 give examples of how to apply these general principles to actual screening data.

STATUS OF IDENTIFICATION PROGRAMS IN THE UNITED STATES

Screening Programs for Children

Identification programs for hearing loss have been implemented in the United States for various age groups including the neonate, the infant, the preschooler, and

Guidelines for calculating the operating characteristics of a screening tool.

Let us now go through the step-by-step procedures for calculating the characteristics of a screening tool. To assist in this process, some screening data are presented. The gold standard was pure-tone audiometry. In this example, a total of 99 patients were screened and then tested using pure-tone audiometry. It is noted that 47 patients failed the screening test, 27 of whom actually had a hearing impairment and 20 of whom did not. On the other hand, 52 patients passed the screening. Of these, the gold standard showed that three had a hearing loss and 49 did not. The prevalence of hearing loss in the population screened $[100(A + C)/(A + B + C + D)]$ is $100(30/99)$, or about 30%.

First, the sensitivity, or the percentage of valid positive test results, is calculated from the data. The formula for computing sensitivity is $100A/(A + C)$. When applied to our data, this gives $100(27/30) = 90\%$. This is excellent.

Next, compute specificity, or the percentage of valid negative test results, using the formula $100D/(B + D)$. This results in $100(49/69) = 71\%$. This is adequate, but not excellent.

In this example, we see that the screening test appears to be a valid tool for the identification of a hearing loss, offering acceptable sensitivity and specificity values. Now, on your own, calculate the operating characteristics of a screening tool for the example in Vignette 6.2.

Gold Standard Test

Hearing Impairment Characteristic

		Present	Absent	Total
Screening Test	Fail	27	20	47
	Pass	3	49	52
	Total	30	69	99

VIGNETTE 6.2.

Computing the characteristics of a screening tool using hypothetical screening data.

Now compute the characteristics of a screening tool for the example shown below. For this example, compute prevalence, sensitivity, and specificity.

Example:

Gold Standard Test

Hearing Impairment Characteristic

Screening Test		Present	Absent	Total
	Fail	160	20	180
	Pass	40	180	220
	Total	200	200	400

How did you do? You can find the answers in the back of the chapter.

the school-age child. Despite the urgency of early identification, however, the majority of screening programs occur at the school-age level. It has been estimated that less than 3% of the newborn population is being screened with the high-risk register, even though this tool has been recommended for universal use for several years. Moreover, only 18 states mandate some type of neonatal screening (3 states mandate universal screening). This is most unfortunate, especially considering the relatively high prevalence of hearing loss and the critical importance of the first 2 years of life for the development of speech and language. In addition, a large number of pediatricians are not familiar with neonatal auditory screening, nor do they recognize its importance. It has been estimated, for example, that only 3% of children from 6 months to 11 years of age receive a screening test at their primary health-care source. Although it is true that more reliable responses can be obtained from infants and young children than from neonates, there is the problem of locating all of the older groups of youngsters for the hearing test. Once newborns leave the hospital, it is not until age 5 years, at the kindergarten level, that these children are available for testing at one common location. Those few screening programs that do exist are conducted in day-care centers, well-baby clinics, and Head-Start programs. These programs, however, attract only a specific segment of children, primarily those from lower socioeconomic levels. Even if a massive national effort were made to screen all preschoolers at these various centers, a large percentage of children would still be missed. Yet screening the preschool child has several distinct advantages over the screening of newborns:

1. Children become easier to test as age increases.
2. Children with a progressive hearing loss and those whose hearing loss was not detected at the newborn screening would stand a good chance of being identified.
3. Children with hearing impairment who have recently moved into the community would have a chance of being identified.

Under our present system, children whose hearing loss was not detected at the newborn identification program or who moved into a community at preschool age are not identified until screening occurs in kindergarten. There is a critical need for a national effort directed at infant and preschool hearing screening programs in every state.

Hearing screening programs using pure tone audiometry are most often conducted in the school system because it affords easy access to the children. However, the availability, accessibility, comprehensiveness, and quality of school screening programs vary significantly from one state to the next. A major problem and source of frustration for audiologists involved in school screening programs is the lack of appropriate follow-up services offered to children who fail the screen.

The incorporation of immittance screening programs is not as universal. It is estimated that at least 24 states incorporate immittance (tympanometry) as part of their screening procedures. Some of the problems associated with mass immittance screening are discussed later in this chapter.

Figure 6.3 shows the percentage of school programs that conduct pure-tone and immittance screening. It is seen that the emphasis for pure-tone and immittance screening in the schools is at the elementary level and that few programs conduct screening in the secondary grades. Moreover, a much larger percentage of school programs use pure-tone screening than immittance screening.

Screening Programs for Adults

There are almost no formalized hearing screening programs in the United States for adult populations. Screenings do occur, however, in the Armed Forces, and most communities conduct health fairs where individuals can have their hear-

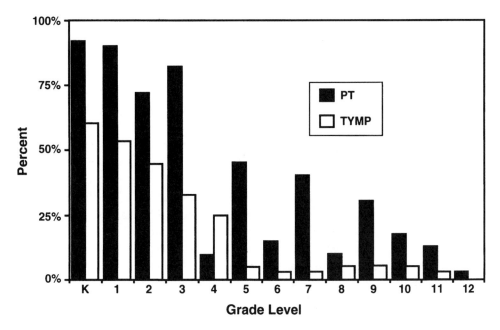

FIGURE 6.3.
Percentage of school programs conducting pure-tone and immittance screening by grade level. (From Roush J: Screening school-age children. *In* Bess FH, Hall JW [eds]: *Screening Children for Auditory Function*. Nashville: Bill Wilkerson Center Press, 1992.)

ing tested. Adult hearing screening programs are also known to take place at community health centers, retirement communities, and nursing homes. Interestingly, evidence suggests that the primary-care physician typically does not screen for hearing even if the patient complains of a hearing loss. There is a critical need for audiologists to educate both consumers and health-care professionals about the importance of hearing health care, including early identification and intervention.

Audiologists and other health professionals have failed to sensitize both the lay public and the educational and medical communities to the effects of auditory impairment on total development and quality of life. The importance of *early* detection of hearing impairment and the effectiveness of the screening methods available are two concepts that have not been presented well to the educational or medical community. Until we begin to educate these other professional groups, we cannot hope to improve our present identification programs.

IDENTIFICATION OF HEARING LOSS

Screening the Neonate

The advantages of detecting sensorineural hearing loss as early as possible in young children are important enough to encourage the implementation of newborn screening programs. It has now been demonstrated unequivocally that children who receive intervention from the age of 3 years or younger show significantly better speech and language outcomes later in life. Early identification and intervention (the word *intervene* means "to come in and modify") also results in substantial cost savings. For example, a deaf infant who receives educational and audiologic management during the first years of life has a better than 50% chance of becoming "mainstreamed" into a regular classroom.

The screening procedures advocated for the newborn nursery have been controversial. Audiologists have not agreed on the most effective and appropriate techniques. The National Joint Committee on Infant Hearing Screening (a committee of representatives from the American Academy of Otolaryngology, the American Academy of Pediatrics, the American Academy of Audiology, the American Speech-Language-Hearing Association (ASHA), the Council on Education of the Deaf, and the Directors of Speech and Hearing Programs in State and Welfare Agencies) endorsed the concept of universal screening and recommended, at a minimum, screening infants who were considered at high risk for hearing loss. Table 6.1 lists the Joint Committee's high-risk criteria (risk indicators) for both newborns and infants. Some risk indicators require periodic audiologic monitoring because their conditions are associated with progressive hearing loss (Table 6.2). Unfortunately, studies have demonstrated that, although the use of a high-risk register can identify some infants with hearing loss, many children with hearing impairment do not manifest any of the risk factors listed in the register.

Behavioral Observation Audiometry

A number of behavioral techniques have been advocated in the high-risk nursery for screening for hearing loss. These techniques make use of a high-intensity wide-band stimulus or a band of noise centered around 3000 Hz. The stimuli are presented while the infant is at rest in a crib. The child's behavioral responses to these stimuli are then observed or recorded. A common behavioral technique of this type once used in neonatal nurseries is the Crib-O-Gram. This test uses a motion-sensitive transducer placed under the crib to detect the infant's responses to the high-level noise presentations. Even subtle respiratory movement can be identified with this device. Behavioral techniques, however, have a number of limitations. The approach generally will identify only those children with the more severe forms of hearing loss. In addition, because of the sound-field approach, it is possible that unilateral sensorineural hearing loss will not be detected. Finally, concern has been expressed about the sensitivity and specificity of this approach, because the response depends as much on the infant's motor state as it does on sensory ability.

Auditory Brainstem Response

The auditory brainstem response (ABR) has been suggested as a reliable indicator of hearing sensitivity in infancy. The advantages of the ABR for newborn

TABLE 6.1.

Listing of Indicators or Risk Factors Associated wtih Sensorineural or Conductive Hearing Loss

Neonates (Birth–28 days)	Infants (29 days–2 years)
1. Family history of hereditary, childhood sensorineural hearing loss	1. Parent/caregiver concern regarding hearing, speech, language, and/or developmental delay
2. In utero infection such as cytomegalovirus, rubella, syphilis, and toxoplasmosis	2. Bacterial meningitis and other infections associated with sensorineural hearing loss
3. Craniofacial anomalies including those with morphologic abnormalities of the pinna and ear canal	3. Head trauma associated with loss of consciousness or skull fracture
4. Birth weight less than 1500 g (3.3 lbs).	4. Stigmata or other findings associated with a syndrome known to include a sensorineural and/or a conductive hearing loss
5. Hyperbilirubinemia at a serum level requiring exchange transfusion	
6. Ototoxic medications including, but not limited to, the aminoglycocides used in multiple courses or in combination with loop diuretics	5. Ototoxic medications including, but not limited to, chemotherapeutic agents or aminoglycocides, used in multiple courses or in combination with loop diuretics
7. Bacterial meningitis	
8. Apgar scores of 0–4 at 1 minute or 0–6 at 5 minutes	6. Recurrent or persistent otitis media with effusion for at least 3 months
9. Mechanical ventilation lasting 5 days or longer (e.g., persistent pulmonary hypertension)	
10. Stigmata or other findings associated with a syndrome known to include a sensorineural and/or a conductive hearing loss	

Adapted from the American Speech-Language-Hearing Association Joint Committee on Infant Hearing 1994 Position Statement—Draft, 1994.

screening include (*a*) the use of less intense, near-threshold stimuli, making it possible to detect milder forms of hearing impairment, (*b*) the ability to detect both unilateral and bilateral hearing losses, and (*c*) the use of a physiologic measurement that depends entirely on a sensory response. Limitations to the technique include the cost and sophisticated nature of the instrumentation, the use of an acoustic click that makes the ABR primarily sensitive to only high-frequency hearing loss, and the fact that the ABR is not a conscious response at the level of the cortex (presence of an ABR does not mean the individual can hear). Nevertheless, the measure is thought to provide a good estimate of hearing status when used carefully,

TABLE 6.2.

Indicators or Risk Factors Recommended for Periodic Monitoring of Hearing

1. Indicators associated with **delayed onset** sensorineural hearing loss include:
   a. Family history of hereditary childhood hearing loss
   b. History of in utero infection such as cytomegalovirus, syphilis, rubella, or toxoplasmosis
   c. Neurofibromatosis type II and neurodegenerative disorders
2. Indicators associated with **conductive** hearing loss include:
   a. Recurrent or persistent otitis media with effusion
   b. Anatomic deformities and other disorders that affect eustachian tube function
   c. Neurodegenerative disorders

Adapted from the American Speech-Language-Hearing Association Joint Committee on Infant Hearing 1994 Position Statement—Draft, 1994.

especially when one considers the limitations of the alternative procedures. A child who fails an ABR screening in the intensive-care nursery must be retested later under more favorable conditions.

Several ABR-based screening systems with automated response collection and evaluation have been designed for use with neonates. Theses devices are portable, automatic, and microprocessor-based. Their primary function is to screen for handicapping hearing loss in newborn infants. These simplified and cost-effective systems employ various automated algorithms to determine whether an infant passes or fails. These devices appear to have considerable promise for use in the high-risk nursery but require further investigation before they can be widely accepted.

Otoacoustic Emissions

As noted in Chapter 2, evoked otoacoustic emissions (OAEs) have been explored as a screening tool to identify hearing loss in neonates. Although there is some disagreement as to the details of such a screening protocol, including whether transient-evoked OAEs (TEOAEs) or distortion-product OAEs (DPOAEs) or both should be used and the appropriate stimulus parameters to optimize screening efficiency, the scientific and clinical communities have recommended that OAEs become an integral part of a universal neonatal hearing screening program for the United States. It has generally been recommended that either OAEs or ABR be used for the initial screening, with all screening failures retested with the alternative measure. Many of the advantages and disadvantages described for the use of ABR as a screening tool also apply to the use of OAEs as a screening measure.

National Institutes of Health (NIH) Consensus Statement

Interest in the early identification of hearing loss among newborns and young infants has increased. Several professional organizations have developed position statements concerning the need for early identification in addition to proposing recommended screening protocols. For example, in 1993, the National Institute on Deafness and Other Communication Disorders sponsored a national meeting on early identification of hearing loss in infants and young children. A task force, composed of members of several different disciplines, developed a consensus statement on early identification following presentations and discussions at the conference. The task force supported universal hearing screening within an infant's first 3 months of life, preferably prior to hospital discharge. A two-stage screening protocol was recommended. First, all infants would be screened with OAEs; those who failed the OAE test would receive an ABR screen at 40 dB nHL. (0 dB nHL represents normal hearing for these systems, just as 0 dB HL does for the audiogram.) Failure at this second stage would lead to a comprehensive diagnostic hearing assessment within 6 months. Periodic infant hearing screening throughout early childhood was also recommended.

The NIH consensus recommendation was met with some controversy. Some advocates of early identification believed that the implementation of a universal screening program was premature because of the limited data on screening healthy newborns in well-baby nurseries (most screening has been conducted in neonatal intensive care units) and because there was limited information on the performance of the two-tier screening protocol. Another major concern with the recommendation of universal newborn screening was the practicability of implementing identification programs in remote/rural communities—communities in which 25% of the births in the United States take place. Nevertheless, more and more hospitals in the United States are initiating screening programs for healthy newborns or high-risk babies using the protocol recommended by the NIH or some modification of the NIH protocol.

Screening the Infant and Preschool-Age Child

Identification Tests and Procedures

Selection of screening techniques will depend on the age, maturity, and cooperation of the child. Generally speaking, a test using sound localization in the sound field will be required for those children between the ages of 4 months and 2 years. Conventional audiometric screening using earphones can usually be employed with children 3 years of age or older. Children between the ages of 2 and 3 years make up the most difficult group for which to select an appropriate test. Some of these children can be conditioned for traditional screening techniques with earphones, whereas others will require the test based on sound localization.

Infant and Prenursery Child (4 Months to 3 Years)

The use of such acoustic stimuli as the human voice, rattles, a teaspoon and cup, and the rustling of tissue paper are often suggested for eliciting a localization (head turn) response. The child is placed on the parent's lap and various stimuli are presented about 2 feet from either ear. If the child fails to localize the signal, a rescreening is recommended. A second failure results in a third test 1 week later. If the child again fails the test, a complete diagnostic examination is conducted.

Sometimes delays in speech/language development are the most sensitive and valid indicators of hearing impairment among preschool children. It has been suggested that primary-care physicians and other allied health personnel screen young children for hearing loss simply by asking the parent three basic questions: (a) How many different words do you estimate your child uses? Is it 100 words, 500 words, or ?; (b) What is the length of a typical sentence that your child uses? Is it single words, two words, full sentences, or ?; and (c) How clear is your child's speech to a friend or neighbor? Would they understand 10%, 50%, 90%, or ? Table 6.3 presents a general guide for referring children with a speech delay.

A more formalized test that probes for delays in speech/language development is known as the Early Language Milestone Scale (ELM). The ELM was designed primarily for physicians and other health-care professionals. It is considered a simple, rapid, cost-effective means of screening for communication disorders in children from birth to 36 months of age; however, it is most sensitive at 24 months of age and higher. The test combines parental report, direct testing, and incidental observation. Important for the primary-care physician is the fact that the test takes only 1–5 min to administer. Sensitivity values as high as 97% and specificity values as high as 93% have been reported when using the ELM with preschool-age children. More representative values for sensitivity and specificity of the ELM are 65–70% and 65–75%, respectively. Nevertheless, asking parents specific questions about speech/language development appears to be a viable alternative for determining the presence of hearing loss among young children.

Preschooler (3–6 Years)

When the child reaches 3 years of age, the more traditional hearing test with earphones can be used for screening. By means of a portable pure-tone audiometer,

TABLE 6.3.
Referral Guidelines for Children with "Speech" Delay

12 Months
No differentiated babbling or vocal imitation
18 Months
No use of single words
24 Months
Single-word vocabulary of ≤10 words
30 Months
Fewer than 100 words, no evidence of two-word combinations, unintelligible
36 Months
Fewer than 200 words, no use of telegraphic sentences, clarity <50%
48 Months
Fewer than 600 words, no use of simple sentences, clarity <80%

From Matkin ND: Early recognition and referral of hearing-impaired children. *Pediatrics in Review* 6:151–156, 1984.

signals may be presented at various frequencies at a fixed intensity level. The child merely indicates to the examiner, usually by raising a hand, if a tone was perceived. The ASHA has recommended that 1000, 2000, and 4000 Hz be used as test frequencies. If immittance testing is not part of the program, the frequency 500 Hz should also be tested (assuming that background noise levels in the test area are acceptable). The Association further recommends a screening level of 20 dB HL for all frequencies tested. A lack of response at any frequency in either ear constitutes a test failure. Children who fail should be rescreened, preferably within the same test session, but no later than 1 week after the original test. The practice of rescreening can significantly reduce the overall number of test failures. Children who also fail the rescreening should be referred for a complete audiologic evaluation.

Procedural Considerations for Preschool-Age Children

In developing a screening program at the preschool level, special attention should be directed toward the groundwork and orientation process that occurs prior to the screening. The success of any screening program depends, to a large extent, on the cooperation of the teachers, the children, and the parents. All three of these parties must be familiarized with the screening process that is to take place.

First, a letter should go to the teacher outlining the need for and the purpose of the screening program. The letter should also review the teacher's responsibilities in preparing the children for the screening. Table 6.4 outlines some suggested prescreening activities with which the teacher can orient the children to the listening task. Such activities performed prior to the identification program can help avoid wasted time during the actual screening. It is also most helpful to provide the teacher with a list of the screening responsibilities of those individuals who will be conducting the screening, as well as of those who will be receiving the screening. This list will serve as an excellent guide and provide the teacher and/or administrator with a better understanding of the entire screening process from start to finish (Table 6.5). Finally, a sample letter to the parents of each child should be included in the packet of materials. The letter should explain the screening program so that the parents will understand the value of screening and support the screening process (Table 6.6).

The person who will be responsible for conducting the screening program should visit the facility and meet with the teacher(s) and administrator(s). Together they should review carefully the sequence of the screening program and discuss any concerns they might have. This is also an excellent opportunity to review with the program officials the sites available for the screening. Needless to say, a quiet room is essential. Other considerations in selecting a testing site have been identified by others. These are:

1. The site will need appropriate electrical outlets (only grounded three-prong outlets should be used) and lighting.
2. The site should be located away from railroad tracks, playgrounds, heavy traffic, public toilets, or cafeterias.
3. The site should be relatively free of visual distractions.

TABLE 6.4.
Recommended Prescreening Activities

I	
Objective:	To introduce children to wearing earphones in hearing testing.
Materials:	Old set of earphones (if possible) or set of earmuffs.
Procedure:	Let each child examine and wear the earphones. Talk about the headband and the muff.
Variation:	Allow the children to put the earphones on each other's ears.

II	
Objective:	To prepare children for the hearing test.
Materials:	Blocks, shoe boxes.
Procedure:	Put a shoe box on the table. Demonstrate holding a block up to your ear. Have one child stand behind you and clap his or her hands. Drop the block in the box when you hear the clap. Have each child take a turn standing in front of the box with the child's back toward you. Tell the children to "listen very carefully" and drop the blocks into the box when they hear the clap.
Variation:	Let the children be the "hand clappers."
Note:	If a child does not seem to understand, guide the child through the activity until he or she can hold the block to the ear and drop it in the box without your help.

III	
Objective:	To prepare the children for the hearing test.
Materials:	Blocks, shoe boxes, bell.
Procedure:	Put a shoe box on the table. Demonstrate holding a block up to your ear. Have one child stand behind you and ring a bell. Drop the block in the box when you hear the bell. Have each child take a turn standing in front of the box with his or her back toward you. Tell the children to "listen very carefully," and drop the blocks in the box when they hear the bell.
Variation:	Repeat the activity and ring the bell softly. Have the children take turns being "bell ringers."
Note:	Encourage the children to listen for the "soft" or "little" sound of the bell as preparation for the hearing test sounds that will be very soft.

4. Ideally, the site should have carpet and curtains to help reduce the room noise.
5. The site should have nearby bathroom facilities to accommodate the needs of the children and screeners.
6. The site should have chairs and tables appropriate for small children.

TABLE 6.5.
Sequence of Screening Responsibilities

Agency Providing Screening	*Program Receiving Screening*
Appoint a person to coordinate all screening activities.	Appoint a program representative to coordinate all screening activities.
Procure the list of all program centers or children needing to be screened.	Prepare a list of all program centers or children needing to be screened.
Establish personnel needs according to the number of children to be screened. Secure the necessary personnel to implement successfully the screening.	
Organize a training session in the use of screening materials, test forms, and test protocol for the screeners.	
Establish mutual screening schedules, including dates and times, allowing ample time to do the necessary prescreening activities.	Establish mutual screening schedules, including dates and times, allowing ample time to do the necessary prescreening activities.
Assist in screening site selection, if needed.	Choose screening sites.
Mail the screening materials and preschool record forms to the recipients. Materials should be in the teachers' hands 3 weeks prior to the screening date to allow ample time for forms to be completed, parent release forms to be mailed, and training in the classroom to be conducted.	Inform teachers about dates, times, sites, and personal responsibilities. All pertinent information should be in writing and given to teachers approximately 2 weeks prior to the screening date.
Conduct screening according to established schedule.	Assist in screening as needed.
Assist in contacting resource agencies for follow-up or serve as the resource.	Contact resource agencies for necessary follow-up for the children failing the screen. Obtain comprehensive speech and language evaluations, therapeutic management, and in-service teacher training assistance.

Table 6.5. — *continued*

Agency Providing Screening	Program Receiving Screening
Type and mail a preschool screening summary report indicating the results of the screening by individual names grouped by classrooms. This report should be completed by the screeners within 2 weeks of the screening date.	
	Receive and review the preschool screening summary report with teachers and staff.
Provide ongoing monitoring of the follow-up activities on all children failing the screening.	Actively pursue follow-up management on all children failing the screening.

Some other suggestions and hints for screening preschool children include the following:

1. One person should be individually responsible for ensuring that the children move through the screening process smoothly and that all children receive the test.
2. Arrangements should be made for the children to have name tags showing their legal names and nicknames.
3. All forms should be accurately completed prior to the screening date. Each child should have his or her own individual preschool record form.
4. When screening children between the ages of 3 and 6 years, it is wise to alternate age groups during the screening day—for example, 3-year-olds followed by 5-year-olds. Three-year-olds are much harder to test and take more time. Another factor to keep in mind is that the little ones tire more easily than older children and need to be screened earlier in the day.
5. Screening activities should run from 8:30 or 9:00 am until 3:00 or 3:30 pm each day. Schedule a full day, even if it means adjustments of schedules and bus runs and special notes of explanation for parents.
6. At all costs, avoid changing screening sites in the middle of the day. Each time you must dismantle a screening site in one center, move, and reassemble in another site, you lose approximately 1 hour plus travel time.
7. If the children are to be away from their own building during their regular lunch period, make arrangements for them to have lunch at the screening site, if possible.
8. If the agency at which the screening is taking place has a speech clinician on staff, ask to have that person available to assist in the screening effort.

TABLE 6.6.
Sample Letter for Teacher to Send Parents Prior to the Screening Test

Dear Parent,

Special arrangements have been made for your child and the others in your child's class to be tested for hearing. This test is a wonderful opportunity and we want to be sure that every parent knows all about it.

Certain learning problems don't ordinarily show up until later school years, when they are harder to remedy. If these special needs can be found early in the school years, the problem can often be solved before it really gets started.

We are very fortunate to have trained, qualified people who will be testing our children during school hours one day in the near future. The testing is provided without any cost to you. Your child will enjoy the "games" that check the ability to listen. There is everything to gain . . . and nothing to lose.

Because of the large number of children to be tested, the procedure will have to be speedy. Therefore, our children will be taking what is called a "screening test," which doesn't draw any conclusions—it just finds the children who may need more careful testing.

The majority of the children will pass with flying colors (and have an enjoyable day doing it). If any problem areas are discovered, someone from the center (school) will get in touch with you to make arrangements to check out the problem completely.

None of us likes to think that our child could have anything that stands in the way of learning. By taking advantage of this screening test, we can make sure. The earlier a problem is found, the less a problem it becomes.

If you have any questions, please contact us.

Teacher

Screening the School-Age Child

The practice of screening school-age children is over 50 years old, and all states conduct some form of hearing screening in the schools. The Joint Committee on Health Problems in Education (consisting of members of the National Educational Association and the American Medical Association) has described some primary responsibilities to be met by a screening program: an awareness of the importance of early recognition of suspected hearing loss, especially in the primary grades; intelligent observation of pupils for signs of hearing difficulty; organization and conduction of an audiometric screening survey; and a counseling and follow-up program to help children with hearing difficulties obtain diagnostic examinations, needed treatment, and such adaptations of their school program as their hearing condition dictates.

Who is Responsible for the Audiometric Screening Program?

Health and education departments are the agents primarily responsible for coordinating audiometric screening programs. Ideally, the state department of education should coordinate the periodic screening of all school children as well as provide for the necessary educational, audiologic, and rehabilitative follow-up. The state department of health, on the other hand, should coordinate the activities of identification audiometry, threshold measurement, and medical follow-up for students who fail the screening tests.

Personnel

The personnel designated to conduct the screening tests have been nurses, audiologists, speech-language pathologists, graduate students in speech and hearing—and even volunteers and secretaries. To assure quality programs, only professionals trained in audiology should be used to coordinate and supervise hearing screening programs. Volunteers and lay groups can best be used for support, such as in the promotion of screening programs. Certified audiologists or speech-language pathologists should administrate screening programs and utilize trained audiometrists or technicians to perform the screening. Public health nurses may serve as organizers and supervisors, but can be of most value in the follow-up phase of the program. A nurse's responsibilities might include (a) counseling parents and children about the child's needs for medical diagnosis and treatment, (b) using all available facilities for diagnosis and treatment, and (c) coordinating information about the child and family with specialists in the health and education field.

Who Should be Screened?

It is not economically feasible to mass screen all children in the schools. A target population must be identified. Most programs have concentrated their annual screening efforts on children of nursery-school age through grade 3. In fact, all of these grades are recommended for screening by the ASHA guidelines. Following grade 3, children may be screened at 3- to 4-year intervals. By concentrating the screening efforts on the first 3 or 4 years, it is still possible to carefully observe other special groups of school children. The following groups of children require more attention than is provided by routine screening:

1. Children with pre-existing hearing loss
2. Children enrolled in special education programs
3. Children with multiple handicaps
4. Children with frequent colds, or ear infections
5. Children with delayed language or defective speech
6. Children returning to school after a serious illness
7. Children who experience school failure or who exhibit a sudden change in academic performance

8. Children referred by the classroom teacher
9. Children who are new to the school

Equipment, Calibration, and the Test Environment

An important component of any identification program is the audiometric equipment used in the screening. The equipment needed for individual pure-tone screening should be simple, sturdy, and portable. Most screening audiometers are portable and weigh as little as 2 or 3 pounds. The performance characteristics of these instruments must remain stable over time. An audiometer that does not perform adequately could result in a higher-than-normal false-positive or false-negative rate. Care should be taken to ensure that all of the equipment used in screening satisfies the national performance standards. Unfortunately, this is not always done. Audiometers used in the schools often fail to meet calibration standards. School audiometers should receive weekly intensity checks with a sound level meter, as well as daily listening performance checks. All aspects of the audiometer should be thoroughly calibrated each year. It is also suggested that spare audiometers be available in case a malfunction occurs during a screening identification program.

Older audiometers will be most subject to instability and malfunction and should receive careful surveillance. Clinical audiologists who use these instruments for threshold measurement (following a screen failure) should know that the masking stimuli generated by many of these portable audiometers are often inadequate.

Once again, screening must be conducted in a quiet environment in order to ensure accurate measurements. Although some modern schools have sound-treated rooms or mobile units with testing facilities, most do not. Screening programs must be conducted in a relatively quiet room designed for some other purpose. Some helpful guidelines for selecting an appropriate room for screening have been outlined in the section on preschool screening. Table 6.7 shows the allowable octave-band ambient noise levels for each test frequency recommended by the ASHA. These ambient noise levels are measured using a sound-level meter with an octave-band filter. (See Chapter 2.)

Identification Tests and Procedures

During the more than 50-year history of identification audiometry in the schools, tests have been developed for screening the hearing of young school-age children. These tests may be classified as either group or individual screening tests. Most of the group tests were designed in earlier years to save time by testing large numbers of children at once. These techniques have never achieved wide acceptance. The majority of screening programs in this country have opted to use individual screening tests. Group screening, as it exists today, has only historical significance.

Table 6.7.

Approximate Allowable Octave-Band Ambient Noise Levels (dB SPL re: 20 μPa) for Threshold Measurements at 0 dB HL (ANSI-1969) and for Screening at the ASHA-Recommended Value of 20 dB HL

	Test Frequency (Hz)			
	500	1000	2000	4000
Octave-band levels:				
For testing with ears covered by earphone mounted in MX-41/AR cushion (ANSI 3.1-1987)	21.5	29.5	34.5	42.0
Plus ASHA screening level re: ANSI-1989	20.0	20.0	20.0	20.0
Resultant maximum ambient octave-band noise level allowable for ASHA screening	41.5	49.5	54.5	62.0

Individual Screening Tests

It is generally accepted that the individual pure-tone screening test is the most effective approach to screening hearing. In 1961, the National Conference on Identification Audiometry (NCIA) wrote a comprehensive monograph on general guidelines for individual pure-tone screening. These guidelines recommended that screening be conducted at frequencies of 500, 1000, 2000, 4000, and 6000 Hz and that the screening occur in a sound-treated environment.

More recently, the ASHA developed its own set of guidelines for pure-tone screening in the schools. The ASHA procedures recognized that sound-treated environments were not readily available in the schools. The ASHA guidelines differ from the NCIA recommendations in that (a) it is not recommended that screening occur in sound-treated rooms, (b) test frequencies of 500 and 6000 Hz are not included in the recommendations, and (c) rescreening of all failures is recommended.

Screening Adult Populations

With the increased awareness of hearing loss in the elderly population, we have witnessed an increased interest in the hearing screening of adult populations. Unfortunately, in primary-care medical practices wherein most older adults are seen regularly, we find that they are seldom screened and referred for audiologic evaluation. There seem to be several reasons for this.

First, the elderly accept their hearing loss as part of getting older and believe that there is simply no recourse for improvement. Second, it is found that primary-care physicians often fail to recognize a hearing impairment. Even when hearing loss is suspected or is reported to the physician, more than half of the patients are not referred for follow-up audiologic services. It appears that the primary-care physician looks upon hearing loss in the elderly in the same way that our society at large does. Deafness is viewed as a common by-product of aging, and little value is seen in rehabilitating the individuals affected by it. Those physicians who do screen for hearing loss rely on such techniques as the case history, or whisper or watch-tick tests, approaches whose validity or reliability have not been tested. Recent studies have shown, however, that primary-care practitioners will, indeed, screen for hearing loss if provided with appropriately validated screening tools and if they are convinced that hearing loss is important to the life quality of their patient. Again, just as with preschoolers, the task confronting the audiologist is one of educating and informing the public and the health-care community.

Pure-Tone Screening

There is no accepted standard or guideline for the identification of hearing loss in the adult population. Some clinicians have suggested that a pure-tone screening level of 20 or 25 dB HL be used for frequencies of 1000 and 2000 Hz and that 40 dB HL be used for 4000 Hz. Others believe that a 20- or 25-dB HL level should also be used for 4000 Hz. Unfortunately, there are limited data to support the validity of a 20- or 25-dB HL criterion at any frequencies for screening adults. We do not know with certainty the sensitivity, specificity, and test accuracy of pure-tone screening when using 20 or 25 dB HL as the cutoff point. Some have suggested that hearing screening in the aged should be done at the test frequencies 1000 and 2000 Hz, with a level of 40 dB HL serving as the pass/fail criterion. Failure for two test conditions (one frequency in each ear or both frequencies in one ear) constitutes a test failure. Data using this guideline are presented later in this section. Regardless of the test protocol, it is advisable to rescreen test failures. The recommendations related to environment, calibration, personnel, and procedural set-up that were discussed above regarding the screening of children can be followed with some modifications for screening the adult population.

Several new tools have been advocated for screening the older adult population. One of these is the Welch-Allyn Audioscope, a hand-held otoscope with a built-in audiometer that delivers a tone at 25 or 40 dB HL for 500, 1000, 2000, and 4000 Hz (Fig. 6.4). To use the audioscope, the clinician selects the largest ear speculum needed to achieve a seal within the ear canal. A tonal sequence is then initiated, with the subject indicating the tone was heard by raising a finger. The audioscope is found to perform very well against the gold standard of pure-tone audiometry when using the 40 dB HL signal at 1000 and 2000 Hz. The sensitivity of the audioscope has been reported to be 94%, and its specificity is between 72% and 90% for identifying a hearing impairment. In addition, the test has been found to have excellent test-retest reliability.

Communication Scales

Communication scales are another screening tool that can be used efficiently with the older adult population. A popular scale at present is the Hearing Handicap

FIGURE 6.4.
An audioscope. (From Lichtenstein MJ, Bess FH, Logan SA: Validation of screening tools for identifying hearing impaired elderly in primary care. *JAMA* 259:2875–2878, 1988.)

Inventory for the Elderly—Screening Version (HHIE-S). This screener is a self-report test that contains 10 items, 5 dealing with the social-situational aspects and 5 with the emotional aspects of hearing loss. Table 6.8 lists the test questions and the instructions for scoring. The test has been reported to identify the vast majority of elderly persons with high-frequency hearing losses exceeding 40 dB HL in the better ear. Again, this tool yields acceptable sensitivity and specificity values. Using a cutoff score of 8, one finds a sensitivity value of 72% and a test specificity of

TABLE 6.8.
Illustration of the Hearing Handicap Inventory for the Elderly—Screening Version (HHIE-S)

Enter: 4 for a "yes" answer, 2 for a "sometimes" answer, 0 for a "no" answer.

1. Does a hearing problem cause you to feel embarrassed when you meet new _____ people?
2. Does a hearing problem cause you to feel frustrated when talking to _____ members of your family?
3. Do you have difficulty hearing when someone speaks in a whisper? _____
4. Do you feel handicapped by a hearing problem? _____
5. Does a hearing problem cause you difficulty when visiting friends, _____ relatives, or neighbors?
6. Does a hearing problem cause you to attend religious services less often _____ than you would like?
7. Does a hearing problem cause you to have arguments with family _____ members?
8. Does a hearing problem cause you difficulty when listening to TV or _____ radio?
9. Do you feel that any difficulty with your hearing limits or hampers your _____ personal or social life?
10. Does a hearing problem cause you difficulty when in a restaurant with _____ relatives or friends?

TOTAL _____

HHIE-S scores may be interpreted as shown below. (Hearing impairment is defined as (a) the inability to hear a 40-dB HL tone at 1000 Hz or 2000 Hz in *each* ear of (b) the inability to hear both frequencies in one ear.)

HHIE-S Score	Probability of Hearing Impairment (%)
0–8	13
10–24	50
26–40	84

Adapted from Ventry IM, Weinstein BE: Identification of elderly people with hearing problems. *ASHA* 25:37–42, 1983; and from Lichtenstein MN, Bess FH, Logan SA: Validation of screening tools for identifying hearing impaired elderly in primary care. *JAMA* 259:2875–2878, 1988.

Table 6.9.

Sensitivity and Specificity of Screening Tests in the Diagnosis of the Hearing-Impaired Elderly

	Sensitivity (%)	Specificity (%)
Audioscope	94	72
HHIE-S score		
>8	72	77
>24	41	92
Combined scores: audioscope fail *and* HHIE >8, *or* audioscope pass *and* HHIE >24	75	86

77%. Although these values are not as high as those reported for the audioscope, they do represent acceptable values for a screening tool. The pencil-and-paper format and the low number of test items are additional advantages of the HHIE-S.

Even though the audioscope and the HHIE-S provide acceptable sensitivity and specificity values, the best test result is obtained when these two tools are used in combination. Table 6.9 summarizes the screening characteristics of the audioscope and the HHIE-S when used in combination. This table shows the sensitivity and specificity for each of the screeners alone and for the two instruments used in combination. Two specific pass/fail criteria seem to afford the most favorable outcome. These criteria are (*a*) audioscope—fail and HHIE-S score > 8 and (*b*) audioscope—pass and HHIE-S score > 24. When these criteria are used, it is seen that the sensitivity is 75%, whereas the specificity is 86%. Although there is some loss of sensitivity compared to that seen when either of the screeners is used alone, there is considerable improvement in specificity. This reduces the potential for over-referrals—an important factor when one is screening on a large-scale basis. Once again, as with most screening protocols, it is recommended that one retest before referral is made.

Another commonly used self-report communication scale is the Self-Assessment of Communication (SAC). Similar to the HHIE-S, the SAC is a 10-item questionnaire that queries an individual's perceptions of communication problems resulting from hearing loss. The SAC was standardized on a sample of adults over the age of 18 years; the post-test probabilities of hearing impairment are similar to that of the HHIE-S. Table 6.10 lists the test questions for the SAC.

Identification of Middle Ear Disease in Children

Electroacoustic Immittance

There is considerable interest in using electroacoustic immittance measures to identify middle ear disease among children. Several factors have contributed to the interest in using immittance as a screening tool. Some factors relate to immittance

TABLE 6.10.
Illustration of the Self-Assessment of Communication

Name _____

Date _____ Raw Score _____ × 2 = _____ − 20 = _____ × 1.25 _____%

Please select the appropriate number ranging from 1 to 5 for the following questions.

Circle only one number for each question. If you have a hearing aid, please fill out the form according to how you communicate when the hearing aid <u>is not</u> in use.

<u>Various Communication Situations</u>

1. Do you experience communication difficulties in situations when speaking with one other person? (for example, at home, at work, in a social situation, with a waitress, a store clerk, with a spouse, boss, etc.)

   1) almost never (or never)   2) occasionally (about ¼ of the time)   3) about half of the time   4) frequently (about ¾ of the time)   5) practically always (or always)

2. Do you experience communication difficulties in situations when conversing with a small group of several persons? (for example, with friends or family, co-workers, in meetings or casual conversations, over dinner or while playing cards, etc.)

   1) almost never (or never)   2) occasionally (about ¼ of the time)   3) about half of the time   4) frequently (about ¾ of the time)   5) practically always (or always)

3. Do you experience communication difficulties while listening to someone speak to a large group? (for example, at a church or in a civic meeting, in a fraternal or women's club, at an educational lecture, etc.)

   1) almost never (or never)   2) occasionally (about ¼ of the time)   3) about half of the time   4) frequently (about ¾ of the time)   5) practically always (or always)

4. Do you experience communication difficulties while participating in various types of entertainment? (for example, movies, TV, radio, plays, night clubs, musical entertainment, etc.)

   1) almost never (or never)   2) occasionally (about ¼ of the time)   3) about half of the time   4) frequently (about ¾ of the time)   5) practically always (or always)

5. Do you experience communication difficulties when you are in an unfavorable listening environment? (for example, at a noisy party, where there is background music, when riding in an auto or bus, when someone whispers or talks from across the room, etc.)

   1) almost never (or never)   2) occasionally (about ¼ of the time)   3) about half of the time   4) frequently (about ¾ of the time)   5) practically always (or always)

6. Do you experience communication difficulties when using or listening to various communication devices? (for example, telephone, telephone ring, doorbell, public address system, warning signals, alarms, etc.)

   1) almost never (or never)   2) occasionally (about ¼ of the time)   3) about half of the time   4) frequently (about ¾ of the time)   5) practically always (or always)

   <u>Feelings About Communication</u>

7. Do you feel that any difficulty with your hearing limits or hampers your personal or social life?

   1) almost never (or never)   2) occasionally (about ¼ of the time)   3) about half of the time   4) frequently (about ¾ of the time)   5) practically always (or always)

8. Does any problem or difficulty with your hearing upset you?

   1) almost never (or never)   2) occasionally (about ¼ of the time)   3) about half of the time   4) frequently (about ¾ of the time)   5) practically always (or always)

   <u>Other people</u>

9. Do others suggest that you have a hearing problem?

   1) almost never (or never)   2) occasionally (about ¼ of the time)   3) about half of the time   4) frequently (about ¾ of the time)   5) practically always (or always)

10. Do others leave you out of conversations or become annoyed because of your hearing?

    1) almost never (or never)   2) occasionally (about ¼ of the time)   3) about half of the time   4) frequently (about ¾ of the time)   5) practically always (or always)

Adapted from Schow RL, Nerbonne MA: Communication screening profile; use with elderly clients. *Ear Hear* 3:135–147, 1982.

in particular, and others relate to screening for middle ear disease in general. These factors include the ease and rapidity with which immittance measurement can obtain accurate information, the relative ineffectiveness of pure-tone audiometry in detecting a middle ear disorder, the high prevalence of otitis media, and the growing awareness of the medical, psychologic, and educational consequences that may result from middle ear disease. Today this popular technique is used routinely, not only in audiology centers but also in public health facilities, pediatricians' and otologists' offices, and schools.

In 1977, a special task force studied the use of immittance measures in screening for middle ear disease. The task force recognized the potential value of immittance screening but concluded, after reviewing the available data, that mass screening with immittance was premature. The task force also recommended the screening of special groups of children, such as Native American children, those with sensorineural hearing loss, developmentally delayed or mentally impaired children, and children with Down syndrome, cleft palate, or other craniofacial anomalies. The task force did not oppose immittance screening as such, but only universal (mass) screening on a routine basis. In fact, recognizing that many screening programs were already in operation and that others were soon to be implemented, the task force developed procedural guidelines to be used in the screening of preschool- and school-age children.

A problem with immittance screening has been the difficulty of developing appropriate pass/fail criteria. The pass/fail criteria developed by the ASHA and the special task force mentioned above have resulted in unacceptably high referral rates (32–36%). The screening criteria known as the Hirtshals program appear to produce a better result. The program uses only tympanometry and does not include the acoustic reflex. At the first screen, all children with normal tympanograms are cleared. The remaining children receive a second screen in 4–6 weeks, and all cases with flat tympanograms are referred. Those children still remaining receive a third screen 4–6 weeks later. Children with normal tympanograms or tympanograms having peaks in the range of −100 to −199 daPa are cleared. Children with flat tympanograms or tympanograms with peaks ≤200 daPa at the third screen are referred. With the Hirtshal screening approach, sensitivity and specificity values are 80% and 95%, respectively. Moreover, the program yields an acceptable referral rate of only 9%.

The ASHA developed a new guideline for screening children that includes a measure for both hearing loss and middle ear disease. The screening protocol involves the use of case history, visual inspection of the ear canal and eardrum, identification audiometry, and tympanometry. For history, the protocol simply considers recent evidence of otalgia (earache) or otorrhea (discharge from the ear). Visual inspection via otoscopy is performed to identify gross abnormalities. For identification audiometry, the ASHA recommends using the pure-tone protocol described earlier. For tympanometry, the recommendations for referral are (a) flat tympanogram and equivalent ear-canal volume outside normal range, (b) low static admittance on two successive occurrences in a 4- to 6-week interval, and (c) abnormally wide tympanometric width on two successive occurrences in a 4- to 6-week interval. Failure of the screen should result in an audiologic evaluation and a medical consultation. The screening protocol recommended by the ASHA is shown in Table 6.11 (referral criteria) and Figure 6.5 (flowchart). Because these guidelines are relatively new, data pertaining to the performance of the protocol are limited. One study examined only the tympanometry component of the revised ASHA guidelines in a large population of 3- and 4-year-old children. The gold standard was pneumatic otoscopy by a validated otoscopist. Resulting sensitivity and specificity were very good. The positive predictive value, on the other hand, was only 69%, meaning that only about two-thirds of the children who failed the screen were classified otologically as abnormal. These data suggest that more research is needed before we can draw any definitive conclusions about these guidelines.

TABLE 6.11.
Referral Criteria for 1990 ASHA Immittance Screening Protocol

I. History
    A. Otalgia
    B. Otorrhea

II. Visual inspection of the ear
    A. Structural defect of the ear, head, or neck
    B. Ear canal abnormalities
        1. Blood or effusion
        2. Occlusion
        3. Inflammation
        4. Excessive cerumen, tumor, foreign material
    C. Eardrum abnormalities
        1. Abnormal color
        2. Bulging eardrum
        3. Fluid line or bubbles
        4. Perforation
        5. Retraction

III. Identification audiometry—Fail air conduction screening at 20 dB HL at 1, 2, or 4 kHz in either ear (ASHA 1985; these criteria may require alteration for various clinical settings and populations)

IV. Tympanometry
    A. Flat tympanogram and equivalent ear canal volume (V_{ec}) outside normal range
    B. Low static admittance (Peak Y) on two successive occurrences in a 4- to 6-week interval
    C. Abnormally wide tympanometric width (TW) on two successive occurrences in a 4- to 6-week interval

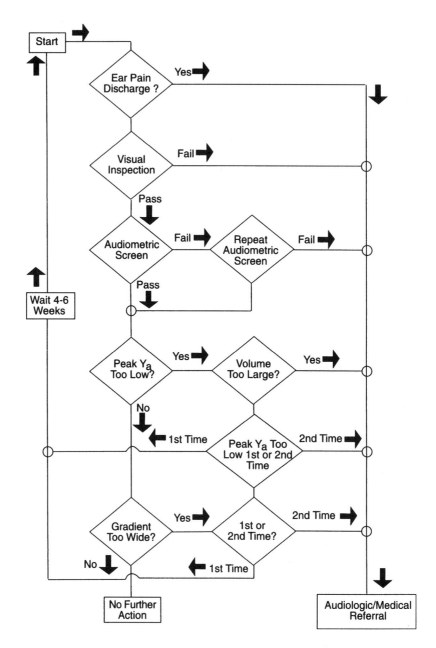

FIGURE 6.5.
Flowchart for establishing the need for audiologic/medical referral using four sources of information: history, visual inspection of the ear, identification audiometry and tympanometry. (From American Speech-Language-Hearing Association: Guidelines for screening for hearing impairment and middle ear disorders. *ASHA* 32:17–24, 1990.)

Acoustic Reflectometry

A relatively new and simple approach for detecting middle ear disease with effusion is known as acoustic reflectometry. This technique is a non-invasive, objective method and reportedly is useful even if a child is crying or if there is partial obstruction of the ear canal.

The hand-held, otoscope-like instrument generates a 80-dB SPL probe tone that begins at a frequency of about 2000 Hz and increases linearly to about 4500 Hz in 100 ms (0.01 s). The microphone in the device measures the combined amplitude of the probe tone and any sound waves reflected off the tympanic membrane (Fig. 6.6). According to the developers, operation is based on the consideration of one-quarter wavelength resonances. Briefly, an acoustic wave traveling in a tube will be completely reflected when it impinges on the closed end of that tube. The reflective wave will completely cancel the original one at a distance one-quarter wavelength away from the closed end of the tube, resulting in zero sound amplitude at this point. Accordingly, the level of reflected sound is inversely proportional to the total sound. Greater reflection produces a reduced sound level at the microphone and suggests that middle-ear impedance is high—as in otitis media with effusion. The degree of reflectivity is numerically displayed on the otoscope. A reading of 0–2 denotes a clear ear, and a reading of greater than 5 implies higher impedance, as with effusion.

Studies on the acoustic reflectometer have reported mixed results; about one-half of the studies report excellent sensitivity and specificity values, and one-half

Figure 6.6.
An acoustic reflectometer.

report unacceptable values. Research, however, has been limited with this device. More research is needed before this screening instrument can receive widespread acceptance.

Hand-Held Tympanometers

In the past several years small portable hand-held immittance screening tympanometers have been developed for screening programs. These hand-held otoscope-like units typically run on rechargable batteries and incorporate a small printer to record a hard copy of the data. The tip of the tympanometer is placed into the ear, and when a pneumatic seal is obtained a microcomputer initiates the miniature pump that varies pressure to the ear canal from +200 daPa to −300 daPa with a 226-Hz probe tone at 85 dB SPL. These hand-held screening instruments record data recommended by the 1990 ASHA Immittance Screening Guidelines. Hence, the data are reported in terms of equivalent ear canal volume, static admittance, and tympanometric width. Although these hand-held instruments appear to have significant potential in screening programs, additional research is needed to determine the usefulness of these systems with different age groups of children.

FOLLOW-UP

Follow-Up Programs for Children

Screening is of little value if follow-up is not provided for the appropriate management of children who fail the screen. This aspect of the conservation program takes as much planning and effort as any other phase of the screening program. Noncompliance has been one of the principal problems of existing hearing screening programs for newborns. In some studies, 25–80% of infants who failed newborn screening have been lost to follow-up despite aggressive recruiting efforts and the offering of cost-saving incentives to parents. In other studies, after early identification of hearing loss, lag times of 8 to 9 months have transpired before infants returned to intervention services. Presently, there are no data on compliance in hearing screening programs for infants beyond the newborn period.

For preschool and school-age programs, the screening coordinator will be responsible for the follow-up under most circumstances. A child who fails the rescreen should receive a comprehensive audiologic test at the screening site as soon as possible. Within a few days following the screening, those steps essential to appropriate follow-up should begin. Letters should be sent to parents indicating whether their child passed or failed the screening test. For those children who failed the screening, the letter should also recommend that the child be referred for medical evaluation. About 6 weeks after the screening, the parents should be asked whether the recommendations were followed.

Frequently, the public health nurse handles this phase of the follow-up program. In some states, audiologists and educators coordinate this activity. Following the medical examination, the child is referred to an audiologic facility for comprehensive testing and counseling. Parent counseling is an important aspect of the follow-up process and too often is overlooked by the supervisors of screening programs. Parents must receive special assistance and guidance in order to understand and cope with the prospect of having a hearing-impaired child. They must receive help before they can help their child.

Finally, the child will need to be referred to educational services that will be used for planning and placement. The follow-up is a lengthy and ongoing process requiring close coordination among all persons involved.

Follow-Up Programs for Adult Populations

If a person fails the screening protocol, he or she should receive an otologic examination and a comprehensive audiologic evaluation. Needless to say, the hearing evaluation will provide information about the extent and nature of the hearing impairment, as well as determine whether the patient could benefit from amplification. If amplification is warranted, the individual should be referred for hearing aid selection and evaluation. Procedures for this particular protocol are outlined in Chapter 7.

SUMMARY

We have defined and justified screening and discussed important considerations and techniques of identification programs. Identification is an important first step in the overall hearing conservation program. The early identification of hearing loss and middle ear disease is the key to effective and appropriate management. There still is much to be learned about our screening programs for the identification of both hearing loss and middle ear disease. In particular, we need to learn more about the feasibility of universal screening of healthy newborns. Such other critical issues as performance of screening tools, accessibility and availability of follow-up services, compliance, and costs need to be further explored. There is also a need for more research on screening with immittance and acoustic reflectometry for middle ear disease in children. There is still only limited information available about the application of the acoustic refectometer as a screening device, and the audiologist, therefore, will need to keep abreast of new developments. Finally, it will also be important to determine the sensitivity, specificity, and test accuracy of pure-tone audiometry for the adult population when using a 20- or 25-dB HL cutoff point.

REFERENCES AND SUGGESTED READINGS

American National Standards Institute: *American National Standards Specifications for Audiometers*. ANSI S3.6-1989. New York, American National Standards Institute, 1989.

American Speech-Language-Hearing Association: Guidelines for acoustic immittance screening of middle ear function. *ASHA* 20:550–555, 1978.

American Speech-Language-Hearing Association: Guidelines for identification audiometry. *ASHA* 27:49–53, 1985.

American Speech-Language-Hearing Association: Guidelines for screening for hearing impairment and middle ear disorders. *ASHA* 32:17–24, 1990.

American Speech-Language-Hearing Association: Considerations in screening adults/older persons for handicapping hearing impairments. *ASHA*, 34:81–87, 1992.

Avery C, Gates G, Prihoda T: Efficacy of acoustic reflectometry in detecting middle ear effusion. *Annals of Otology, Rhinology, and Laryngology* 95:472–476, 1986.

Bess FH, Hall JW: *Screening Children for Auditory Function*. Nashville: Bill Wilkerson Center Press, 1992.

Coplan J, Gleason JR, Ryan R, Burke MG, Williams ML: Validation of an early language milestone scale in a high risk population. *Pediatrics* 70:677–683, 1982.

Downs M: Early identification of hearing loss: where are we? Where do we go from here? *In* Mencher GT (ed): *Early Identification of Hearing Loss*. Basel, S Karger, 1976.

Harford ER, Bess FH, Bluestone CD, Klein JO (eds): *Impedance Screening for Middle Ear Disease in Children*. New York, Grune & Stratton, 1978.

Joint Committee on Infant Hearing 1994 Position Statement, 1994. Draft.

Kileny PR: ALGO-1 automated infant hearing screener: preliminary results. *In* Gerkin KP, Amochaev A (eds): *Hearing in Infants: Proceedings from the National Symposium. Seminars in Hearing*. New York, Thieme-Stratton, 1987.

Lichtenstein MJ, Bess FH, Logan SA: Validation of screening tools for identifying hearing impaired elderly in primary care. *JAMA* 259:2875–2878, 1988.

Lous J: Screening for secretory otitis media: evaluation of some impedance programs for long-lasting secretory otitis media in 7-year-old children. *International Journal of Pediatric Otorhinolaryngology* 13:85–97, 1987.

Matkin ND: Early recognition and referral of hearing-impaired children. *Pediatrics in Review* 6:151–156, 1984.

Northern JL, Downs MP: *Hearing in Children*, ed 4. Baltimore, Williams & Wilkins, 1991.

Roush J: Screening school-age children. *In* Bess FH, Hall JW (eds): *Screening Children for Auditory Function*. Nashville: Bill Wilkerson Center Press, 1992.

Sackett DL, Haynes RB, Guyatt, GH, Tugwell P: *Clinical Epidemiology: A Basic Science for Clinical Medicine*, ed 2. Boston, Little Brown, 1991.

Ventry IM, Weinstein BE: Identification of elderly people with hearing problems. *ASHA* 25:37–42, 1983.

Walton WK, Williams PS: Stability of routinely serviced portable audiometers. *Language, Speech, Hearing Services in the Schools* 3:36–43, 1972.

Weber BA: Screening of high-risk infants using auditory brainstem response audiometry. *In* Bess FH (ed): *Hearing Impairment in Children.* Parkton, MD, York Press, 1988.

Welsh R, Slater S: The state of infant hearing impairment identification programs. *ASHA* 35:49–52, 1993.

Wilson WR, Walton WK: Public school audiometry. *In* Martin FN (ed): *Pediatric Audiology.* Englewood Cliffs, NJ, Prentice-Hall, 1978.

Answers to Problem in Vignette 6.2

Prevalence—50%

Sensitivity—80%

Specificity—90%

PART III

MANAGEMENT STRATEGIES

CHAPTER SEVEN

AMPLIFICATION AND REHABILITATION FOR THE HEARING IMPAIRED

OBJECTIVES

Following completion of this chapter, the reader should be able to:

- List and describe the devices currently available to assist in the rehabilitation of the hearing impaired, including conventional hearing aids, assistive listening devices, classroom amplification, cochlear implants, and vibrotactile systems.
- Understand the basic components, function, and electroacoustic characteristics of hearing aids.
- Describe the general approaches used to select and evaluate conventional hearing aids.
- Understand some of the principles and techniques used in the management of children and adults with hearing impairment.

Probably the most significant problem experienced by the hearing-impaired adult is difficulty understanding speech, especially against a background of noise. Individuals with severe or profound sensorineural hearing loss also have trouble hearing their own speech. This typically results in speech production problems as well, making the overall communication process even more difficult. The intent of rehabilitation for the hearing-impaired adult is to restore as much speech-comprehension and speech-production ability as possible. For the child with congenital hearing impairment, however, the problem is more complicated since the symbols of our language system have not yet been learned. In these circumstances, the emphasis is on helping the child to acquire this complex language system and to use language appropriately so that communication skills might be gained. The focus is more on habilitation than on rehabilitation. That is, the objective is not to restore a skill that once existed, but to help the child develop a new skill—the ability to communicate.

In this chapter, we will review different approaches for developing and/or improving the communicative abilities of children and adults with hearing impairment. This process is usually referred to as aural rehabilitation or aural habilitation. A central core of any rehabilitation/habilitation program is the use of a hearing aid, an amplification device designed to help compensate for the hearing deficit. A substantial portion of this chapter focuses on various aspects of amplification systems.

AURAL REHABILITATION/HABILITATION PROCESS

The aural rehabilitation process involves at least two phases. The first phase is the identification of the problem. Before an intervention strategy can be developed, one must know about the type and degree of hearing loss as well as the impact of the impairment on communicative, educational, social, or cognitive function. For the adult with hearing impairment, the measurement of the patient's audiogram, the administration of speech-recognition tests, and the use of self-report surveys or questionnaires can provide much of this information. Pure-tone and speech audiometry have already been discussed (see Chapter 4). Self-report surveys are often used to assess in detail the social, psychological, and communicative difficulties experienced by the hearing-impaired. The Hearing Handicap Inventory for the Elderly—Screening version (HHIE-S), discussed in Chapter 6, is an example of such a survey, but in an abbreviated format. For the child with hearing impairment, additional assessment considerations might include the extent of parental support and the evaluation of skills in language, speech, auditory training, and speechreading (lipreading).

After the problem has been identified, the next phase of the rehabilitation process is intervention. For the hearing-impaired, the nature of the intervention package is determined, in large part, by the identification phase. Consider, for example, just the degree and type of hearing loss, ignoring other factors such as age and social or emotional difficulties. First, regarding type of hearing loss, the most appropriate candidates for amplification are those with sensorineural hearing loss. Occasionally, individuals with chronic conductive hearing loss not amenable to medical or surgical intervention will be fitted with a hearing aid. Most often, though, the individual with sensorineural hearing loss due to cochlear pathology is the type of patient fitted with a rehabilitative device, such as a hearing aid.

Generally, as the degree of sensorineural hearing loss increases, speech-understanding difficulties increase. The need for intervention increases in proportion to the degree of speech-understanding difficulty. Thus, those with mild hearing loss (pure-tone average of 20–30 dB HL) generally have less need for intervention than do those with profound hearing loss (> 85 dB HL). Conventional hearing aids provide the greatest benefit to those hearing-impaired persons whose average hearing loss is between 40 and 85 dB HL. For milder amounts of hearing loss, the difficulties experienced and the need for intervention are not great enough for full-time use of a conventional hearing aid. Part-time use of a hearing aid, or another type of device known as an assistive listening device, is usually recommended for these patients. For the profoundly impaired, on the other hand, the difficulties in communicating and the need for intervention are great. Unfortunately, the conventional hearing aid is of limited benefit in such cases. For patients with profound impairments, alternative devices, such as vibrotactile systems and cochlear implants, are sometimes explored. Currently, however, high-powered conventional aids are still the most common alternative for the profoundly impaired. Because amplification provides limited benefit for this group, though, the fitting of the hearing aid is usually accompanied by extensive training in several areas, including speechreading (lipreading), auditory training, and/or manual communication (finger spelling and sign language).

Consider also the time of onset of the hearing loss. Of course, the intervention approach will be much different for a congenitally hearing-impaired child than for someone who acquired the hearing loss later in life (after communication has developed). With a congenital onset, the emphasis will focus on such critical issues as early amplification, parental guidance, and a comprehensive habilitation package designed to facilitate communication development.

In summary, the intervention phase of aural rehabilitation/habilitation typically begins with the selection and fitting of an appropriate rehabilitative device, such as a hearing aid. This is followed by extensive training in communicative skills with the device.

Many of the procedures used in the identification phase of the rehabilitation process have been reviewed in earlier chapters. This chapter focuses on the intervention phase. The remainder of this chapter is divided into three sections. The first section reviews many of the rehabilitative devices available, emphasizing the conventional hearing aid. Methods of selecting and evaluating hearing aids are also reviewed in the first section. The final two sections review training methods and philosophies for rehabilitation/habilitation of children and adults.

Amplification for the Hearing-Impaired

Classification of Conventional Amplification

There are five basic types of hearing aid available today. These are (*a*) body aid, (*b*) eyeglass aid, (*c*) behind-the-ear (BTE) aid, (*d*) in-the-ear (ITE) aid, and (*e*) in-the-canal (ITC) aid. Figure 7.1 shows each type of instrument. When electroacoustic hearing aids were first developed several decades ago, the body aid was the only type available. In the ensuing years, the other types of instruments were developed. In 1960, eyeglass hearing aids were the most popular, accounting for 44% of all hearing aids sold, with the remaining 56% divided evenly between body and BTE instruments. As indicated in Figure 7.2, BTE hearing aids became the most common type of hearing aid sold in the two-decade period from 1962 through 1982. Since 1983, however, the trend has been for ITE aids to capture an increas-

Figure 7.1.
The different types of hearing aids. *1*, body aid; *2*, eyeglass; *3*, in-the-ear aid; *4*, in-the-canal aid; and *5*, behind-the-ear aid.

ingly larger portion of the hearing aid market. Since 1987, about 80% of the hearing aids sold in the United States have been ITE instruments; the bulk of the remaining 20% of instruments sold have been of the BTE type. (The sales percentages for ITEs shown in Figure 7.2 actually represent the combination of all types of ITE hearing aids, including the ITE and ITC types shown in Fig. 7.1.) In 1992, 55% of the ITE aids sold were full custom ITE aids like the type shown as no. *3* in Figure 7.1, and 30% were the ITC type, shown as no. *4* in this figure. The increasing popularity of the ITE and ITC hearing aids is a result of both consumer pressures to improve the cosmetic appeal of the devices and rapid developments in the field of electronics. High-fidelity electronic components and the batteries to power them have been drastically reduced in size, making the ITE devices possible. In fact, several companies began producing even smaller hearing aids, referred to as either completely-in-canal (CIC) or totally-in-canal (TIC) instruments, in the early 1990s. These instruments are inserted very deep into the ear canal; only a thin wire or

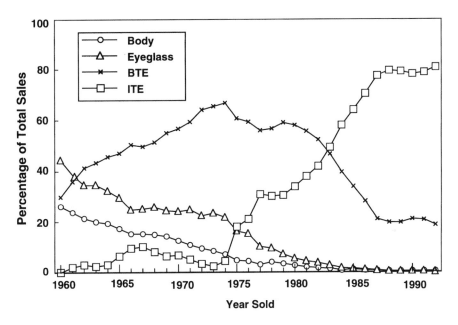

FIGURE 7.2.
Sales trends for various hearing aid types since 1960. *BTE*, behind-the-ear; *ITE*, in-the-ear.

thread is visible in the lateral portion of the ear canal when these devices are inserted.

Operation Of Amplification Systems

Components and Function

Although the outer physical characteristics of the types of hearing aids shown in Figure 7.1 differ, the internal features are very similar. The hearing aid, for example, is referred to as an electroacoustic device. It converts the acoustic signal, such as a speech sound, into an electrical signal. The device then manipulates the electrical signal in some way, converts the electrical signal back to an acoustic one, and then delivers it to the ear canal of the wearer. A microphone is used to convert the acoustic signal into an electrical signal. The electrical signal is usually amplified or made larger within the hearing aid. It may also be filtered to eliminate high or low frequencies from the signal. A tiny loudspeaker, usually referred to as a receiver, converts the amplified electrical signal back into a sound wave. Up to this point, the hearing aid could be thought of as a miniature public-address system with a microphone, amplifier, and loudspeaker. Unlike a public-address system, though, the hearing aid is designed to help a single person, the hearing aid wearer, receive the amplified speech. The microphone is positioned somewhere on the hearing-aid wearer, and the amplified sound from the receiver is routed directly to the wearer's ear. For ITE and ITC hearing aids, the sound wave is routed from the receiver to the ear canal by a small piece of tubing within the plastic shell of the instrument. For the other types of hearing aids, an earmold is needed. The earmold (or shell for the ITE and ITC hearing aids) is made of a synthetic plastic or rubber-like material from an impression made of the outer ear and ear canal. The earmold is custom-made for the patient's ear and allows the output of the hearing aid to be coupled to the patient's ear canal. As a result, only the patient receives the louder sound and not a group of people, as with a public-address system. (See Vignette 7.1.)

Electroacoustic Characteristics of Hearing Aids

The primary purpose of the hearing aid is to make speech that is inaudible to the hearing-impaired person audible, and to do so without causing discomfort. Modern-day conventional hearing aids have several electroacoustic characteristics that are used to describe the hearing aid's performance. Probably the two most important of these characteristics are the amount of amplification provided, referred to as the gain of the instrument, and the maximum possible sound pressure level that can be produced, referred to as the saturation sound pressure level (SSPL). Currently, these characteristics can be measured in several ways. For instance, there is a standard issued by the American National Standards Institute, ANSI S3.22–1992, that describes a set of measurements that must be made on all hearing aids sold in the United States. It is not necessary in an introductory text such as this, however, to review the ANSI standard in detail. Rather, the concepts underlying gain and SSPL and their importance in fitting the hearing aid to the patient are critical.

Gain, for example, is simply the difference, in decibels, between the input level and the output level at a particular frequency. Consider the following example. A 500-Hz pure tone is generated from a loudspeaker so that the sound level at the hearing aid's microphone is 60 dB SPL. The output produced by the hearing aid under these conditions is 90 dB SPL. The acoustic gain provided by the hearing aid is 30 dB. The gain is simply the difference between the 60-dB SPL input and the 90-dB SPL output. The gain of the hearing aid can be measured at several frequencies. Most hearing aids provide some amplification or gain over the frequency range 200–5000 Hz. When the gain is measured across this whole frequency range by changing the frequency of the input signal and holding the input level constant, a frequency response for the hearing aid is obtained. The frequency response displays how the output or gain varies as a function of frequency. The concepts of gain and frequency response are illustrated in Figure 7.3. Because the gain is seldom constant at all frequencies, an average gain value is frequently calculated and reported. In the current ANSI standard, the gain is measured at three frequencies, 1000, 1600, and 2500 Hz, and the values are averaged. These frequencies are used because of their importance to speech understanding and because the hearing aid usually has its greatest output in this frequency region.

A feature shared by nearly all hearing aids is a volume control wheel that allows the user to adjust the gain of the hearing aid. The frequency response of the hearing aid can be measured while the position of the volume control is varied.

VIGNETTE 7.1.

Basic components of an electronic hearing aid.

The top part of the schematic drawing shows the basic components of a contemporary electronic hearing aid. As illustrated here, the hearing aid is like a miniature head-worn public-address (PA) system with a microphone, amplifier, and loudspeaker (or receiver). The amplifier needs a portable power supply to do its job and this is supplied by a battery. In addition, a volume control allows the user to adjust the loudness so that sound is comfortably loud in different environments. The microphone and receiver are known as transducers in that their primary job is to convert waveforms from one form of energy to another. The microphone, for example, converts sound waves into electrical voltage waveforms. The amplifier then makes this incoming electrical waveform larger, and the receiver converts it back to a sound wave.

Although the components shown in the top portion of the drawing are fundamental to almost all electronic hearing aids, most hearing aids also come equipped with two additional controls. These are illustrated in the bottom portion of the drawing and are listed as the "tone control" and the "output limiting control." These two controls are generally adjusted by the audiologist and not by the hearing aid wearer. The tone control functions like a bass or treble control on a stereo in that the audiologist can adjust it to change the amount of amplification in the low or high frequencies. The output-limiting control allows the audiologist to regulate the maximum possible sound level produced by the hearing aid to assure that loud sounds are not made uncomfortably or hazardously loud.

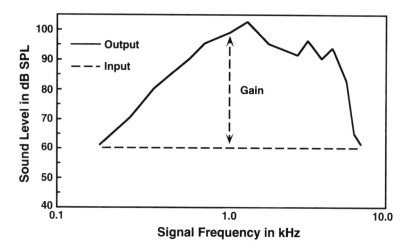

FIGURE 7.3.

Calculation of hearing aid gain. The *output curve* represents the frequency response of the hearing aid for a constant 60-dB *input*.

Usually, at least two sets of measurements are obtained: one with the volume control in the full-on position, and one designed to approximate a typical or "as worn" volume setting. The volume control is designed to provide an approximately 30-dB variation in gain. It is typically assumed that a hearing aid wearer will select a volume setting about in the middle of this 30-dB range—that is, about 15 dB below the full-on position. If the frequency response is measured with the volume control of the hearing aid in the full-on position, the gain is referred to as "full-on" gain. When the volume control is in the middle of the usable range, the gain approximates "use" gain, or "as worn" gain.

As mentioned, a second fundamental electroacoustic characteristic of the hearing aid is the SSPL. SSPL is measured to determine the maximum possible acoustic output of the hearing aid. Consequently, a high-level input signal is used (90 dB SPL), and the volume control is set to the full-on position. Under these conditions, the hearing aid is likely to be saturated. Saturation is a characteristic of all amplifiers, and the hearing aid is no exception. The amplifier is simply incapable of producing output exceeding a certain value, known as the saturation level.

The gain and SSPL of a hearing aid are inter-related, as illustrated in Figure 7.4. The function shown in this figure is known as an input-output function because it displays the output along the ordinate as a function of the input level along the abscissa. For this hypothetical input-output function, the volume control is assumed to be in the full-on position. Note that low input levels (50–60 dB SPL) reveal output values that exceed the input by 25 dB. That is, the gain (output minus input) is 25 dB at low input levels. At high input levels (90–100 dB SPL), on the other hand, the output remains constant at 110 dB SPL. This is the SSPL of the hearing aid. The instrument simply can't produce an output higher than 110 dB

FIGURE 7.4.
Input-output function for a hearing aid.

SPL. Because the hearing aid is saturated, the gain at these higher input levels is lower. The gain for the 90- and 100-dB inputs is 20 and 10 dB, respectively. Because of this interaction between gain and SSPL, gain is usually measured for input levels of 50–60 dB. These are also levels that approximate those of conversational speech, the input signal of greatest interest.

Candidacy for Amplification

How does one know whether an individual is a good candidate for amplification? We have already indicated that the ideal candidate for amplification is one who displays a sensorineural hearing loss. Many audiologists use the degree of hearing loss as a "rule of thumb" for determining hearing aid candidacy. Figure 7.5 shows a general guideline based on the average (500–2000 Hz) pure-tone hearing loss in the better ear. As hearing loss increases, the need for assistance increases, reaching a maximum for moderate amounts of hearing loss. Potential benefit from amplification, however, is lowest at the two extremes, mild and profound impairment. Those individuals with the mildest hearing losses and those with the most profound hearing deficits are usually the candidates who will benefit the least from a hearing aid. There are many exceptions to this pure-tone–based "rule of thumb." Because of this, there is now a tendency to move away from these pure-tone guidelines and to consider anyone with a communicative difficulty due to hearing impairment a candidate for amplification.

There are other considerations in determining hearing aid candidacy. Some of these factors are the patient's motivation for seeking assistance, the patient's acceptance of the hearing loss, and the patient's cosmetic concerns. Even if a significant hearing loss is present, some patients put off seeking assistance for several years. The reasons for this delay are not altogether clear, although the cost of the hearing aid and the failure of the primary-care physician to refer for a hearing aid are con-

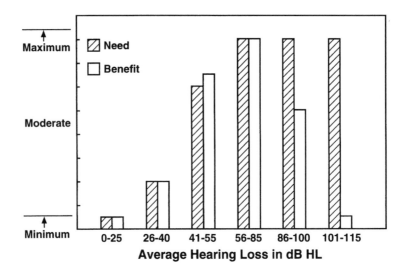

FIGURE 7.5.
Illustration of the need for and potential benefit from amplification as a function of degree of hearing loss.

TABLE 7.1.
Factors That Influence a Patient's Decision to Obtain Amplification[a]

Factor	Percentage Reporting Strong or Moderate Influence
Communication problems at home	82
Communication problems in noisy listening situations	81
Communication problems in social settings	81
Communication problems at work	77
Encouragement from spouse	77

[a]Adapted from Mueller HG, Grimes A: Amplification systems for the hearing impaired. *In* Alpiner JG, McCarthy PA (eds): *Rehabilitative Audiology: Children and Adults:* Baltimore, Williams & Wilkins, 1987 p 119.

sidered contributing factors. Table 7.1 summarizes factors that influence patients to pursue amplification. Note that communication problems at home, in noisy situations, or in social settings are the major motivating factors for seeking a hearing aid.

Acceptance of a hearing loss is another consideration in determining hearing aid candidacy. Some individuals simply deny that a hearing problem exists. This is particularly true for persons with very mild losses, those who fear loss of employment, and those who have suffered gradual onset of hearing loss.

Finally, one cannot overlook cosmetic concerns when considering a patient's candidacy for amplification. Amplification is still considered stigmatic. Although the acceptance of hearing aids is improving, many hearing-impaired individuals are concerned about the stigma associated with amplification, especially the more conspicuous instruments (body and BTE aids).

Hearing Aid Selection and Evaluation

Once it has been established that an individual can benefit from amplification, an appointment for hearing aid selection and evaluation is usually scheduled. In the selection phase, some important clinical decisions must be made. For example, what type of hearing aid would be most appropriate for a given hearing-impaired person? Recall from Figure 7.1 that a number of different types of hearing aids are available. The audiologist and patient need to decide whether the patient will benefit most from a body-type hearing aid, a BTE instrument, or one of the ITE systems (ITE or ITC). As noted earlier, most hearing aids sold today are BTE, ITE, or ITC units. BTE hearing aids have several distinct advantages over body aids, the most important of which are cosmetic appeal, improved sound localization, and better speech understanding in noise when two aids are worn. Importantly, very few young children wear ITE or ITC systems because of the frequent need to recast the earpiece because of a growing ear canal. Currently, about 75% of hearing aids selected for children are BTE systems. Sometimes it is appropriate to use a hearing aid that includes a bone conduction transducer. Bone conduction hearing aids are used most often in patients with pinna deformities such as those discussed in Chapter 5.

Another important clinical decision that must be made in the selection phase is whether to recommend one hearing aid (monaural amplification) or two hearing aids (binaural amplification). For years, there has been considerable controversy over the true benefits of binaural amplification. Although one would intuitively think that binaural amplification is superior to monaural amplification, it has traditionally been difficult to demonstrate any objective advantages for two hearing aids. More recently, however, there has been mounting evidence in favor of binaural fittings, and this has affected clinical practice. In 1980, for example, 75% of patients were fit monaurally and 25% binaurally. A decade later, in 1990, about 50% of the hearing aid wearers in the United States were fit monaurally and 50% binaurally. The percentage of binaural fittings of hearing aids, moreover, has continued to increase into the 1990s. The primary reason that binaural amplification is not more widespread is undoubtedly the added cost to the patient of buying two hearing aids rather than one. Nonetheless, there is mounting clinical evidence that failure to fit hearing aids on both ears of patients with bilateral hearing loss can result in temporary, and perhaps permanent, decreases in auditory function in the unaided ear. The deterioration over time of auditory perceptual function in the hearing-impaired ear left unaided has been referred to as an "auditory deprivation" effect.

In addition to avoiding these possible deprivation or adaptation effects, some of the reported advantages to binaural amplification include better sound localization, binaural summation (a sound is easier to hear with two ears than with one), and improvement in speech recognition in noise. Experienced hearing aid users often favor binaural amplification and report that two aids offer more balanced hearing, better overall hearing, improved speech clarity in noise, improved sound localization skills, and more natural and less stressful listening. Accordingly, binaural amplification is being recommended with increasing regularity. Some clinical research indicates, however, that the benefits of binaural fittings over monaural ones increase as the amount of hearing loss increases. Monaural fittings may be appropriate for many persons with mild hearing impairment.

Several other factors must be considered in the selection process but are beyond the scope of an introductory text. Briefly, the audiologist must consider the type of microphone (directional versus omnidirectional), earmold material (soft silastic versus hard acrylic), and type of earmold or shell (e.g., vented versus unvented). Additional choices include whether the instrument is programmable and whether a remote control unit is available for adjusting volume on the hearing aid. For children, an additional consideration is the adaptability of the instrument to various classroom amplification systems.

Modern-day hearing aids provide a wide range of electroacoustic characteristics that can be tailored to the patient's individual needs. The process of selecting a hearing aid with the appropriate electroacoustic characteristics for a particular patient is referred to as hearing aid selection. This process has undergone major changes in recent years. Today, most audiologists use a prescriptive approach to hearing aid selection. Using information obtained from the patient, such as the pure-tone thresholds, the appropriate gain can be prescribed according to some underlying theoretical principles. From the mid-1970s through the mid-1980s, at least a dozen different prescriptive hearing aid selection methods were developed. Although they differ in detail, these methods have the same general feature that more gain is prescribed at those frequencies for which the hearing loss is greatest. As an example, one of the simplest approaches makes use of the so-called "half-gain rule." One simply measures the hearing threshold at several frequencies and multiplies the hearing loss by a factor of one-half. Thus, for a patient with a flat 50-dB hearing loss from 250 through 8000 Hz, the appropriate gain would be 25 dB (0.5 × 50 dB) at each frequency. A person having a sloping hearing loss with a 40-dB HL hearing threshold at 1000 Hz and an 80-dB HL threshold at 4000 Hz would require gains of 20 and 40 dB, respectively, using this simple one-half gain rule. Regardless of the prescriptive method used, once the prescription is made, the audiologist searches among existing hearing aids to find the one with the most appropriate gain characteristics. For ITE and ITC hearing aids, the instrument is simply ordered using the prescribed gain values.

SSPL can also be prescribed for the patient. Usually additional information is required from the patient. One common approach is to measure the loudness discomfort level (LDL) of the patient for tones or narrow bands of noise. The LDL is a measure of the maximum sound level that the patient can tolerate at each frequency. It would not be desirable for the hearing aid's acoustic output to exceed the maximum tolerable level of the patient because this might cause the patient to reject the hearing aid. The SSPL of the hearing aid is frequently adjusted to a value slightly lower than the LDL. In this way, the audiologist can be assured that the acoustic output of the hearing aid will not exceed the maximum tolerance level of the patient.

Once the appropriate prescription has been made and the hearing aid has been selected, the next process, the hearing aid fitting, is conducted. In this process, the hearing aid is inserted into the patient's ear, and its acoustic performance on the wearer is evaluated. This is most commonly accomplished using real-ear measurements of the sound pressure level generated in the ear canal, in close proximity to the eardrum, with and without the hearing aid in place. This is made possible by using a tiny microphone connected to a long, thin tube made of flexible plastic. The tube can be safely inserted into the ear canal, yet is strong enough to resist being squeezed shut when the hearing aid is inserted into the ear canal over the thin tube. When sound pressure level measurements are made at several frequencies in the patient's ear canal with and without the hearing aid, the difference between these two measurements provides a measure of the real-ear insertion gain of the hearing aid. The measured insertion gain is compared with the target gain generated by the particular prescriptive method chosen by the audiologist (e.g., half-gain rule), and the hearing aid's settings are adjusted until a reasonable match is observed. Similar adjustments should also be made in the maximum output of the hearing aid to assure that real-ear sound pressure levels measured in the aided conditions for high-level input signals (90 dB SPL) do not exceed the LDL.

After fine tuning the gain and maximum output of the hearing aid to match the targeted values, the hearing aid is evaluated. Again, there are several hearing aid evaluation procedures from which the audiologist can choose. These alternatives, however, have a common goal: evaluation of the benefit provided by the hearing aid when it is worn by the hearing-impaired patient. In that the primary benefit to be derived from use of the hearing aid is improved understanding of speech, the hearing aid evaluation usually involves the measurement of the patient's speech-recognition performance with and without the hearing aid. This is done using loudspeakers with the patient positioned in the sound field. Standardized tape-recorded speech materials are preferred for testing. (See Chapter 4.) The patient is typically presented with a sample of continuous speech or speech-shaped noise at a level approximating conversational levels (65 or 70 dB SPL).

While listening to this stimulus, the patient adjusts the volume control on the hearing aid to a comfortable setting. Next, speech-recognition testing is conducted, with the materials being presented at the same overall level (65–70 dB SPL). Speech-recognition testing is often performed both in quiet and in a background of noise or multitalker babble. This is done to permit evaluation of the benefit provided by the hearing aid for a range of conditions representative of those in which the hearing aid is to be worn. With this in mind, a speech-to-noise or speech-to-babble ratio of +6–8 dB is recommended for use. This range of values represents "typical" noisy conditions encountered by most patients. The speech-recognition measures are also often obtained in quiet and in noise under identical stimulus conditions while the hearing aid is not worn by the patient. The difference in performance between the aided and unaided measures provides a general indication of the benefit provided by the hearing aid under various listening conditions. These direct measures of the effects of the hearing aid on speech-recognition performance have sometimes been referred to as "objective" measures of benefit (see Vignette 7.2).

VIGNETTE 7.2.

Effects of a hearing aid on speech understanding in quiet and in noise.

The *left-hand panel* in the figure shows the distribution of various speech sounds at conversational levels on the coordinates of the audiogram. We will refer to this type of plot in this chapter as the "speech audiogram." Note that the full range of speech sounds is audible to an individual with normal hearing in quiet conditions. Also notice that many of the speech sounds, such as /f, s, t/, are low in intensity and high in frequency.

In the *middle panel*, a high-frequency sensorineural hearing loss, not unlike that found in many elderly individuals, has been superimposed on the speech audiogram. Notice that many of the high-frequency, low-intensity consonants are no longer heard by the individual with this hearing loss, although many low- and mid-frequency speech sounds (such as vowels and nasal sounds) remain audible. A frequent complaint of individuals with this very common type of hearing loss is that they can hear speech but they can't understand it. When presented with the words "wife, white, wide, wipe, wise," for example, the individual may only hear the word "why" repeated several times. The high-frequency consonant at the end of each word is not heard and the words are misperceived.

In the *right-hand panel*, the speech sounds have been amplified by a well-fit hearing aid. In this case, a well-fit hearing aid would amplify the high frequencies to make the high-frequency consonants audible to the patient while not amplifying

VIGNETTE 7.2.—*continued*

the low frequencies, where hearing is essentially normal. With the audibility of all of the speech sounds in conversational speech restored by the hearing aid as shown in this panel, the hearing aid wearer will regain the ability to understand speech as well as a normal-hearing listener. Depending, in part, on how long they have become accustomed to hearing speech through their hearing loss, the time required to perform normally will vary from patient to patient.

In noise, however, the microphone of the hearing aid amplifies the noise as much as the speech. That is, the speech-to-noise ratio is not improved by the conventional hearing aid. If the conversational speech of the person in front of the listener is 6 dB greater at the input to the hearing aid (microphone) than the background of babble produced by the other attendees at a cocktail party, then this 6-dB speech-to-noise ratio will remain at the output from the hearing aid. The speech will be made audible by the hearing aid, but so will the noise. Consequently, conventional hearing aids are generally not considered to work as well in noise as in quiet.

In addition to these objective measures of hearing aid benefit, the hearing aid evaluation should also include some "subjective" measures of performance and benefit. Most commonly, self-assessment surveys or inventories of hearing handicap and hearing aid performance have been used. The self-assessment scale, generally consisting of about 25 items, is administered prior to hearing aid delivery and at several intervals following use of amplification (e.g., 30 days, 3 months, 6 months). Such scales generally show reliable reductions in hearing handicap following use of amplification. Hearing aid performance scales, on the other hand, are designed to be used only after the hearing aid has been worn by the user. Items in the survey typically seek to assess hearing aid performance in a variety of situations and environments. Interpretation of a hearing aid's performance requires one to compare results from a given hearing aid wearer with normative data, although relative indications of hearing aid performance are still possible without norms (e.g., patient performs better with hearing aid in quiet rather than in noise, or with visual contact with talker than without visual contact).

Hearing Aid Orientation

Once the hearing aid has been selected and evaluated, the patient is counseled about the measured benefits, the limitations of hearing aids, the cost of the instrument(s), and so forth. If the patient decides to purchase the hearing aid, the audiologist may either dispense the hearing aid or refer the patient to another party who sells it. As noted in Chapter 1, an increasing percentage of audiologists today are directly involved in the dispensing of hearing aids. Hearing aids are typically sold on a 30-day trial basis; dissatisfied patients are given a refund at the end of that trial period. During the trial period, the patient is encouraged to visit the audiologist two or three times for a series of hearing aid orientations. During the hearing aid orientations, the patient is instructed in the use and care of the hearing aid, counseled about its limitations, given strategies to maximize its benefit, and given an opportunity to voice any complaints about its function. Frequently, modification of the earmold or the earpiece (shell) of the aid is needed to make the hearing aid fit more comfortably in the patient's ear. The hearing aid may require some electronic adjustments as well. After the 30-day trial period, the hearing aid user is encouraged to return for further evaluation in a year, or sooner if he or she experiences difficulty.

Alternative Rehabilitative Devices

Assistive Listening Devices

As mentioned previously, full-time use of a hearing aid is not necessary or beneficial for many hearing-impaired individuals. Many people with mild hearing loss require only part-time use of a hearing aid or alternative device. For many of these individuals, a practical alternative is a class of devices known as assistive listening devices. These devices are typically electroacoustic devices designed with a much more limited purpose in mind than that of the conventional hearing aid. Two of the most common purposes for which these devices were developed are use of the telephone and listening to the television. Several telephone handsets have been developed, for instance, that can amplify the telephone signal by 15–30 dB. These devices are effective for people with mild hearing loss who have difficulty communicating over the telephone.

Many of the assistive listening devices physically separate the microphone from the rest of the device so that the microphone can be placed closer to the source of the desired sound. Recall that the microphone converts an acoustic signal into an electrical one so that it can be amplified by the device. If the microphone on the assistive listening device is separated by a great distance from the rest of the device, the electrical signal from the microphone must somehow be sent to the amplifier. This is accomplished in various ways, with some devices simply running a wire, several feet in length, directly from the microphone to the amplifier. Other devices convert the electrical signal from the microphone into radio waves (FM) or invisible light waves (infrared) and send the signal to a receiver adjacent to the amplifier and worn by the individual. The receiver converts the FM or infrared signal back to an electrical signal and sends it to the amplifier to be amplified. The FM and infrared systems are frequently referred to as wireless systems because they eliminate the long wire running directly from the microphone to the amplifier. The wireless feature of these assistive listening devices makes them more versatile and easier to use, but it also makes them more expensive. These assistive listening devices overcome the primary disadvantage of the conventional hearing aid; they improve the speech-to-noise ratio. By separating the microphone from the rest of the device and positioning it closer to the sound source (e.g., the talker's mouth or the loud-speaker of the television set), the primary signal of interest is amplified more than the surrounding background noise. On a conventional hearing aid, the ear-level microphone amplifies both the speech and the surrounding noise equally well. That is, the speech-to-noise ratio is not improved; all sound at the position of the microphone is simply made louder by the conventional hearing aid. (See Vignette 7.3.)

Separating the microphone from the rest of the device, however, has its draw-backs. It is only a reasonable alternative when the sound source is fairly stable over time. If the microphone is positioned near the loudspeaker of the television, for example, the voice of a talker seated next to the impaired person will not be amplified. The impaired individual is forced to listen to the sound source closest to the microphone. For assistive listening devices, this is not a serious drawback, because they have a limited purpose.

Selection and evaluation of assistive listening devices is not as formalized as it is for hearing aids. Most clinics today have a room designated as the "assistive lis-tening device area." This room or area is set up to simulate the conditions under which the devices are to be used. Typically, the room takes on the atmosphere of a living room or family room, with television, stereo, and telephones available. After the patient's needs have been assessed through a written or oral questionnaire, sev-eral assistive devices are tried by the patient in the simulated environment under controlled conditions. If the patient finds the device beneficial, it is dispensed by the audiologist, or the patient is referred to an appropriate source for its purchase.

Assistive devices of various types also benefit the severely or profoundly impaired. In addition to those devices mentioned above, some nonauditory devices have been developed. Devices have been produced that flash lights in response to various acoustic signals occurring in the home, such as the ringing of the doorbell or the telephone. Other special telephone devices enable text to be sent over phone lines (in printed form) so that a profoundly impaired person can carry on a tele-phone conversation by sending and receiving text messages. Special keyboard-like devices are needed at both ends of the phone line to enable such communication.

Classroom Amplification

A discussion of hearing aids would not be complete without a review of the special amplification systems designed for education. Classroom amplification is a term used to describe a hearing aid device that provides amplified sound to a group of children. Classroom amplification gained added importance with the advent of Public Law 94–142, a federal mandate regarding the education of all handicapped children. The law required that schools provide hearing-impaired children with adequate services and funding. This included habilitative/rehabilitative services, such as selection and evaluation of personal hearing aids and group systems, audi-tory training, speech training, speechreading, and any other services deemed neces-sary for the child's educational development.

Hearing aid microphone at 1 meter from sound source

Hearing aid microphone at 1/2 meter from sound source

Hearing aid microphone at 1/8 meter from sound source

VIGNETTE 7.3.

Improving the speech-to-noise ratio with an assistive listening device or classroom system.

In this vignette, we will make use of the same "speech audiogram" concept used in Vignette 7.2. The *left-hand panel* below shows the speech audiogram for conversational speech with a background noise (several other people talking) as it has been amplified by a hearing aid. This is the same as the right-hand panel of Vignette 7.2. with the addition of background noise. The level of the noise is indicated by the *heavy dashed line*. The speech and noise levels shown here represent those measured through the hearing aid with the listener in the middle of a living room or classroom full of people at about 1 m from the desired talker.

In the *middle panel*, the microphone has been detached from the hearing aid and is now positioned about half a meter from the primary talker. (The hearing aid's microphone really can't be detached. We're just pretending that it is to illustrate the concept behind assistive listening devices.) According to the inverse-square law (see Chapter 2), as the distance to the sound source is halved (from 1 m to a half meter), the sound level increases by 6 dB. Notice that the speech is now 6 dB higher than it was in the *left-hand panel*, whereas the diffuse background noise (*dashed line*) coming from a variety of sources, including reflections from walls and the ceiling, remains unchanged. Thus, the speech-to-noise ratio has improved 6 dB.

In the *right-hand panel* we have positioned the microphone still closer to the sound source, about 1/8 m (4–5 inches) from the primary talker's mouth. As a result, the speech level from the talker has increased another 12 dB (two more halvings of the distance), and the speech-to-noise ratio has been improved a total of 18 dB compared with that in the *left-hand panel*.

VIGNETTE 7.3.—*continued*

As noted in Vignette 7.2, the conventional hearing aid does not improve the signal-to-noise ratio, but simply amplifies the acoustic signals, speech and noise alike, that arrive at the microphone (*left panel*). By moving the microphone closer to the desired sound source (*middle* and *right panels*), whether a talker or a loud-speaker, the speech signal level is increased while the background noise remains unaffected. The result is an improved speech-to-noise ratio and better communication. This is the primary operational principle behind many assistive listening devices, as well as similar classroom-amplification systems.

Why should a child need a special educational amplification system? A primary concern is the acoustic environment that children are exposed to in the classroom. Children are continually bombarded with excessively high noise levels that interfere with their ability to understand the teacher. These noise levels originate from sources outside the school building (aircraft, car traffic), within the school building (adjacent classrooms and hallways, activity areas, heating/cooling systems), and within the classroom itself (students talking, feet shuffling, noise from moving furniture). These various noise sources contribute to noise levels ranging from 40 to 67 dB SPL (A).[a] Such high noise levels result in an unfavorable signal-to-noise (S:N) or speech-to-noise ratio reaching the child's ear. Recall that a S:N ratio represents the difference, in decibels, between speech (from the teacher) and the overall ambient noise (within the classroom). For example, a S:N ratio of +10 dB means that the teacher's speech is 10 dB more intense than the noise in the classroom. Ideally, a S:N ratio of +20 dB is necessary if a hearing-impaired child is to understand speech maximally. Noise surveys in classrooms have shown that S:N ratios typically range from −6 dB to +6 dB, a listening environment that precludes maximal understanding even for normal-hearing children.

Classroom noise is not the only variable that contributes to a difficult listening environment. Reverberation time, a term used to denote the amount of time it takes for sound to decrease by 60 dB following the termination of a signal, also contributes to an adverse acoustic environment. When a teacher talks to the child, some of the speech signal reaches the child's amplification system within just a few milliseconds. The remainder of the signal, however, strikes surrounding areas and reaches the child's ear after the initial sound in the form of reflections. The strength and duration of these reflections are affected by the absorption quality of the surrounding surfaces

---

[a] Sound level meters have three weighting networks—A, B, and C—which are designed to respond differently to noise frequencies. The A network weighs (filters) the low frequenices and approximates the response characteristics of the human ear. The B network also filters the low frequencies, but not as much as the A network does. The C scale provides a fairly flat response. The federal government recommends the A network for measuring noise levels.

and the size (volume) of the classroom. If an area has hard walls, ceilings, and floors, the room will have a long reverberation time. In contrast, an acoustically treated room with carpeting, drapes, and an acoustic tile ceiling will have a shorter reverberation time. Generally, as reverberation time increases, the proportion of reflected speech sound reaching the listener increases and speech recognition decreases. In addition, the smaller the room size, the greater the reverberation. Many classrooms for the hearing-impaired have reverberation times ranging from a very mild value of 0.2 s to more severe reverberation, with times greater than 1 s.

These factors, noise and reverberation, are known to adversely affect speech recognition. As the noise levels and reverberation times increase, the S:N ratio becomes less favorable and there is a significant breakdown in speech understanding. Further, as the distance between the talker and listener increases, the S:N ratio worsens. Figure 7.6 illustrates this phenomenon by showing the speech-recognition scores for sentence materials in a group of normal-hearing children who listened to speech with noise levels and reverberation times similar to those in a classroom. The reverberation time is 0.46 s, and the S:N ratio at 6 feet is +6 dB. Note that speech recognition deteriorates with increasing distance. At 6 feet, speech recognition is seen to average about 90%, whereas at 24 feet, it averages 40%. Table 7.2 shows how noise and reverberation can produce a hardship for young hearing-impaired children. These data represent the unaided speech-recognition scores of hearing-impaired children in a quiet environment, and under different S:N ratios and reverberation times. It is seen that as the noise levels increase, speech recognition decreases. Further, as reverberation increases, speech recognition decreases. At a S:N ratio of +6 dB (a common listening condition in the classroom) with a reverberation time of 0.4 s, the mean recognition score is 52%; when reverberation time is 1.2 s, recognition is only 27%. It is not surprising that a hearing-impaired child will find it hard to learn under such adverse conditions.

FIGURE 7.6.
Typical speech-recognition scores for normal-hearing children at different speaker-to-listener distances. At 6 feet the signal-to-noise ratio is +6 dB and the reverberation time is 0.46 s.

TABLE 7.2.

Mean Word Recognition Scores for Hearing-Impaired Children with Hearing Aids under Various Noise and Reverberant Conditions[a]

Reverberation Time (seconds)	Signal-to-Noise Ratio (dB)			
	Quiet	*+12*	*+6*	*0*
0.0 (nonreverberant)	83	70	60	39
0.4	74	60	52	28
1.2	45	41	27	11

[a]Adapted from Finitzo-Hieber T, Tillman TW: Room acoustic effects on monosyllabic word discrimination ability for normal and hearing impaired children. *Journal of Speech and Hearing Research* 21: 440–448, 1978.

Several types of special educational amplification systems have been designed to overcome the adverse effects of the classroom environment by offering a better S:N ratio. These system types include hard-wire systems, FM wireless systems, infrared systems, and a system that combines the FM wireless system with a personal hearing aid. The concept behind these systems is similar to that described for the assistive listening devices. The microphone is moved closer to the desired sound source, the teacher. A brief description of each of these systems follows.

Hard-Wire System. In this system, a microphone worn by the teacher is wired to an amplifier. Each student then wears headphones or insert-type receivers that are connected to the amplifier by wires, so that the teacher and the students are, in effect, "tethered" together (Fig. 7.7 *top*). The primary advantage of a hard-wire system is the high fidelity and high level of output available through earphones. These systems are inexpensive and are simple and easy to operate. The obvious disadvantage is the restricted mobility of both the teacher and students.

FM Wireless Systems. About 75% of all classrooms for the hearing-impaired use either FM devices or a combination of an FM system and a personal hearing aid. A microphone transmitter is worn around the teacher's neck, and a signal is broadcast to an FM receiver worn by the child (Fig. 7.7 *bottom*). Most FM receivers have an environmental microphone so that the child can monitor his or her own voice, the voices of his or her peers, and other environmental sounds. When the environmental microphone is used, however, the S:N ratio is compromised because of the distance between the talker and the microphone. The advantage to this system is the mobility allowed. In other words, the teacher and the students are free to move around the room and the students will continue to receive amplification.

Infrared Systems. Infrared group amplification is seldom used in classroom settings but is used widely as an assistive device in theaters, churches, and other public facilities. As mentioned earlier, the system employs an infrared emitter that transmits the speech signal from the input microphone to individually worn infrared-receiver/audio-amplifier units. It is very similar in design to the FM system shown in Figure 7.7 (*bottom*), except that infrared light waves are used to send the signal

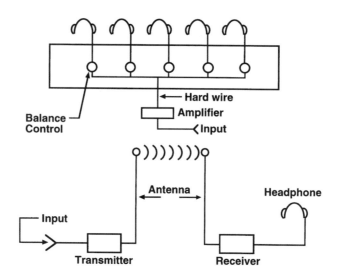

FIGURE 7.7.

Two classroom amplification systems. *Top,* Hard-wire. *Bottom,* FM. The personal hearing aid could replace the headphones shown at bottom to produce a dovetailed system.

from the transmitter to the receiver rather than FM radio waves. Infrared systems, however, are somewhat limited in power output.

Combining the FM Wireless System with the Personal Hearing Aid. A number of attempts have been made to combine the personal hearing aid with the FM system. This approach, commonly referred to as dovetailing, is done to take advantage of the benefits of both systems: the improved speech-to-noise ratio offered by the FM system and the custom fitting of the personal hearing aid. A commonly accepted method for combining the FM system with the personal hearing aid is the use of an electrical connection from the student-worn receiver to the child's hearing aid amplifier. Most modern-day BTE aids can be designed to accept an electrical plug from the student's FM receiver unit. This combined system can use FM input alone, FM input plus the signal from the microphone of the personal hearing aid, and input from the microphone of the personal hearing aid alone.

Advances in micro-miniature FM technology have resulted in the development of a BTE FM device. The BTE system houses, at ear level, both the FM receiver and the hearing aid circuitry, thus eliminating the need for cords, neckloops, and body-worn receivers. The BTE FM device looks like a conventional BTE hearing aid.

Cochlear Implants

A relatively recent clinical development was the emergence in the 1980s of the cochlear implant as a viable alternative to conventional amplification for individuals with profound hearing impairment. Several types of cochlear implants are available commercially today. They all share a common conceptual framework but differ in its implementation. The cochlear implant is a device that is surgically implanted, with its stimulating electrodes (wires) inserted directly into the cochlea. The implant contains from 1 to 22 electrodes. The electrodes are used to stimulate the auditory nerve directly with electric current, bypassing the damaged cochlear structures. As in the conventional hearing aid, a microphone is used to convert the acoustic signal into an electrical one. The electrical signal is then amplified and processed in various ways in a separate, body-worn component known as the stimulator. The stimulator is about the size of a body-worn hearing aid or a package of cigarettes. The output of the stimulator is then sent to an electromagnetic receiver worn behind the ear. This external receiver generates a magnetic field which, in turn, activates a similar internal receiver implanted surgically just under the skin and behind the ear. The implanted internal receiver converts the magnetic signal into an electrical one and directs it to the electrode(s) penetrating the cochlea. This electrical signal, when routed to the electrode(s), stimulates the remaining healthy auditory nerve fibers of the damaged inner ear. Figure 7.8 illustrates a typical arrangement for a single-electrode cochlear implant and compares this device with a conventional hearing aid. As can be seen, many features are shared by these two devices.

Many contemporary cochlear implants, however, are multiple-channel and multiple-electrode devices. The "channels" essentially refer to adjacent bands in the frequency domain analogous to a series of band-pass filters. The sound picked up by the microphone is analyzed and sorted into several frequency-specific packets of information, or channels of information, by the processor. The output of each channel is then routed to a corresponding electrode that is positioned in a specific location along the length of the cochlea. Thus, low-frequency channels are connected to electrodes in the more apical region of the cochlea, whereas high-frequency channels are connected to electrodes in more basal locations. This system is an attempt to restore tonotopic mapping (see Chapter 3) to the damaged cochlea.

At present, the ideal candidates for cochlear implants are persons who acquired profound bilateral sensorineural hearing loss after acquiring language. Although the results of clinical trials with these devices have varied markedly between patients, the best performance appears to be achieved with the multi-electrode devices. There are examples of so-called "star" patients who perform remarkably well with the device by itself; however, most people fitted thus far appear to derive the greatest benefit from the device when it is used as an aid to speechreading. Its primary usefulness as an aid to speechreading appears to lie in making gross cues of timing and voicing available to the patient. At a minimum, cochlear implants appear to provide an awareness of sound to the once-silent world of the deafened patient. At its present stage of development, however, the cochlear implant is an alternative for only a very small percentage of the hearing-impaired population: those without usable residual hearing sensitivity.

Vibrotactile Devices

Many profoundly hearing-impaired persons can receive little or no meaningful information through the ear. This is true whether the ear is stimulated with an

A CONVENTIONAL HEARING AID

B COCHLEAR IMPLANT

FIGURE 7.8.
Illustration of the similarities between A, conventional behind-the-ear hearing aid and B, cochlear implant device. The components of each system are numbered identically to highlight the similarities.

acoustic signal in the case of the conventional hearing aid or an electrical one in the case of the cochlear implant. Often this results in the use of alternative means of communication using normally functioning senses. Manual communication, or sign language, takes advantage of the normal sight of most of the hearing-impaired population, including those with profound impairments. Adoption of manual communication as a primary means of communicating, however, restricts one to communicating with the small percentage of the population able to converse in sign language. Other senses have also been explored for use as alternative means of encoding the acoustic signal. Tactual (touch) stimulation is used by various vibrotactile devices as an alternative to auditory stimulation. A microphone again converts the acoustic signal to an electrical one, as in the hearing aid and cochlear implant. This electrical signal is used by the vibrotactile device to activate a series of vibrators. The vibrators, when activated by the electrical signal, make contact with the skin and stimulate the patient's sense of touch. The most common clinical vibrotactile devices are single-channel instruments. They stimulate the skin at a constant rate or frequency and increase the amplitude of vibration as the intensity of the acoustic signal increases. The vibrators for most clinical devices are worn on the hand, wrist, arm, or thigh. Multichannel devices, which attempt to mimic the auditory system's tonotopic organization (see Chapter 3) by routing sounds of different frequencies to vibrators at separate locations on the skin (along the length of the wrist or the length of the waist, for example) have been developed and are undergoing clinical evaluation. Generally, however, vibrotactile devices are primarily used as aids to speechreading.

Device Management

The prosthetic device, whether a hearing aid, FM classroom device, cochlear implant, or vibrotactile aid, is one of the most important aspects of rehabilitation for the majority of hearing-impaired individuals. It is essential that every precaution be taken to assure that the device is always in good working order.

For the vast majority of hearing-impaired individuals, the conventional electroacoustic hearing aid is the prosthetic device of choice. Care must be taken to avoid dropping the instrument or exposing the aid to severe environmental conditions, such as excessive moisture or heat. If dampness reaches the microphone or receiver, it can render the unit inoperable. It is also important to check the earmold or canal portion of the device periodically for blockage by cerumen and signs of wear from extended use, such as a cracked earmold or tubing. Perhaps the most common problem that interferes with adequate hearing aid performance is the battery or battery compartment area. Old batteries that have lost their charge, inappropriate battery size, inadequate battery contact, and improper battery placement are all problems that can contribute to a nonworking hearing aid.

Consistent amplification for the young child with hearing impairment is essential. Yet numerous school surveys have revealed that about one-half of children's hearing aids do not perform satisfactorily. The most common problems seen among hearing-impaired children are weak batteries, inadequate earmolds, broken cords, bad receivers (sometimes the wrong receiver), and high distortion levels. Even the FM-wireless systems are susceptible to faulty performance. About 30–50% of these systems have been reported to perform unsatisfactorily in the classroom setting. The solution to inconsistent and inadequate amplification is the implementation of a daily hearing-aid check using a form like the one shown in Vignette 7.4. In addition, the school audiologist must conduct a periodic electroacoustic analysis of every child's hearing aid.

REHABILITATION OF THE CHILD WITH HEARING IMPAIRMENT

Management of the child with hearing impairment is a monumental challenge to the clinical audiologist. In learning to understand the spoken language of others and to speak it, there is no adequate substitute for an intact auditory system. Without normal or near-normal hearing, it is extremely difficult to acquire an adequate communication system. Because so much of the language-learning process occurs within the first few years of life, there has been considerable emphasis on early identification and intervention for young hearing-impaired children. The various approaches to early identification were outlined in Chapter 6 and will not be restated here. Suffice it to say that it is generally believed that the earlier one can identify the hearing loss, preferably during the first year of life, the sooner intervention can begin and the better the chances for a favorable outcome. Generally speaking, hearing-impaired children who exhibit the best spoken language and show the most satisfactory progress in school are those who have had the benefit of early identification and intervention. Early intervention is essential to the successful development of speech and language. The intervention must include adequate parent-infant management, wearable amplification, speech and language training, and development of perceptual and cognitive skills.

Choosing the Appropriate Communication Mode

An important issue facing audiologists, teachers, and school officials is determining which educational approach is most appropriate for a given hearing-impaired child. Presently, two primary modes of instruction are recommended in the educational system: auditory-oral communication and total communication. The auditory-oral approach places emphasis entirely on the auditory system for developing receptive and expressive forms of communication, whereas total communication emphasizes a combination of audition, vision, finger spelling, and signs for achieving the same goal. These approaches will be discussed in greater detail in Chapter 8. Although most would agree that oral language maximizes the options available to the child, the reality is that not all children are able to learn spoken English. Even in total communication programs, decisions are sometimes made

Vignette 7.4.

Sample monitoring form for a personal hearing aid worn by a hearing-impaired child.

Student_____

Teacher_____ Aid make/model_____

School_____ Serial no. _____

Classroom_____

Electroacoustic check   ___Y ___N

Date of inspection_____

Overall condition: ___Satisfactory ___Marginal ___Unsatisfactory ___Missing

Recommendations_____

_____

_____

Examiner_____

Problem Checklist

Item	Inspected?: Yes	No	Comments
Battery	___	___	_____
Battery compartment	___	___	_____
Microphone	___	___	_____
Power switch	___	___	_____
Gain control	___	___	_____
Telephone switch	___	___	_____
Tone control	___	___	_____
Amplifier	___	___	_____
Cord	___	___	_____
Receiver	___	___	_____
Earmold	___	___	_____
Clip/case	___	___	_____
Harness	___	___	_____
Other	___	___	_____

As-worn setting:

    Volume control_____

    Tone control_____

    Receiver type_____

about whether to emphasize oral language or manual communication. How then does one determine which mode of communication is most beneficial?

Two approaches have been proposed for audiologists who must determine whether a hearing-impaired child would be better off in an auditory-oral or a total-communication program of instruction. One is the Deafness Management Quotient (DMQ). The DMQ uses a weighted point system (total of 100 points) to quantify a number of factors about the child and the child's environment. These factors include the amount of residual hearing (30 points), central auditory system intactness (30 points), intellectual factors (20 points), family constellation (10 points), and socioeconomic issues (10 points). A child scoring greater than 80 points would be recommended for an auditory-oral program. Unfortunately, it is very difficult to quantify objectively the recommended factors, and more importantly, the DMQ has not been adequately validated. An alternative index, known as the Spoken Language Predictor (SLP), was proposed and validated. Similar to the DMQ, the SLP incorporates five factors considered important to a child's success in an auditory-oral program. The factors are weighted, and a point score (total of 100 points) is derived. The factors include hearing capacity (30 points), language competence (25 points), nonverbal intelligence (20 points), family support (15 points), and speech-communication attitude (10 points). Children with scores of 80–100 are judged to have excellent potential for developing spoken language. Not only can the SLP be of use in deciding on placement, but it can also verify the appropriateness of placement for an older child already enrolled in a program.

Let us now review some of the appropriate management strategies for hearing-impaired children. The approaches to be discussed can accommodate either an auditory-oral or a total communication emphasis.

Parent-Infant Management

It is recognized that the first 3 years of life are critical to the child's general development, especially with respect to communication. It is also recognized that the parents of young handicapped children often lack the skills necessary to optimize family-infant interactions, which could facilitate the child's communication development. Awareness of this situation has led to parent-infant intervention programs. In addition to espousing early identification and intervention, most parent-oriented programs include family support for parents and members of the child's extended family. Information sharing or exchange, demonstration teaching (in which the family explores a variety of strategies to assist the child in achieving communication), and educational advocacy for the parents are also frequently included. The latter entails helping the parents to become effective consumers of services and knowledgeable child advocates.

An important component of a parent-infant curriculum is audiologic management and amplification. Here the emphasis is on helping the child to develop his or her auditory potential. Emphasis is placed on further clarification of the nature of the hearing loss, selection of amplification, and the development of full-time hearing aid use. Teaching parents the importance of care and maintenance of hearing aids is also an important dimension. Another element of effective parent-infant management is auditory training—that is, an organized sequential approach to the development of listening skills. Here the emphasis is on developing a program of auditory training experiences that will guide the parents through a developmental sequence for their child that parallels the development of auditory perceptual skills in the normal-hearing infant. The hierarchy of skills can be divided into the following levels:

1. Auditory perception of both environmental sounds and the human voice
2. Awareness of environmental sounds and the human voice as conveyors of information and association of sounds with their physical sources
3. Development of an auditory-vocal feedback mechanism in which the child monitors his or her own speech
4. Comprehension of meaning in syllables, words, phrases, and sentences
5. Increasing verbal comprehension and the emergence of auditory memory and sequencing skills

Another important component of parent-infant management is vocal play strategies for speech habilitation. The initiation and maintenance of vocal behavior is a major area of the early-intervention program that is critical to young children. Full-time use of amplification is important so that the hearing-impaired child can hear his or her own speech as well as the speech of others. The use of an auditory program to enhance the use of the auditory feedback mechanism is also important. Further, parents are taught to use vocal play interaction techniques that are necessary for the development of prelinguistic speech skills. Parents must also learn to develop strategies that facilitate social and communicative turn-taking.

Finally, there are the verbal interaction techniques of language programming. At this point the focus is on teaching the parent communicative interaction styles, particularly verbal interaction patterns, that enhance the child's acquisition of language. Linguistic development is maximized by training parents to incorporate those principles of adult-child interaction patterns that are reported to occur during the language acquisition of normal children.

Amplification

The importance of amplification to the hearing-impaired child cannot be overemphasized. The personal hearing aid and other amplification devices are the primary link many of these children have to an auditory society. If these children are to develop speech and language in a manner somewhat similar to that of the normal-hearing child, everything possible must be done to capitalize on whatever residual hearing exists. Toward this end, the child receives amplification (usually binaural) soon after identification. The audiologist then offers periodic hearing evaluations and modifies the hearing aid fitting(s) as more is learned about the child's hearing sensitivity.

Language: Characteristics, Assessment, and Training

Language may be defined as a set of systematic rules used to designate experience and facilitate social interaction. It is the primary means by which humans communicate with one another. Although a comprehensive review of language is beyond the scope of this book, a general knowledge of the dimensions of language is important to the understanding of management issues. Most would agree that there are three components of language: form, content, and use. The form of language is simply the pattern of sounds, syllables, words, and sentences that are used to express thoughts and ideas. For example, the endings /t/ and /d/ in "talk*ed*" and "pray*ed*" both express past tense, yet the phonetic forms of the past-tense morphemes (a morpheme is the smallest grammatical unit of language) are quite different (/t/ vs. /d/). To learn language, children must be able to identify and process such subtle nuances. Form can be further categorized into phonology, morphology, and syntax. Phonology is the sound system of a given language. Morphology is concerned with the structure of words (i.e., past tense, plurals, possessives). Syntax addresses the relationship of words with larger units of language, such as phrases, clauses, and sentences. The second aspect of language is content, or what is being communicated. This is often referred to as the semantic level of language. The content is concerned with the knowledge of objects, the knowledge of relationships between or among objects, and the knowledge of relationships among other things. The final component of language is use, which is how one communicates. This has been referred to as pragmatics. It is learning to transmit information appropriately and intentionally. It is achieving a goal by communicating. For example, a child can point to a cookie and say "more," indicating communicative intent. Hence, the pragmatic component of language is present in the absence of syntax. The development of language is a complex interaction that occurs among these three components of language: form, content, and use.

Given what we have discussed about language, it is not surprising to learn that children with hearing loss experience great difficulty in learning language through speech. This difficulty increases with increasing hearing loss. Most research dealing with the language characteristics of hearing-impaired children has focused on the "form" component, primarily because errors in form (phonemes, morphemes, and syntax) are easier to quantify. Studies have shown that hearing-impaired children with high-frequency hearing losses experience difficulty with morphologic markers, such as plurals and possessives. In addition, it is well recognized that hearing-impaired children have trouble learning vocabulary, acquiring words that express relationships between other words, and learning syntactic structures.

Many commercially available instruments are designed to assist the clinician in the ongoing evaluation of a child's language development. These evaluative approaches explore a wide range of language skills but, for the most part, do not cover some of the experiences encountered in day-to-day situations. Hence, clinicians always need to develop informal nonstandardized tasks to obtain information in areas not covered by the standard diagnostic tools.

A number of approaches have been used in language intervention, most of which have focused on the syntactic forms of language. These approaches can be classified as analytic or natural methods for teaching language. Analytic methods have concentrated on the form of a child's language, and most techniques categorize the various parts of speech grammatically. These approaches are also characterized by extensive drills and exercises. An example of the analytical method is the Fitzgerald key, which emphasizes the analysis of relationships among discrete units through the visual aid of written language. Students classify words from a sentence as to whether they belong in a "who," "what," or "where" category. The natural approach, sometimes referred to as the experiential method, holds that language is learned through experiences, not systematic drills and exercises. This content/unit approach emphasizes identifying areas of interest for the child, which then serve as the basis for teaching vocabulary and practicing spoken and written language.

More recently, language-intervention approaches have begun to consider modern language theory and to develop strategies that attempt to integrate syntactic, pragmatic, and semantic levels. The reader interested in learning more about language intervention techniques with the hearing-impaired can consult the suggested readings at the end of this chapter.

Speech Production: Characteristics, Assessment, and Training

We noted earlier that significant hearing losses make it difficult not only to understand speech but also to produce speech. Nevertheless, it is the general consensus that many hearing-impaired children, even those with profound losses, can develop speech skills. Hearing-impaired children manifest a variety of speech production errors categorized as either segmental (i.e., phonemic) or suprasegmental (i.e., related to intonation and prosody). The most common segmental errors include the omission of word-final sounds and substitution errors for both consonants and vowels. Suprasegmental errors include inadequate timing, which results in very slow, labored speech, and poor control of the fundamental frequency, causing abnormal pitch and distorted intonation. Predictably, as the frequency of errors increases, overall intelligibility decreases.

Assessment of speech production is not as easy as one might predict, since many of the tools were designed for normal-hearing children. The evaluation of segmental errors is usually conducted with commonly available picture identification tests. Since most of these tests do not consider many of the unavoidable problems of testing the hearing-impaired, it is not unusual for the clinician to develop informal tests that will focus on specific segmental errors frequently seen among the hearing-impaired population. Assessment of intelligibility of speech is also important for the planning of an intervention program. Some clinicians record spontaneous speech samples, which are then judged by a group of listeners to evaluate a child's intelligibility.

Perhaps the most popular method for teaching speech to the hearing-impaired child is an approach advocated by Daniel Ling. Very briefly, this method focuses on using the child's residual hearing to monitor speech production, as well as to understand the speech of others. The approach to speech acquisition attempts to dupli-cate the process that normal-hearing children experience. The teaching of speech is carried out primarily at the phonetic and phonologic levels, with emphasis on the phonetic domain. At the phonetic level, there is emphasis on nonsense syllable drills (i.e., /ta, ta, ta/, or /ti, ta, to/). Several stages are proposed in which target behaviors are established using criterion-referenced skills. A child must complete each phase satisfactorily before moving on to the next level. These stages include undifferenti-ated vocalizations; suprasegmental voice patterns; a range of distinctly different vowel sounds; consonants contrasted in manner of production; consonants con-trasted in manner and place of production; consonants contrasted in manner, place, and voicing; and consonant blends. The following additional strategies have been suggested to supplement the Ling approach.

1. Production by imitation—the child produces the target sound using auditory clues only
2. Production on demand—the child produces the target sound from visual cues
3. Discrimination—the child selects the speech pattern from a closed set of alterna-tive speech patterns
4. Self-evaluation—the child evaluates his or her own speech production

REHABILITATION OF THE HEARING-IMPAIRED ADULT

The rehabilitation techniques employed with the hearing-impaired adult are quite different from the approaches used with children. There are similarities, how-ever. The individual must receive a careful assessment to determine the nature and extent of the problem; amplification plays a major role in the rehabilitation process; and the techniques and strategies used in rehabilitation are determined by the infor-mation elicited in the assessment phase.

Assessment Issues

In the introduction to this chapter, we talked about the importance of the assessment phase and how it is used to establish a rehabilitative program. The assessment phase typically consists of a comprehensive case history, pure-tone audiometry, immittance measurements, speech-recognition tests, a communication-specific self-assessment questionnaire, and, occasionally, a measure of speechread-ing ability. Because we have already reviewed in some detail the basic assessment battery (case history, pure-tone audiometry, immittance measurements, and speech recognition), we will focus here on questionnaires and speechreading skills in the planning of rehabilitation programs.

Assessment with Communication Scales

Communication scales need to be a part of every assessment approach. These scales usually assess how the hearing impairment affects everyday living—that is, the way in which the hearing deficit affects psychosocial, emotional, or vocational performance. Such information can be of value in determining the need for and probable success of amplification, irrespective of the degree of hearing loss and the specific areas in which the rehabilitation should occur. Most scales have focused on communication-specific skills. Examples of questions that could be included in such a scale are: "Do you have difficulty hearing when someone speaks in a whisper?" and "Does a hearing problem cause you difficulty when listening to TV or radio?"

The answers to such questions illuminate listening problems. Once the areas of difficulty have been identified, possible solutions can be considered. For example, if the individual reports difficulty only when listening to a television or radio, an assistive listening device might be considered. If, on the other hand, a patient reports difficulty in a variety of listening situations and notes a tendency to withdraw from social activities because of the hearing loss, the individual would be a good candidate for a personal hearing aid. Counseling for this patient and the patient's relatives might also be indicated. Furthermore, the audiologist may wish to develop techniques for improving speechreading and auditory training skills in situations that present listening difficulty. Numerous communication scales are available to the audiologist, and it is not possible to review all of them in an introductory book. Two commonly employed scales are the Hearing Handicap Scale (HHS) and the Hearing Performance Inventory (HPI). The HHS was designed to measure objectively the impact of hearing loss on an individual's independent living skills. There are two forms, each containing 20 items, and the test requires no more than 5 minutes to administer. Examples of typical questions are: "Can you understand if someone speaks to you in a whisper and you cannot see his face?" and "Do you hear all right when you are in a streetcar, airplane, bus, or train?" The response format to the various questions is:

Almost always
Usually
Sometimes
Rarely
Almost never

The HPI is a more comprehensive scale than the HHS and probes hearing-impaired patients across several dimensions rather than only one. These dimensions include speech comprehension, signal intensity, response to auditory failure, social effects of hearing loss, personal effects of hearing loss, and occupational difficulties. Examples of items on the HPI are: "You are home reading in a quiet room. Do you hear the telephone ring when it is in another room?" and "At the beginning of a conversation, do you let a stranger know that you have a hearing problem?" In this inventory, the patient is queried about a specific listening environment and responds to each item with "practically always," "frequently," "about half the time," "occasionally," or "almost never." The original version of the HPI was quite long, taking about 60 minutes to administer and score. A shortened version (about 35 minutes) is also available. The HPI affords valuable information regarding the impact of hearing loss on communication and identifies the general listening situations in which the patient experiences trouble. It is also useful as a formal performance measure that can be used at the initial assessment and to track progress during rehabilitation.

Assessment of Speechreading Skills

The ability to use vision as an aid to understanding spoken English is another important area of assessment. Several tests are available for assessing a patient's speechreading or lipreading skills. One such test is the Denver Quick Test of Lipreading Ability, a group of 20 short, simple statements (Table 7.3). The test is scored in terms of percentage correct, with each test item representing 5%. The test can be used to assess speechreading abilities in a vision-only mode as well as in a combination mode of both vision and hearing. Performance in the vision-only mode can offer valuable diagnostic information. A low score on the Denver Test would suggest that the patient needs speechreading instruction—that is, instruction in paying attention to visual cues for the purpose of complementing auditory input. The use of both modes offers insight into how the patient will perform under realistic conditions and should also be helpful in determining how well the individual will perform with amplification.

TABLE 7.3.
Examples of Items on the Denver Quick Test of Lipreading Ability[a]

1. Good morning.
2. How old are you?
3. I live in (state of residence).
4. I only have one dollar.
5. There is somebody at the door.
6. Is that all?
7. Where are you going?
8. Let's have a coffee break.
9. Park your car in the lot.
10. What is your address?
11. May I help you?
12. I feel fine.
13. It is time for dinner.
14. Turn right at the corner.
15. Are you ready to order?
16. Is this charge or cash?
17. What time is it?
18. I have a headache.
19. How about going out tonight?
20. Please lend me 50 cents.

[a]From Alpiner JG, Schow RL: Rehabilitative evaluation of hearing-impaired adult. *In* Alpiner JG, McCarthy PA (eds): *Rehabilitative Audiology: Children and Adults,* ed 2. Baltimore, Williams & Wilkins, 1993.

Management Strategies with the Hearing-Impaired Adult

Importance of Counseling

Counseling should be a central focus of any management strategy for the hearing-impaired adult. In fact, the hearing-impaired adult should receive counseling both before and after the provision of a hearing aid. Counseling is a vital part of the assessment phase, since it is during this phase that information about the patient's communication problems is determined. The first component of the counseling process is to explain to the patient, in lay terms, the nature and extent of the hearing loss. If the audiologist believes that the patient can benefit from amplification, counseling is needed to discuss with the patient the value of a hearing aid and what can be expected from it. Possible modification of the patient's motivation and attitudes may also be appropriate at this juncture. The audiologist will have information from the assessment data on the patient's feelings about wearing a hearing aid. Often the patient has no real interest in a hearing aid but is simply responding to the will of a spouse or "significant other." Others have received misleading information about hearing aids from friends or from advertisements. Some patients are concerned about whether the hearing aid will show because of the stigma commonly associated with deafness in the United States. (See Vignette 7.5.) Under such circumstances, the objective of the audiologist is to help the hearing-impaired individual realize that many of the fears or concerns about hearing loss or hearing aids are unwarranted. The individual should be counseled that the use of amplification can help in a variety of listening situations. Counseling is also sometimes appropriate for relatives and friends who have developed erroneous impressions about hearing loss and amplification. For example, a patient with a high-frequency sensorineural hearing loss will typically experience difficulty in understanding speech. Relatives and friends sometimes interpret this difficulty as a sign of senility, inattention, or even stupidity. It is helpful for the audiologist to counsel relatives and friends about the nature and extent of hearing loss as well as the psychosocial complications associated with a hearing deficit. Reviewing such information with loved ones helps them to understand better and to be more tolerant of the listening difficulties caused by a significant hearing impairment. The audiologist may also choose to offer suggestions for enhancing communication. The significant other can be counseled in the use of deliberate, unhurried speech, good illumination of the speaker's face, and care to ensure that the lips are clearly visible.

Once the hearing aid has been purchased, or just prior to a purchase, the patient is counseled about the use and care of a hearing aid. The audiologist reviews the manipulation of the various controls, the function of the battery compartment, the trouble-shooting techniques in cases of malfunction, the proper care of the earmold or shell, and the warranty of the hearing aid. A potential difficulty is that patients often have unrealistic expectations for a hearing aid, especially in the initial stages of use. The audiologist must take care to advise the hearing-impaired patient about the limitations of amplification and to help the individual adjust to very difficult listening situations, such as competing speech or the presence of a competing background noise. Finally, some patients will need special help in the

VIGNETTE 7.5.

"The hearing aid effect."

Examine the two top pictures. How would you rate the person on the left on a continuum from bright-to-dull or from smart-to-dumb or from pretty-to-ugly? How about the person on the right at the top?

Now, examine the two pictures below. How would you rate these two individuals on the same continua listed above?

Notice that the two people pictured in the top set of "photographs" are the same as the two in the bottom set, but the one wearing the hearing aid has changed. When researchers have had large groups of subjects rate their impressions of real photographs similar to these drawings along continua similar to those listed above and have counterbalanced the design so that each person is pictured wearing a hearing aid by the conclusion of the testing, the results indicate that the presence of a hearing aid on the individual in the photo leads to lower ratings on many continua. This negative image associated with the wearing of a hearing aid is called "the hearing aid effect." It has been documented in adults and children alike and is part of the stigma hearing aid wearers must overcome.

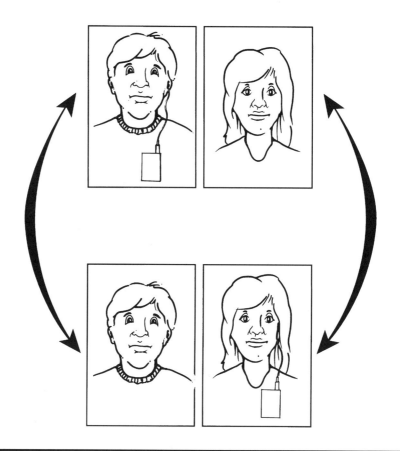

manipulation of hearing aid controls. This is a common problem among the elderly and will be discussed in more detail later in this chapter.

Throughout the entire rehabilitation cycle, counseling is seen as a continuing process. The audiologist spends time listening, advising, and reacting to the needs and concerns of the hearing-impaired individual.

Instruction for Speechreading and Auditory Training

The two primary training aspects of aural rehabilitation for the adult are speechreading and auditory training. Speechreading refers to the ability of a person, any person, to use vision as a supplement to audition when communicating. All persons, regardless of the degree of impairment, can benefit from visual cues. At one time, speechreading was referred to simply as "lipreading." The change in label to "speechreading" has come about in recognition of the fact that more than just the talker's lips provide important visual cues to understanding speech.

Speechreading should be viewed not as a replacement for auditory coding of speech, but as an important supplement. Using visual information alone, about 50–60% of a "spoken" message can typically be understood by the average person. However, individuals vary widely in this ability.

Acquisition of speechreading skills can take hours of training. There are two basic approaches to speechreading training: analytic and synthetic. Analytic methods begin with training on individual speech sounds and progress to words, phrases, sentences, and continuous discourse, in sequence. The synthetic approach begins training at the phrase or sentence level. The synthetic approach appears to be the one more widely used by audiologists. Training usually begins with simple, commonly encountered questions such as, "What is your name?" or "What time is it?" It then progresses to less frequently encountered statements and continuous discourse.

Auditory training refers to training the hearing-impaired individual to use his or her hearing as well as possible. The approaches pursued vary with the onset of the hearing loss. Typically, a hierarchy of skills is developed at the phoneme and word level, beginning with detection of the sound or word (can the patient hear anything when the sound is spoken?). The next goal is discrimination of the targeted sound or word (is it the same or different from some other sounds or words?), followed by the development of skills in the identification of the sound or word (which one of several words or sounds was it?). The final goal is often to develop proficiency in the open-set recognition of the speech sound or word (what sound or word was it?). Auditory training is encouraged for all individuals wearing a hearing aid for the first time. It takes time and training to learn to understand speech with a hearing aid. Many hearing-impaired individuals have never heard speech or have heard it through the distortion of the hearing loss—in many cases, for a period of several years—before seeking assistance. Fitting the hearing aid or other rehabilitative device will not bring about an instant restoration of normal function. Recent research indicates, for instance, that at least 3–6 months may be required for many hearing aid wearers to attain maximum levels of speech-communication performance with their hearing aids. In fact, many patients will probably never perform *completely* as well as a normal-hearing person does. With continued training, however, they can come much closer to achieving this objective. Auditory training is designed to maximize the use of residual hearing, whereas speechreading is meant to supplement the reduced information received through the auditory system. Extensive training in both areas can result in very effective use of the rehabilitative device chosen for the patient.

Listening Training, Speech Conservation, and Speech Tracking

Another role of the audiologist is to help the hearing-impaired patient develop or maintain good listening skills and to assist the patient in maintaining good speech production skills. Listening training refers to helping the patient to attend better to the spoken message. Some people simply have poor listening skills, and this problem is exacerbated in the presence of a hearing loss. The emphasis in listening training is on teaching the impaired listener to be alert, attentive, and ready to receive the spoken message. Training should focus on eliminating or avoiding distractions, learning to focus on the speaker's main points, attending to nonverbal information, keeping visual contact with the speaker, and mentally preparing oneself to listen to the speaker.

As hearing loss increases, it becomes more difficult for an individual to monitor his or her own speech production. This inability results in faulty speech characterized by poor vocal quality, nasality, segmental errors, and suprasegmental errors. Under such conditions, learning the effective use of kinesthetic (sensation of movement) cues is essential for creating an awareness of the segmental elements of speech. The patient must become physically aware of the kinesthetic qualities of each phonetic element in speech. Auditory training and speechreading can also help in preserving the perception of subtle nuances in the speech message. Techniques for developing an awareness of the rhythm, quality, intonation, and loudness of one's own speech are needed by the hearing-impaired. Finally, the importance of listening is critical to this population, and the enhancement of listening skills should be part of any speech conservation program.

Speech tracking refers to a procedure in which connected speech is presented by a reader, and a listener repeats the message, word-for-word or syllable-for-syllable. Both the speaker and the listener participate in the procedure, with the impaired listener attempting to immediately imitate the speaker. The technique has great face validity since the material approximates normal communication more closely than single words do. Tracking ability is measured in terms of the number of words tracked per minute. Rate of speech tracking improves with rehabilitative training (speechreading and/or auditory training) and with the use of amplification or alternative rehabilitation devices. Speech tracking can be used as a tool in aural rehabilitation, especially for measuring the effects of rehabilitation or training.

Special Considerations for the Hearing-Impaired Elderly

We have noted on several occasions throughout this text that a large number of elderly people exhibit significant hearing impairments. Typically, the hearing impairment in the aged is a mild-to-moderate, bilateral, high-frequency sensorineural hearing loss with associated difficulty in understanding conversational speech (see Chapter 5). The loss usually begins around 50 years of age and progresses with each succeeding decade. In addition, speech understanding difficulties become greater when the listening task is made more difficult. Such hearing loss adversely affects both the functional health status and the psychosocial well-being of the impaired individual. It is generally thought that hearing loss can produce withdrawal, poor self-concept, depression, frustration, irritability, senility, isolation, and loneliness.

Despite the high prevalence of hearing loss among the elderly and the accepted psychosocial complications, the hearing-impaired elderly are not usually referred for audiologic intervention. Frequently, they are not considered candidates for amplification until they reach advanced old age. The reasons for this are not clear. Some elderly persons believe that their deafness is simply another unavoidable aspect of the aging process. This feeling lessens the person's felt need to seek rehabilitation, or the ability to justify it. This belief, combined with an inadequate knowledge and low expectations of rehabilitative measures, appears to discourage these individuals from seeking assistance. Even those who do seek assistance often fail to use their hearing aids to the fullest. In fact, some stop using their amplification systems soon after purchase.

The special problems of the hearing-impaired elderly require that the audiologist educate physicians and laypersons about the benefits of hearing aids. It is also important that audiologists recognize the special needs of this population. For example, during the assessment phase, one must determine whether there are any limitations in upper body movement or if arthritis exists. These conditions can interfere with an individual's ability to reach, grasp, or manipulate a hearing aid. Such information is most helpful in deciding on the type of hearing aid to be recommended. For example, a small ITC hearing aid with micro controls would be inappropriate for an individual who has arthritis affecting the hands and arms. (See Vignette 7.6.) Another important consideration in the assessment phase is the visual acuity of the patient. Like hearing, vision declines with increasing age. Since visual acuity is important for receiving auditory-visual information, it is prudent for the audiologist to assess the visual abilities of an elderly patient. This can be done simply by posing questions to the hearing-impaired person about visual status. Examples of such questions might include:

1. Do you have problems with your vision? If so, what kind?
2. Do you wear eyeglasses? Do they help you to see?
3. Are you able to see my mouth clearly?

Some audiologists actually test for far-visual acuity using the well-known Snellen eye chart.

A check of mental status is also appropriate for the elderly population. Many elderly individuals exhibit declines in cognitive function that would reduce the likelihood of successful use of a hearing aid. Formal tests are available to assess mental status. In lieu of these, however, the audiologist can simply pose questions that will offer information about the patient's cognitive functioning (i.e., memory, general knowledge, orientation). If there are problems with mental status, the audiologist

VIGNETTE 7.6.
Remote controls for hearing aids.

One alternative to overcome manual dexterity and vision difficulties experienced by many elderly persons while using hearing aids is the remote control. The hearing aid remote control is a hand-held device not unlike the remote controls used with many modern-day televisions, videocassette recorders (VCRs), or stereo systems. The remote control communicates with the hearing aid and adjusts its settings via infrared transmission. An example of one type of remote control is shown in the drawing below. Their larger size makes it easier both to manipulate and to see than the corresponding controls on a BTE or ITE hearing aid. The remote controls can include on/off switches, volume controls for one or two hearing aids, and, for multiple-memory programmable hearing aids, a memory selector (much like the channel selector on a TV remote control), which lets the wearer choose the set of hearing aid settings he or she wishes to listen through.

will need to work closely with a significant other to assure appropriate use and care of the hearing aid.

Other factors that need to be considered before amplification is recommended to an elderly person include motivation, family support, financial resources, and life style. Special attention is also important for the elderly during the hearing aid orientation program. Greater care is required to explain the various components of a hearing aid. Furthermore, the audiologist should schedule elderly patients for periodic follow-up visits to monitor the patients' progress and to review questions and concerns that they may have about their amplification devices. When considering amplification for this group, one must recognize that they could benefit from many of the assistive listening devices described earlier in this chapter. Many of the problems exhibited by this group center around using the telephone, watching television, and understanding speech in group situations, such as church or public auditoriums.

To summarize, the hearing-impaired elderly have unique problems and concerns that require the special consideration of the audiologist throughout the rehabilitation process. If the audiologist attends to these needs and concerns, there is a far greater probability that use of a hearing aid will be successful.

SUMMARY

In this chapter, we have reviewed and discussed the more pertinent aspects of amplification and rehabilitation of hearing-impaired children and adults. It was noted that the hearing aid is the most important rehabilitative tool we have available to us for the management of the hearing-impaired. Numerous types of amplification systems, including personal hearing aids, assistive listening devices, and classroom systems, are available for the habilitation/rehabilitation of hearing-impaired individuals. Further, we have detailed in this chapter some of the varied rehabilitative approaches used for hearing-impaired children and adults.

SUGGESTED READINGS

Alpiner JG, Schow RL: Rehabilitative evaluation of hearing-impaired adults. *In* Alpiner JG, McCarthy PA (eds): *Rehabilitative Audiology: Children and Adults,* ed 2. Baltimore, Williams & Wilkins, 1993.

Bloom L, Lahey M: *Language Development and Language Disorders.* New York, John Wiley & Sons, 1978.

Byrne D: Theoretical prescriptive approaches to selecting the gain and frequency response of a hearing aid. *Monographs in Contemporary Audiology* 4:1–40, 1983.

Clark JG, Martin FN: *Effective Counseling in Audiology. Perspectives and Practice.* Englewood Cliffs, NJ, Prentice Hall, 1994.

Fitzgerald MT, Bess FH: Parent/infant training for hearing-impaired children. *Monographs in Contemporary Audiology* 3:1–24, 1982.

Geers AE, Moog JS: Predicting spoken language acquisition of profoundly hearing impaired children. *Journal of Speech and Hearing Disorders* 52:84–94, 1987.

Hawkins D, Yacullo W: The signal-to-noise ratio advantage of binaural hearing aids and directional microphones under different levels of reverberation. *Journal of Speech and Hearing Disorders* 49:278–286, 1984.

High WS, Fairbanks G, Glorig A: Scale for self-assessment of hearing handicap. *Journal of Speech and Hearing Disorders* 17:321–327, 1964.

Hodgson WR (ed): *Hearing Aid Assessment and Use in Audiologic Habilitation,* ed 3. Baltimore, Williams & Wilkins, 1986.

Giolas TE, Owens E, Lamb SH, Schubert ED: Hearing performance inventory. *Journal of Speech and Hearing Disorders* 44:169–195, 1979.

Kretschmer RR, Kretschmer LW: Communication/language assessment of the hearing-impaired child. *In* Bess FH (ed): *Hearing Impairment in Children.* Parkton, MD, York Press, 1988.

Ling D: *Speech and the Hearing-Impaired Child: Theory and Practice.* Washington, DC, Alexander Graham Bell Association for the Deaf, 1976.

Mueller HG, Grimes MA: Hearing aid selection and assessment. *In* Alpiner JG, McCarthy PA (eds): *Rehabilitative Audiology: Children and Adults,* ed 2. Baltimore, Williams & Wilkins, 1993.

Moeller MP, Brunt MA: Management of preschool hearing-impaired children: a cognitive-linguistic approach. *In* Bess FH (ed): *Hearing Impairment in Children.* Parkton, MD, York Press, 1988.

Moeller MP, Carney AE: Assessment and intervention with preschool hearing-impaired children. *In* Alpiner JG, McCarthy PA (eds): *Rehabilitative Audiology: Children and Adults,* ed 2. Baltimore, Williams & Wilkins, 1993.

Mueller HG, Grimes A: Amplification systems for the hearing impaired. *In* Alpiner JF, McCarthy PA (eds): *Rehabilitative Audiology: Children and Adults.* Baltimore, Williams & Wilkins, 1987.

Mueller HG, Hawkins DB, Northern JL: *Probe Microphone Measurements. Hearing Aid Selection and Assessment.* San Diego, Singular, 1992.

Norlin PF, Van Tassell DJ: Linguistic skills of hearing-impaired children. *Monographs in Contemporary Audiology* 2:1–32, 1980.

Northern JL, Downs MP: *Hearing in Children,* ed 4. Baltimore, Williams & Wilkins, 1991.

Pascoe DP: *Hearing Aids. Who Needs Them?* St. Louis, Big Bend Books, 1991.

Sanders DA: *Management of Hearing Handicap: Infants to Elderly,* ed 3. Englewood Cliffs, NJ, Prentice Hall, 1993.

Schwartz DM, Bess FH: Amplification techniques for hearing-impaired children. *In* Bluestone CD, Stool S (eds): *Pediatric Otolaryngology,* ed 2. Philadelphia, WB Saunders, 1990.

Skinner MW: *Hearing Aid Evaluation.* Englewood Cliffs, NJ, Prentice-Hall, 1988.

Studebaker GA, Bess FH (eds): The Vanderbilt Hearing Aid Report. *Monographs in Contemporary Audiology*, 1982.

Studebaker GA, Bess FH, Beck LB (eds): *The Vanderbilt Hearing Aid Report II.* Parkton, MD, York Press, 1991.

CHAPTER EIGHT

EDUCATION FOR THE HEARING IMPAIRED

Following completion of this chapter the reader should be able to:

- List and describe the legislative provisions for children with hearing impairment.
- Describe the different educational programs and settings available for children with hearing impairment.
- Describe the educational achievements exhibited by today's children with hearing impairment.
- Understand the impact of varying degrees of hearing loss on educational performance.
- Develop an appreciation for the role of audiology in the educational setting.

Previous chapters referred to the importance of the auditory system for acquiring information about the world. It was noted that significant hearing loss can result in serious developmental complications, such as delays in development of language, speech production and understanding, and cognition. It was also mentioned that, in the absence of hearing, the symbol system we traditionally use for developing and verbally expressing thoughts and ideas is not automatically perceived and learned. Given this background, it should come as no surprise to learn that children with hearing impairment often exhibit significant lags in educational achievement.

Education is a process of imparting to individuals information that will better prepare them for life and enable them to use their native abilities in a meaningful and constructive manner in society. When one considers the method by which information is imparted, it becomes apparent that auditory input from teacher to pupil and from pupil to pupil is critical to acquiring an education in the typical manner. Vision also plays a vital role, but is secondary to hearing. One need only watch a television program without the sound to gain some realization of what children with hearing impairment experience in the classroom. Communication through hearing, so natural and automatic that it is taken for granted by most people, is reduced dramatically between a teacher and a child with hearing impairment.

Many students enrolled in an introductory audiology class are likely to be faced with the responsibility of working with a child with hearing loss later in their careers. This chapter, as a result, focuses on educational programming and the educational difficulties experienced by children with hearing impairment.

LEGISLATIVE PROVISIONS FOR HANDICAPPED CHILDREN

In 1975, Part B of the Education of the Handicapped Act (EHA) (known as the Education for All Handicapped Children Act—Public Law 94–142) was passed by Congress and signed into law. Public Law (PL) 94–142 focused on the rights and protection of handicapped children and their parents. As noted in Chapter 1, this act became known as the Individuals with Disabilities Education Act (IDEA) in 1990. Briefly, the law had four major functions. First, it guaranteed the availability of a special-education program to all handicapped children and youth who require it. This was true without regard for factors, such as geographic residence, that contributed to many inequities of opportunity in the past. Second, the law assured fair and appropriate decision-making in providing special education to handicapped children and youth. Third, PL 94–142 established, at every level of government, clear management, auditing requirements, and procedures for special education. Fourth, the law assisted the special-education efforts of state and local governments through the use of federal funds. Importantly, the law does not mandate special education for every handicapped child, but only for those who by reason of one or more disabilities require it. Many children are able to enroll in regular classes without program modification and should do so. The law further implies that special education is "special" and includes only instruction aimed at meeting the unique needs of a handicapped child. The law also makes clear that handicapped children may require related services that might not be available from the school system itself. These services would be provided through contractual relations with other agencies, either public or private, and with outside specialists. The act demonstrates a clear and logical progression: the child is handicapped and special education and/or related services are needed by the child; special education is the specially designed instruction program to meet the child's unique needs; and related services are those additional services necessary to enable the child to benefit from special-education instruction.

In 1986, amendments were proposed that authorized the extension of the EHA to infants and toddlers, 0–2 years of age. Known as Part H of the EHA, this newly created legislation was designed to assist states in the development and implementation of comprehensive, coordinated, interdisciplinary programs of early intervention services for handicapped infants, toddlers, and their families. Children experiencing delays in language and speech development are among those covered by Part H of the EHA. Early intervention services are defined as "developmental services which include ... speech pathology and audiology ... and are provided by qualified personnel, including speech and language pathologists and audiologists" (1). Other services targeted by the bill include early identification, screening, and

assessment services; psychological services; medical services for diagnostic or evaluation purposes only; and any other services deemed appropriate for helping infants
and toddlers benefit from early intervention. In addition, the bill strengthens portions of the original act by developing better incentives for states to serve the 3- to
5-year-old population. Finally, not only does the bill help to expand the services to
young infants and toddlers, but it also helps to ensure that states use appropriately
trained personnel.

In considering this bill, now known as IDEA, Part H, PL 102–119 (formerly PL
99–457), Congress recognized a need to:

1. Enhance the development of handicapped infants and toddlers and to minimize
   their potential for developmental delay;
2. Reduce the educational costs to our society, including our nation's schools, by
   minimizing the need for special education and related services after handicapped
   infants and toddlers reach school age;
3. Minimize the likelihood of institutionalization of handicapped individuals and
   maximize the potential for their independent living in society; and
4. Enhance the capacity of families to meet the special needs of their infants and
   toddlers with handicaps. (1)

Implementation of this law involves, in part, a multidisciplinary evaluation to
determine eligibility and to develop an individualized educational plan (IEP)
designed to detail the child's educational management program. The IEP will be
discussed in more detail later in this chapter. Other components of the law include
nondiscriminatory evaluation, rights of the parents to be involved in the decisions
affecting their child, and education in the least restrictive environment.

Another important legislative initiative for individuals with disabilities is the
Rehabilitation Act of 1973 (Title V, Section 504, Subpart D: Preschool, Elementary, and Secondary Education). This law, later amended in 1978, was developed to
protect disabled individuals from discriminatory action—that is, a person with a
handicap should have the same rights and benefits (e.g., accessibility to public facilities) as one who does not have a handicap. Hence, the bill, sometimes referred to
as the Bill of Rights for individuals with handicaps, offers special provisions
beyond that of instructional services. For example, these services might include
availability of special devices such as fire alarms, public announcement systems,
and telephone services for children with hearing impairment.

Finally, in 1990, the Americans with Disabilities Act (ADA) was passed in an
effort to prevent discrimination against individuals with handicapping conditions,
particularly in the area of employment. To this end, President Reagan's National
Council on Disability created a bill, the ADA, designed to afford the handicapped
equal opportunities in employment, public accommodations, transportation, and
state and local services in telecommunications.

All of the above legislation has significantly improved the life quality of individuals with hearing impairment. It has created an environment in which individuals with hearing loss can compete effectively in all aspects of our society.

THE CULTURE OF DEAFNESS

Historically, hearing health care professionals have treated deafness as a pathologic medical condition. The audiologist's general goal has been to "mainstream" the deaf child into a normal-hearing world, to provide the child with speech (English) or some other means of communication, and to help the child and the child's family to make educational and social decisions. Today, however, there is a strong movement toward considering the deaf not just a group of people with a medical condition, but a cultural and linguistic minority. That is, there is a move to acknowledge the cultural values of the deaf population and to view the differences between deaf and normal-hearing people as cultural differences, not as deviations from the norm. Deaf people now promote the deaf culture to get hearing people to understand deaf people as they understand themselves. The book *Deaf in America: Voices from a Culture* made the following statement:

> The traditional way of writing about deaf people is to focus on the fact of their condition—that they do not hear—and to interrupt all other aspects of their lives as a consequence of this fact.... In contrast to the long history of writings that treat them as medical cases, or as a people with disabilities who compensate for their deafness by using sign language, we want to portray the lives they live, their art in performances, their everyday talk, their shared myths, and the lessons they teach one another. We have always felt that the attention given to the physical condition of not hearing has obscured far more interesting facets of deaf peoples' lives. (2)

The above statement offers some valuable insight into the differences between hearing and deaf views of deafness. For hearing health care professionals, the emphasis appears to be placed on the handicap, the audiologic data, or the mode of communication, whereas deaf people are more concerned with social, linguistic, and cultural aspects of the deaf experience. Hence, it is important for all hearing health care professionals to recognize and understand the attitudes and feelings of deaf people. Audiologists must be cognizant of and sensitive to the characteristics and problems of deaf people and not just view the deaf as persons affected by a pathologic condition, but rather as a group of people with specific language and behavior patterns and a proud history.

COMMUNICATION MODES USED IN EDUCATIONAL INSTRUCTION

In Chapter 7, we discussed briefly the different modes of communication used for educational instruction: auditory-oral and total communication. It is not our intent here to suggest that one mode of communication is better than another. Unquestionably, the two most common approaches used in education are the auditory-oral and total communication methods. Recall that the auditory-oral method, sometimes referred to as the oral-aural approach, emphasizes use of the child's existing residual hearing to develop oral communication. Some of the advocates of this method use early amplification with no emphasis on vision for receiving information. Others emphasize vision over hearing or stress the combined use of hearing and vision equally. Whatever modification is used, this approach does not permit the use of signs or finger spelling. The only means of expression allowed is speech.

The other popular approach to educational instruction is the method known as total communication. Total communication combines the auditory-oral method with signs and finger spelling. That is, the emphasis is on receiving the information by all possible means, including amplification, vision, signs, and finger spelling. Similarly, expression can occur by speech or through signs and/or finger spelling. Like advocates of the auditory-oral approach, proponents of total communication believe that the method should be introduced in early infancy, if possible, and that parents should be intensively involved. The difference, of course, is that with total communication, the parents assist the child in the development of language using all means available.

At this point, a brief discussion of manual communication is warranted, since it is an important component of the total approach. Variations of the auditory method will also be presented to help the reader contrast the different instructional approaches used in children with hearing impairment. At the outset, it is important to realize that the language development of children depends on the nature of the language presented to the child (English or American Sign Language) and the type of communication system used (manual vs. oral). As shown in Figure 8.1, language is coded into three basic forms, American Sign Language (ASL), Manually Coded

FIGURE 8.1.
Summary of the various approaches used to teach communication/language skills to children with hearing impairment. Note that the approaches fall on a continuum according to how closely they resemble the English language. *ASL*, American Sign Language; *MCE*, Manually Coded English; *OE*, Oral English; *PSE*, Pidgin Sign English; *SE*, Signed English; *SEE II*, Signed Exact English; *SEE I*, Seeing Essential English; *F*, Finger Spelling; *A*, Auditory; *AVO*, Auditory-Visual-Oral; *CS*, Cued Speech. (From Quigley SP, Paul PV: *Language and Deafness*. San Diego, College-Hill Press, 1984.)

English (MCE), and Oral English (OE). Each of these forms varies according to how closely it resembles the structure of the English language. Note that for MCE and OE, several additional subdivisions further complicate the classification scheme.

One means by which a word or idea can be presented manually is through a sign. There are four basic features common to all signs. These include general position, configuration, orientation (direction of the palms), and movement of the hands. These four features are combined in various ways to formulate signs of different meanings. Figure 8.2 shows examples of signs. Although the different signs in this figure all use the same handshape, the movement, position, and palm orientation alter the meaning. The manual communicator has the flexibility to use finger spelling only, sign only, or a combination of the two. The sign language used in the United States is generally referred to as ASL, to differentiate it from some of the more recent modifications devised to make signs conform more closely to the syntax of the English language. ASL has its own vocabulary and grammatical structure, and it is the major communication mode used among deaf adults. In fact, many believe that ASL should be taught as the primary language to all children with hearing impairment and that English should be taught as a second language. ASL users do not typically speak while signing and, hence, sound is not used as an information source.

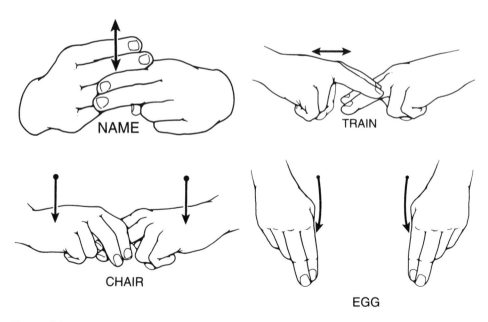

FIGURE 8.2.
Examples of a group of signs. Note that, although each sign has a similar handshape, there are differences in movement, placement, and orientation of the hands. (From Schleper D: *Communicating with Deaf People: An Introduction*. Washington, DC, National Information Center on Deafness, Gallaudet University, 1987.)

MCE represents those approaches that incorporate gestures, signs, finger spelling, or some combination of these to approximate English. Varying forms of MCE that attempt to bring ASL closer to English include Pidgin Sign English (PSE), Signed English (SE), Signing Exact English (SEE II), Seeing Essential English (SEE I), and finger spelling. With the exception of finger spelling, each of the above systems is based on ASL, but employs the word order of English. PSE is a sign system used by deaf adults to approximate English using sign and finger spelling. The term "pidgin" means simplified speech used for communicating between two people with different languages. Hence, PSE is often used to communicate with hearing persons, who are usually not familiar with ASL and deaf persons. SE, originally designed for preschool children, consists of both signs and finger spelling. Each of the approximately 3500 signed words in the SE system parallels the meaning of a separate word entry in a standard English dictionary. Morphologic sign markers are used to represent the regular and irregular plurals and thus more closely approximate English than does PSE. SEE II is one of the more widely contrived systems that adds morphemes such as prefixes and suffixes that are not included in the basic signs. Examples include the morphemes -*ed*, as in "talk*ed*," and -*ly*, as in "friend*ly*." A common way to accomplish this is through finger spelling. SEE I was developed before SEE II and in fact was one of the first attempts to use signs in a structure that replicated English. SEE I has a vocabulary of about 5000 words, and signs are used to represent word forms and even word parts such as roots, prefixes, or suffixes. Compound words were made by putting two words together. For example, the sign for understand was made by joining the signs of under and stand. SEE I and SEE II differ in that they use different rules for establishing sign boundaries. SE, SEE II, and SEE I have some common characteristics: (*a*) they borrow from the ASL vocabulary, (*b*) they were developed for use by hearing parents of deaf children and teachers, and (*c*) they attempt to use signs for such elements of speech as pronouns, affixes, and verb tenses.

Finger spelling simply involves spelling a word letter by letter, representing each letter by a specific sign that corresponds to a letter in the English alphabet. As noted earlier, finger spelling is often used in combination with sign. The hand is held at about chest level, and different finger configurations are then formed. The presentation rate is somewhat similar to that of speech. Figure 8.3 shows the American manual alphabet used in the United States. Note that there are 26 handshapes representing the different letters in the English alphabet. Those who desire a more detailed coverage of manual communication are referred to the Suggested Readings at the end of this chapter.

It is seen from Figure 8.1 that the approach that most closely represents English is OE. This approach emphasizes the key role of acoustic input as a means of developing skill in both understanding and producing connected speech as the primary mode of communication. Major characteristics of this approach include maximum emphasis on hearing, comprehensive intervention well beyond the traditional setting, and emphasis on connected speech. Early full-time use of amplification with periodic re-examination of hearing to monitor the child's auditory capacities with

FIGURE 8.3.
The American Manual Alphabet (shown as signs appear to person reading them). (From Schleper D: *Communicating with Deaf People: An Introduction.* Washington DC, National Information Center on Deafness, Gallaudet University, 1987.)

and without hearing aids is crucial to this method. In general, language is best learned by hearing it, just as it is with normal-hearing persons. Approaches that focus on residual hearing (*A*) are referred to as auditory, auditory-oral, or acoupedics, whereas techniques that employ vision (lipreading) as part of training are referred to as auditory-visual-oral (AVO).

Another approach classified as oral is cued speech (CS). CS is a system that incorporates eight hand configurations and four hand positions near the lips to aid hearing and speech reading. The basic premise is that the hand cues can supplement speechreading and audition by signaling differences between sounds. For example, the words *bee* and *me* look alike to the speech reader. A hand cue made simultaneously at the lips signals the difference between the two "look-alike" words.

The auditory-oral method was easily the most widely used method of instruction until the mid-1970s. Since that time, however, total communication has become the more popular method and is used in about 80% of the educational programs in the United States, regardless of grade level. This approach gained widespread acceptance following research that showed that deaf children, exposed to manual communication by deaf parents, exhibited better educational performance than deaf children of hearing parents. At the same time, the two groups of children showed essentially no differences in their speech. In Chapter 7, we discussed the approaches used to determine whether a child with hearing impairment would benefit most from an auditory-oral or a total communication program of instruction.

EDUCATIONAL SETTINGS

What are the different settings used to educate children with hearing impairment? There are numerous types of programs, both public and private, designed to serve children with hearing impairment of all ages. One of the most well-recognized educational programs is the residential school. Residential programs maintain facilities for room and board as well as instruction and recreation. Most residential schools are operated by state governments. There are, however, some well-known private residential programs throughout the United States. Today, many children commute on a daily basis to residential facilities, especially if the school is in a metropolitan area. Also found in large metropolitan areas are private and public day schools for the hearing-impaired. In these schools, the children with hearing impairment commute on a daily basis as normal-hearing children do. Day classes are another type of instructional format for children with hearing impairment. Here, classes for the hearing-impaired are conducted in public schools at which most of the children have normal hearing. Instruction may take place entirely in classrooms containing only hearing-impaired students, or the children may be "mainstreamed." Mainstreaming refers to the integration of children with hearing impairment into regular classrooms on a full-time or part-time basis. Special classes (resource rooms) are arranged for areas in which the child needs individualized tutorial assistance, but most of the student's time is spent in regular classrooms. Finally, there are itinerant programs, in which a child with hearing impairment attends regular classrooms full time but receives support services from an itinerant teacher. Typically, the itinerant teacher moves from one school to another throughout the week, offering support services to those children with special needs.

It is of interest to consider how these placement alternatives have changed over the past several decades. First, there are many more children with hearing impairment in public day classes today than there were in the 1970s and even in the 1980s. Paralleling the increase in public day classes was a decrease in the public residential schools and public day schools for the hearing-impaired. Also noteworthy is the decrease in all types of private schools throughout the United States. Since about 1974, there has been a trend toward an increase in the role of the public schools in educating the hearing-impaired, mostly through day-school programs (public day classes). This trend is no doubt due to the mandate of Public Laws 94–142 and 99–457.

A number of postsecondary educational opportunities are available for the deaf and hard-of-hearing population in the United States. Foremost is Gallaudet University, which was for many years the only higher educational program in the world developed specifically for persons with hearing impairment. The establishment of the university was spearheaded by the efforts of Edward Minor Gallaudet and Amos Kendall, two resourceful professionals who were committed to serving the hearing-impaired population. The university was named after Edward Gallaudet's father, Thomas Gallaudet, a pioneer in deaf education. (See Vignette 8.1 for a discussion of pioneers in deaf education.) Today, Gallaudet serves as a major source of leadership to the individuals with hearing impairment in the United States. In addition to offering liberal arts and graduate education for the hearing-impaired, Gallaudet also trains professionals, such as school administrators, audiologists, speech-language pathologists, teachers, and researchers, to serve the hearing-impaired population. There is no comparable postsecondary program for individuals with hearing impairment in the United States.

Vignette 8.1.
Pioneers in deaf education.

Charles Michael de l'Pée

One of the most prominent names in the history of deaf education worldwide is that of Abbé de l'Pée, the individual credited with making education of the hearing-impaired a matter of public concern. He was also interested in making education available to the indigent population. Charles Michael de l'Pée was born in Versailles, France, in 1712. He was well educated and pursued the priesthood as his chosen profession. His interest in deafness stemmed from his knowledge of twin sisters who were severe-to-profoundly hearing-impaired. Because of his concern for these sisters, he agreed to instruct them, and soon his success gained him widespread recognition. From this time on he devoted his life to working with the hearing-impaired. He established a school, and educators from all over the world came to study his technique. Also, de l'Pée helped develop and expand sign language for the hearing-impaired and served as an advocate for manual communication.

Alexander Graham Bell

Alexander Graham Bell is recognized as one of the great teachers of the deaf in the United States. He was born March 3, 1847, in Edinburgh, Scotland. At 24 years of age, he came to the United States to visit a school for deaf children. He was most impressed with how hearing-impaired children utilized lipreading and speech. This initial experience motivated Bell to become more involved with the hearing-impaired. Bell spearheaded the development of the auditory-oral method for teaching the deaf in the United States. In 1872, he opened a training school for teachers of the deaf in Boston, Massachusetts. His plan to develop an auditory-oral training school was greatly opposed by advocates of the manual approach. His desire to develop a mechanical means of making speech visible to the hearing-impaired led Bell to experiment with the electrical transmission of sound. He hoped to develop a means of amplification for the hearing-impaired. These experiments resulted in the development of the telephone. Bell later married Mabel Hubbard, a deaf woman who helped start the auditory-oral approach in the United States. Throughout his later years, Bell maintained his interest in the education of the hearing-impaired and served as an advocate for the hearing-impaired population.

Edward Minor Gallaudet

Edward Minor Gallaudet was the son of Thomas Hopkins Gallaudet, a pioneering teacher of the hearing-impaired in the United States and the man for whom Gallaudet University in Washington, D.C., was named. Edward Minor Gallaudet studied under his father and served as the first president

VIGNETTE 8.1.—*continued*

of Candle School, a private school for the hearing-impaired. The school was later renamed Gallaudet College in honor of his father, Thomas Hopkins Gallaudet. Candle School became the preparatory department at this college. Edward Minor Gallaudet studied both oral and manual techniques; he supported the combined method but was convinced that manual communication was the most appropriate and natural approach for the educational instruction of hearing-impaired children.

Irene R. Ewing

Irene W. Ewing is considered one of the modern pioneers in the education and audiologic management of children with hearing impairment. During the war years between 1939 and 1945, nurseries, clinics, and hospitals in Great Britain kept a steady and careful watch over the general development of their young infants and children. Children with abnormal responses or behavior were quickly noted and referred to appropriate clinics. Children who exhibited abnormal responses to sound were typically referred to Ewing's clinic for deaf children at Manchester University. The worldwide reputation of this program for children with hearing impairment came about primarily because of Ewing's persistent and undaunted efforts as a teacher and as one who had a unique ability to impart knowledge to others. She demonstrated worldwide the benefits of early identification and intervention, the importance of parent-home training for the development of speech, and the techniques for testing young children with hearing loss. From her clinic's opening in 1919 until her retirement in 1949, she encouraged and aided successive groups of students with her own enthusiasm and conveyed something to them of her steadfast principles on educating children with hearing impairment. She also encouraged others to pursue a professional career in deaf education. Her efforts won worldwide renown, and her advice and consultation were sought throughout the United Kingdom and the world.

Technical schools for the hearing-impaired also exist in this country. Perhaps the best known is the National Technical Institute for the Deaf (NTID), a technical school of higher education that serves deaf students in association with the Rochester Institute of Technology in Rochester, New York. The educational programs can lead to certificate programs, associate degrees, or bachelor's degrees. The NTID is also involved in carrying out research concerned with the deaf and hard-of-hearing populations.

Finally, it is important to note that a number of state universities and community colleges throughout the United States have federally funded programs providing vocational or liberal arts training to the hearing-impaired. In fact, some of these programs serve as feeder programs for the NTID and Gallaudet University.

EDUCATIONAL ACHIEVEMENT OF CHILDREN WITH HEARING IMPAIRMENT

One only needs to contrast the manner in which a normal-hearing child develops oral speech and language with the situation of the child with hearing loss to appreciate the learning difficulties that children with auditory deficits experience. The typical normal-hearing child comes to kindergarten or first grade with a wide array of auditory experiences and a well-developed language symbol system. The child with hearing loss, on the other hand, has had limited auditory experiences and was most likely not even identified as suffering from hearing loss until 3 years of age. Therefore, the child with hearing loss will have been wearing hearing aids for only 1 or 2 years. The child with a significant hearing impairment will have had far fewer learning-readiness experiences prior to entering first grade. Thus, we find that children with hearing loss lag behind normal-hearing children in educational achievement.

Indeed, the influences of both education and communication are reflected in the incomes earned by the deaf population. Those deaf persons with the most education generally earn the highest incomes. Those using only manual communication or gestures report the lowest median earnings. Of those deaf individuals in the upper half of the income range, about 90% use speech to communicate at work, with about half of these persons using speech combined with one or more other modes of communication and half using speech exclusively.

Although we find that unemployment rates among the deaf are higher on the average than in the hearing population, underemployment is a much more serious problem. For example, less than 10% are employed in professional, technical, or managerial positions, and less than 1% are employed in sales. Almost 75% are engaged in clerical, craft, or machine operator positions—the latter being the single largest occupation. Some of the reasons for underemployment will become apparent as we review the educational difficulties experienced by children with varying degrees of hearing loss. The case illustrations of five different school-age children with hearing impairment presented in Vignettes 8.2 through 8.6 also provide some insight into the problem.

VIGNETTE 8.2.

Case illustration of a child with bilateral moderately severe to profound sensorineural hearing loss.

This 10-year-old male was identified at the age of 17 months as having a moderately severe to profound bilateral sensorineural hearing loss. Binaural amplification was introduced within a month; the accompanying figure shows an audiogram obtained after 2 months of amplification (*left panel*). Thresholds obtained in a sound field (*S-S*) reveal a severe-to-profound hearing loss. When the child wears a hearing aid, the sound field thresholds (*A-A*) improve markedly compared with unaided thresholds. A more recent pure-tone audiogram is shown in the *right panel*. Data for aided thresholds are also presented.

VIGNETTE 8.2—*continued*

He was enrolled in an auditory-oral parent-infant training program as soon as amplification was introduced. His parents were taught speech, language, and auditory stimulation techniques and were excellent in carrying out auditory training at home. The child progressed rapidly and was making single-word approximations accompanied by jargon at 1 year post amplification.

At 3 years of age, he was enrolled in a half-day oral-acoustic nursery for hearing-impaired children. He wore an FM-wireless system during school hours. By 5 years of age, he was using simple sentences to communicate (orally), and he was mainstreamed into a private pre-kindergarten classroom with support services from the local school. The support services consisted of individual speech and language therapy as well as assistance in the curricular areas of reading, math, science, and social studies.

The subject continues to be mainstreamed in a private school, with supportive speech and language therapy. He is presently in the third grade and functioning at grade level in reading comprehension and math. He is functioning below age level in the areas of vocabulary development and language associated with logical thinking skills (i.e., sequencing events, predicting outcomes, verbal analogies, and multiple meanings).

Intelligibility of speech production is good, with approximately 90% of his speech understood by peers, teachers, and family members. The child orally presents essays and other assignments on a par with other children in his class.

He probably will require speech/language therapy throughout his school years, as well as special assistance with academic subjects. However, this is a case in which appropriate early identification combined with proper educational management and parental determination has led to a life in the mainstream.

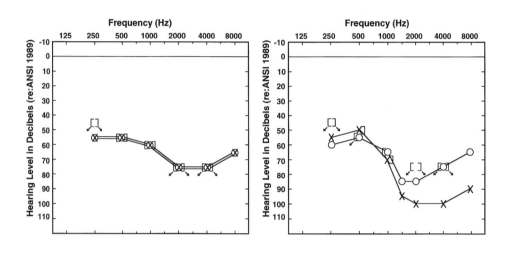

VIGNETTE 8.3.

Case illustration of a child with bilateral moderate-to-severe sensorineural hearing loss.

This 11-year-old female was identified as having a bilateral moderate-to-severe sensorineural hearing loss at age 5 years and was referred to a hearing clinic. The etiology of the hearing loss is unknown. Her audiogram at age 5 is shown in the accompanying figure (*left panel*). The most recent audiogram indicated a moderate-to-severe sensorineural hearing loss in the right ear and a moderate-to-profound sensorineural hearing loss in the left ear (*right panel*).

The child was enrolled in both a self-contained kindergarten classroom in a local school system and in a parent-infant training program. Her communicative skills were fair, and she responded well to amplification. Her speech was judged to be partially intelligible, and her language skills were similar to those of a 3- to 4-year-old. She has continued in a self-contained classroom with additional individual speech/language therapy. She is presently in a second-grade self-contained classroom. Her reading skills are at age level, and she is functioning at grade level in math and social sciences. When compared with normal-hearing children, expressive language skills are at the 7-year-old level.

Mainstreaming has been considered but has not been implemented because of concerns regarding her ability to work independently. In addition, mainstreaming has been prevented because of a lack of qualified personnel to provide the necessary support services. It is probable that she will be mainstreamed, at least partially, when she is older and more able to work independently.

Vignette 8.4.

Case illustration of a child with unilateral severe-to-profound sensorineural hearing loss.

This child is a 6-year-old male with a severe-to-profound sensorineural hearing loss in the left ear and normal hearing in the right ear. Pertinent medical history includes maternal diabetes and syphilis, meningitis at 1 year of age, and head trauma at 5 years of age. He is currently attending first grade and receives preferential seating (child seated to the right side of the teacher so that the good ear is fully exposed to the teacher). The teacher indicated that the child would be retained in the first grade for the next year. She reported that he is a "slow learner," although he is more capable than he demonstrates. He also attends a reading resource class and receives articulation therapy.

Prior to a 2-week trial with an FM system, the teacher rated his ability to understand and/or follow directions as "fair" in small group situations and as "very poor" in large group situations. The teacher also rated his ability to concentrate on tasks as "poor."

Use of an FM wireless system reportedly resulted in a marked improvement in his performance. His ability to understand and follow directions in small and large group situations, as well as his ability to concentrate on tasks while using the FM wireless system, was now rated by the teacher as "good." In addition, the teacher felt that peer acceptance of the FM wireless system was excellent. According to the teacher, the FM wireless system was especially useful in classroom learning situations.

Both the teachers and the parents were counseled about the dangers that unilaterally hearing-impaired children can encounter in such routine activities as crossing busy streets and bike riding in heavy traffic. In addition, the teachers and the parents were counseled about the need for practicing good hearing health care. Monitoring the child for possible conductive hearing loss resulting from effusion in either ear and progressive sensorineural hearing loss was emphasized. Furthermore, the practice of using ear protection in any high-noise environment was recommended as a conservation measure.

VIGNETTE 8.5.

Case illustration of a child with bilateral minimal hearing loss.

This child is a 6-year-old male with a long history of middle ear disease with effusion. He has had persistent otitis media for several years and a history of myringotomy with insertion tubes beginning at the age of 6 months. The child has had seven or eight sets of tubes during the first 6 years of life. He was hospitalized a total of 22 times for difficult-to-resolve otitis media, and he underwent mastoidectomy and tympanoplasty on the right side.

The audiogram shows that the child has a very mild bilateral hearing impairment through the speech frequency range and a somewhat precipitous drop in the high frequencies. The child experienced considerable difficulty understanding speech in a background of noise. That is, when tested in a sound field situation in the presence of background noise (+6 dB S:N ratio), the child was only able to understand 76% of the speech material.

He is currently enrolled in kindergarten, where he is having considerable difficulty. There is serious question as to whether he will progress to the first grade. He is reportedly immature and hyperactive. Language skills, especially vocabulary, are delayed by 1–2 years.

Based on these results, a number of recommendations were made: (*a*) that he continue with otologic management for middle ear disease with effusion, (*b*) that he receive support in the form of an FM system for use in the academic setting (this system was recommended to improve the S:N ratio in the noisy classroom environment), (*c*) that the Board of Education be notified of the child's circumstance so that his audiologic and academic needs can be monitored, and (*d*) that the child be seen by the audiologist on a 6-month basis to monitor progress.

VIGNETTE 8.6.

Case illustration of a child with unilateral conductive hearing loss.

This child is a 5-year old female with a history of early otitis media. The child underwent myringotomy with insertion tubes at 1 year of age, a second set at 2 years of age, and a third set at 2.5 years of age. When this audiogram was taken, the child did not have tubes. At 5 years the child presented with a perforation in the left ear and underwent tympanoplasty to repair the eardrum. An ear infection shortly after the tympanoplasty compounded the child's conductive problem. The child is currently enrolled in a headstart program, where she is experiencing difficulty understanding speech and is delayed in speech and language by approximately 1 year.

Based on these results, the following recommendations were made: (*a*) that the child receive a comprehensive speech/language evaluation and that periodic evaluations occur every 6–8 months, (*b*) that the child be evaluated for the use of an FM system to help her in the classroom, (*c*) that the child be placed in a special education class in the fall, and (*d*) that the child receive classroom seating preference.

Children with Severe-to-Profound Hearing Losses

In general terms, there appears to be an association between the severity of hearing loss and the degree of educational retardation. The milder the hearing loss, however, the more difficult it is to predict the educational potential of the child. Since the 1920s, it has been acknowledged that deafness causes an educational lag of 4–5 years. This lowered achievement is thought to result from the difficulty children experience in acquiring language and communication skills. Delayed speech and language in the important preschool years cannot help but be reflected when a child learns to read, since reading achievement is an important indicator of linguistic competence. Reading is a basic learning tool that directly influences the mastery of all other academic content. For years, educators of deaf children have been concerned with the apparent "plateau effect" that begins at about 9–10 years of age and persists through the teens. This effect is reflected in very minimal gains in reading level over several years of instruction. For example, the average gain in reading level between 10 and 16 years of age among deaf students is less than a year. One can expect most profoundly hearing-impaired children to be retarded 7–8 years in reading vocabulary by the age of 18 years. There are, however, many exceptions.

There have been a number of national surveys of the hearing-impaired population. In a 1974 census of deaf individuals who could not hear and understand speech and who had lost that ability by 19 years of age (or never had it), it was found that 52% had not completed high school, and 25–33% had not completed the ninth grade. Although such data should be interpreted with caution because the census reports years of school completed and not achievement level, it does offer insight into some of the educational difficulties experienced by the deaf population. Figure 8.4 shows the results from the 1990 nationwide norms on the Stanford Achievement Test (SAT) for reading comprehension and mathematics computation for children with hearing impairment and for children with normal hearing. Note that for reading comprehension (*upper panel*), the average child with hearing impairment increased only about two grade equivalents in 8 years of education between 9 and 17 years of age. Moreover, whereas children at 8 years of age are delayed about 2 years in grade level compared with normal-hearing children, the children at 15 years of age have fallen even farther behind and are delayed more than 7 years. In contrast, computational scores are seen to be less affected by hearing impairment, approaching the eighth-grade level at age 17 years. These data clearly illustrate the educational lag that is common to deaf and partially hearing children enrolled in our special programs.

Children with Mild-to-Moderate Hearing Losses

Thus far, our discussion has focused on the impact of severe-to-profound hearing losses on education. What about children suffering from the milder forms of hearing loss, sometimes referred to as the hard-of-hearing or the partially hear-

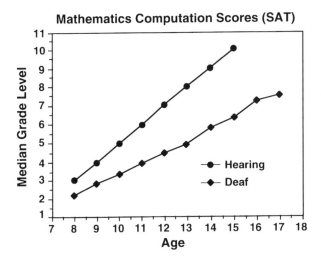

FIGURE 8.4.

Median Stanford Achievement Test (SAT) scores in grade levels for the 1990 population. *Top panel* shows reading comprehension levels as a function of age in years for both normal-hearing children and children with hearing loss. *Bottom panel* shows mathematics-computation scores for the same two groups. (From deVilliers, PA: Educational implications of deafness: language and literacy. *In* Eavey RD, Klein JO [eds]: *Hearing Loss in Childhood: A Primer, Report of the 102nd Ross Conference on Pediatric Research.* Columbus, OH, Ross Laboratories, 1992.)

ing-impaired population? Once again, we find that even those with milder hearing losses can experience difficulty in school. In 1968, researchers examined the educational potential of 116 children with hearing impairment using subtests of the Stanford Achievement Test. Table 8.1 summarizes the results from this study and shows the differences between expected performance (computed from the birthdates of the children) and actual performance for children with varying

TABLE 8.1.

Differences Between Expected and Actual Performance of Children on the Stanford Achievement Test

Average Hearing Threshold Level (Better Ear) in dB	No. of Children	IQ	Word Meaning[a]	Paragraph Meaning[a]	Language[a]	Subtest Average[a]
<15	59	105.14	−1.04	−0.47	−0.78	−0.73
15–26	37	100.81	−1.40	−0.86	−1.16	−1.11
27–40	6	103.50	−3.48	−1.78	−1.95	−2.31
41–55	9	97.89	−3.84	−2.54	−2.93	−3.08
56–70	5	92.40	−2.78	−2.20	−3.52	−2.87

[a]Negative values represent a deficit in measured grade level compared to normal-hearing children.

From Quigley SP: *Some Effects of Hearing Impairment upon School Performance.* Springfield, IL, Division of Special Education Services, Department of Special Education Development and Education, 1968.

degrees of hearing loss on the subtests of word meaning, paragraph meaning, and language. Several important points are evident from this table. First, it is noted that there is a slight trend toward decreasing IQ with increasing hearing loss. Second, all groups of children with hearing impairment, even those with losses as mild as 15–26 dB, lagged in educational performance. This is indicated by the appearance of negative numbers in the table. Third, one can see by looking at the subtest averages that the discrepancy between expected performance and actual performance increases with increasing hearing loss. The average difference between expected performance and actual performance for all groups was −1.25 grades. These data, although not universally acknowledged as valid, demonstrate that children with slight hearing impairments are not realizing their educational potential.

The data in Table 8.1 prompted other investigators to explore the impact of milder hearing losses on educational achievement. Foremost in this effort has been the work of Davis and coworkers published in 1981 and in 1986. Davis and coworkers conducted two comprehensive studies on the educational abilities of hearing-impaired children in the schools. In the first study, data were taken from the school files of more than 1000 children with mild to moderately severe hearing impairments. The findings of this retrospective study revealed that the children with mild-to-moderate degrees of hearing loss (three-frequency pure tone average of ≤ 50 dB) did not show significant educational problems. Those with average hearing losses of more than 50 dB, however, exhibited significant deficits in academic achievement, and these problems increased over time. In contrast, most of the hearing-impaired children, even those with mild losses, demonstrated difficulties with language.

In a follow-up investigation, a prospective study was performed on a group of 40 children with mild to moderately severe hearing losses. Rather than rely on test scores from the school files, as before, the researchers administered the same battery of educational achievement tests to all subjects in the sample. Importantly, and in contrast to the previous study, it was not possible to predict educational performance solely on the basis of hearing level. That is, it was possible for a child with minimal hearing loss to exhibit as much (or even more) difficulty with a given task as a child with a mild-to-moderate hearing loss. The difficulties experienced by these children could be lumped into three general areas: verbal skills, academic skills, and social development. Verbal skills appeared to be affected most, and this area was also reported to be the most closely associated with hearing loss. These researchers emphasized the heterogeneity of the hearing-impaired population and concluded that "children with any degree of hearing loss appear to be at risk for delayed development of verbal skills and reduced academic achievement" (3).

Another important finding of this study was that many of these children exhibited behavioral problems. Many were also concerned about peer acceptance. One of the children from the study related the following: "I don't have very many friends. Oh, people say, 'Hi, Kris, hi, Kris,' but only 'Hi, Kris,' never anything— you know—go out for lunch or go out on dates or anything like that. The only friends I almost have are my teachers and my counselors" (3).

Children with Unilateral Sensorineural Hearing Losses

Not only are children with mild hearing loss at risk, but it appears that children with unilateral sensorineural hearing loss also experience difficulty in the schools. The auditory, linguistic, and psychoeducational skills of a group of school-age children with unilateral sensorineural hearing loss have been examined extensively. Some of the important findings of this recent research include the following:

1. In a survey of 60 children with unilateral hearing loss, 35% were found to have failed at least one grade in the schools, and an additional 13% needed special resource assistance.

2. Children with unilateral sensorineural hearing loss exhibited greater difficulty than children with normal hearing in understanding speech in the presence of competing background noise.

3. Children with unilateral sensorineural hearing loss experienced significantly greater problems with localization of sound.

4. Children with severe-to-profound unilateral hearing loss exhibited lower IQs than did children with milder unilateral loss.

5. Children with unilateral sensorineural hearing loss who failed a grade in elementary school exhibited verbal IQs that were significantly lower than those of unilaterally hearing-impaired children who had not failed a grade.

6. Children with right ear impairments are at greater risk for academic failure than children with left ear impairments.

7. Teachers rated children with unilateral losses as having greater difficulty in peer relations, less social confidence, greater likelihood of "acting out" or withdrawn behavior in the classroom, greater frustration and dependence on the teacher, and more frequent distractibility.

Prior to this research, the prevailing belief had been that unilaterally hearing-impaired children do not experience any problems in the schools. It had always been assumed that one good ear is sufficient to enable a child to achieve satisfactorily in school.

Children with Mild Conductive Losses from Otitis Media

For almost two decades, there has been a growing awareness of the potential psychoeducational complications associated with recurrent otitis media (ROM) during the early developmental years. Although many of the research studies conducted in this area have flaws in design, the vast majority of such studies imply a link between a history of ROM, associated hearing loss, and some area of child development. Otitis-proneness in children has been linked to learning disabilities, academic problems, lower intelligence levels, behavior and attention problems, difficulties in understanding speech in a background of noise, and delayed language development.

How is it that the mild, fluctuating hearing loss associated with otitis media could possibly interfere with the development of auditory, linguistic, and psychoeducational skills? Recall from Chapter 5 that children with otitis media experience hearing loss averaging about 30 dB through the speech-frequency range. During the early developmental period for speech and language, the otitis-prone child could experience an inconsistent, and perhaps a somewhat distorted, auditory signal. In fact, many of the speech sounds that have low speech energy, such as /f/, /s/, /θ/, /k/, /p/, /h/, /z/, and /v/, may well be missed altogether in the presence of a mild 30-dB hearing loss. Similarly, important acoustic information, such as morphologic markers (i.e., plural -s, past tense -ed) and inflections, could be especially difficult to identify.

The loss of acoustic energy explains, in part, how these children could experience trouble in the developmental years. Once the otitis-prone years have passed, can the child make up for the lost input? Unfortunately, there is some evidence to suggest that some children do not. Otitis media can produce both delays in language and an inattention to language. Once the otitis media resolves or the episodes become less frequent, the child can recover basic language skills, but the habit of not attending to language may persist. Some of the more basic language components, such as syntax and semantics, may not be as seriously affected as discourse and narrative skills. The latter require some amount of attention to language. Figure 8.5 summarizes the possible sequence of events that could occur from repeated bouts of early otitis media.

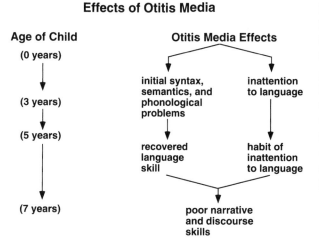

Effects of Otitis Media

FIGURE 8.5.
Hypothetical model to explain how later language functioning might be affected by early persistent otitis media. (From Feagans L: Otitis media: a model for long term effects with implications for intervention. *In* Kavanagh JF [ed]: *Otitis Media and Child Development.* Parkton, MD: York Press, 1986.)

FACTORS AFFECTING THE EDUCATIONAL STATUS OF CHILDREN WITH HEARING IMPAIRMENT

The Terminology Dilemma

Leading commentators over the past two decades have frequently deplored the growing tendency for issues of all kinds—political, social, religious, ethnic, minority, and many others—to become polarized. This unfortunate predilection seldom benefits either of the opposing groups, because it tends to lock them into such rigidly exclusive positions that flexibility and compromise are not often possible. For example, the terms *liberal* and *conservative* in social and political affairs can no longer be accurately described or defined along traditional lines, for the majority of individuals are likely to cross over these boundaries, depending on the particular issue involved. So it is with the use of the terms relating to individuals with hearing impairment. Despite attempts to emphasize the various inter-relating factors that determine the functioning level of an individual with hearing loss, laypeople, as well as many professionals, continue to dichotomize individuals with hearing impairment as either deaf (those who cannot hear) or hard of hearing (those who can hear, at least partially). Thus, children with degrees of hearing loss designated as mild, moderate, severe, and profound could in fact spend their lives in one or the other category with its subsequent lifestyle pattern. The determinant would then be not the degree or severity of hearing loss but other factors, most of which were present in the earliest years of life. The terms "deaf" and "hard of hearing" are not mutually exclusive, since a child may begin life deaf but become hard of hearing. Of course the reverse could also happen if the hearing mechanism suffers further damage. The following definitions of hearing impairment, deaf, and hard-of- hearing may be useful:

Hearing impairment. A generic term indicating disability that may range in severity from very mild to profound; it includes the subsets of deaf and hard of hearing.

Deaf. Of or pertaining to one whose disability precluded successful processing of linguistic information through audition with or without a hearing aid.

Hard-of-hearing. Of or pertaining to one who generally, with the use of a hearing aid, has residual hearing sufficient to enable successful processing of linguistic information by way of audition. The term "partially hearing" is sometimes used synonymously with hard-of-hearing.

Although the above definitions are likely to be inappropriately used and interpreted, they represent a thoughtful and reasonable approach to a very complex issue in this field. There is a need to recognize that "hearing-impaired" includes all gradients of severity of hearing loss. The term has too often been used redundantly in the phrase "the deaf and the hearing-impaired." To be deaf is to be impaired in hearing, but hearing-impaired is often used as if it were synonymous with hard-of-hearing or partially hearing.

Such definitions suffer the same fault that has been inherent in most other definitions; the majority of children with hearing impairment cannot be classified either as deaf or hard-of-hearing early in life. Nor will the label necessarily remain appropriate from that time forth. The distinction made in the definitions relates to the present auditory capabilities. Many individual variables determine the borderline between the residuum of hearing for which aural linguistic processing is not possible and that for which it is possible. It is not unusual, for example, for a child with only a moderate hearing impairment to function more like a deaf child whose hearing loss is in the profound range. Thus, although some levels of hearing impairment do preclude linguistic processing by audition, for many severely impaired persons, the more important factor is the age at which auditory experience through individual amplification is initiated and how successfully it is monitored and maintained.

Degree of Hearing Loss

In general, the more severe the hearing impairment, the greater the likelihood that a child will be enrolled in a special education program. In fact, about 80% of children enrolled in special programs have losses greater than 55 dB in the better ear.

The serious nature of the educational handicap of hearing loss requires that parents and professionals diligently seek every possible advantage needed by children with hearing impairment. However, although many will enthusiastically ascribe to this established principle, it is not always put into practice. For example, although early detection and intervention and use of amplification are pretty much universally endorsed regardless of the particular method supported, the majority of children enrolled in special education programs have not had such opportunities.

Age of Intervention

The rubella epidemic that swept across the United States during 1964–1965 sharply increased awareness of childhood deafness and its challenges to educators. During the late 1960s, several well-known programs were developed for parents and their deaf babies between the ages of birth and 3 years. These programs emphasized parent counseling and training instead of focusing the training efforts on the child. The theory was that formal procedures were not yet suitable for such young children. By demonstration and example, parents were tutored in principles of communicating with their children. They were shown the importance of amplification and adaptation to use of hearing as a primary source of language input in the first years of life, which for all children is the most natural time for language acquisition. Although several highly successful programs were organized and conducted, such facilities were not always within the reach of many children with hearing impairment and their parents. Most children with hearing loss are affected at birth or before the age of 3 years. Congenital and other forms of prelingual hearing impairment are the most handicapping educationally as evidenced by the need for special education facilities. If the impairment had occurred following language acquisition, many of these children might have been enrolled in regular education.

Given the fact that more than 9 of every 10 children enrolled in special schools and classes are known to have incurred hearing impairment either at birth or before 3 years of age, the proportion of those who are actually enrolled in some type of formal intervention program designed for children in the period of birth to 3 years of age is probably small. Hence, most children who require special education for hearing impairment are known to have a hearing loss before 3 years of age, but they do not find their way into formal organized programs for infants and preschoolers in the same proportions as do older children with hearing impairment. This is not necessarily due to late identification of hearing loss. Studies show that after early identification of hearing loss, lag times of 9–12 months transpire before an infant is begun on intervention services.

Communication Patterns

In general, speech—either alone or in combination with other modes—is the communication pattern most frequently used by parents and hearing-impaired students in their interaction. The children use signs somewhat more than their parents do, and they use speech a bit less. Speech alone is used by about 40% of the parents and by 31% of the children, whereas signs alone are used by 5% of parents and 9% of children. Speech alone and speech supplemented with gestures account for about 50% of the parent-to-student communication and for 40% of student-to-parent communication. In general, the communication patterns of children with hearing impairment yield the following conclusions: (*a*) children who have hearing loss vary widely in their communication patterns, (*b*) combinations of methods rather than a single method are the rule in the classroom, but far less so at home, (*c*) speech alone is the single most common pattern at home, whereas a combination of speech signs, finger spelling, writing, and gestures is the single most common pattern at school, and (*d*) there is relatively little consistency between patterns of communication used at home and in school.

In the view of most educators, there should be consistency in the communication patterns used by parents and teachers, regardless of the particular educational philosophy held. Much improvement could be made through more intensive efforts for parent participation in the education process for children with hearing impairment.

Ethnic Background

In general, Caucasians score higher on reading comprehension tests than either African-American or Hispanic students, a fact thought to be a consequence of socioeconomic and cultural elements as well as possible differences among these populations in access to medical, education, and other remedial services. For Hispanic students, the problem is compounded by the fact that Spanish is the primary language spoken in the home and English is the primary language spoken in the schools. Very few programs for children with hearing impairment in this country can adequately deal with the problems raised by bilingual spoken language acquisition, not to mention the issues of signing and written language. No doubt, as the numbers of minorities increase among children with hearing impairment, this issue of ethnicity will become increasingly important.

Presence of An Additional Handicapping Condition

It is generally estimated that about one-third of all children with hearing impairment have at least one additional handicapping condition that has educational impact. Close to 10% have at least two additional handicaps in combination. Some of these conditions include visual impairment, brain damage or injury, mental retardation, epilepsy, learning disabilities, and emotional/behavioral problems. These children are more likely to be placed in special education settings only. Clearly, such handicapping conditions will adversely affect the child's ability to learn in the schools.

To summarize to this point, hearing impairment in childhood is a serious barrier to the normal educational process. However, this problem is related not just to one or two but to many interacting variables. When this cluster of variables is for the most part favorable, even severely and profoundly impaired children can achieve remarkably well in comparison to hearing children.

AUDIOLOGY IN THE SCHOOLS

We have just seen that children with varying degrees of hearing loss undergo considerable hardship in school and typically lag behind their normal-hearing peers in terms of academic achievement. The audiologist can play an important role in the management of these children in the schools. The following discussion focuses on the role of the audiologist in the educational setting.

Models for Delivering Audiologic Services to the Schools

The delivery of audiologic services within the educational environment varies considerably from one local educational agency (LEA) to the next. Educational systems offer programs ranging from comprehensive audiologic management to only minimal services. Although numerous models exist for the provision of audiologic management to the schools, there are three commonly employed approaches. These models are the *parent-referral* approach, the *cooperative interagency* approach, and the *audiology approach within the schools*.

Parent-Referral Model

The parent-referral model is the most traditional approach to the delivery of audiologic services in the schools. The LEA provides identification and intervention services, while the more comprehensive assessment and evaluation services are supplied by agencies or parties outside of the LEA. The success of this model depends highly on the parents, who become responsible for the management and follow-up of their child. Once the parents have been notified by the school that their child has been identified by the screening process as needing further testing, they must then make arrangements on their own for an audiologic or medical evaluation. The results of these evaluations are given directly to the parent, with feedback supplied to the LEA.

The advantages to this model are that services are provided at a minimal cost to the LEA and that the school system uses resources that already exist within the community, avoiding unnecessary duplication of services. Unfortunately, there are more disadvantages to the parent-referral model than advantages. The LEA has no control over the management of a child and must rely on the cooperation of the parent, the hearing and speech center, and the physician to supply the necessary information and recommendations. Since the LEA does not monitor referred children, many complications can arise. For example, there is no mechanism for ensuring that diagnostic reports will be sent to the school within a reasonable period or that they will be sent at all. In addition, the received reports may be incomplete or perhaps inappropriate in that the information provided may not assist the school or teacher in helping the child educationally. Seldom does the report supply sufficient information relative to the child's educational placement and/or management. Even if such information is available, the model provides no assurance that the child will receive appropriate follow-up. Finally, the parent-referral model is only conducive to an annual evaluation and not to continuous audiologic management.

Cooperative Interagency Model

A more desirable alternative to the provision of audiologic services in the schools is a contractual arrangement between the LEA and a community hearing and speech center. Once the child is identified, the school notifies the parents and the contracting agency. Although dependent on the contracted services, the agency ordinarily provides audiologic management of the child and maintains constant feedback to an LEA designate, usually the coordinator of the program for the hearing-impaired. In some instances, an audiologist coordinates the referral and management activities. The parent initiates a referral to the physician, if necessary, at the recommendation of the school. The physician, in turn, provides feedback to the parent, school, and contract agency.

The success of this model depends on the types of services contracted. The more knowledgeable the administrator, the more comprehensive the contract will be and the more success the program will have. The agreement works best when an audiologist from the agency is solely responsible for coordinating the audiologic services. The contact person at the LEA and the teachers must have one person to whom they can refer questions or problems.

The model offers several advantages and eliminates some of the disadvantages associated with the parent-referral model. It is particularly useful for educational systems with small numbers of hearing-impaired children (such as schools in rural areas). Duplication of services is avoided, and, as with the parent-referral model, the LEA does not need to be concerned with the high cost of equipment and facilities. At a time when funding is a primary concern in education, this must be considered a distinct advantage. This model also has several limitations. Unless responsibilities and lines of authority are clearly defined and monitored on a continuing basis, communication can break down. Since the LEA is paying for the audiologic services, there is a tendency for the educational administration to dictate the type and extent of services to be provided. Open lines of communication, willingness to cooperate with the LEA staff, and general agreement on services to be delivered are essential. Another potential difficulty is the LEA's loss of control over expenditures, although this problem can be eliminated by carefully defining in the contract how funds will be expended.

School Audiology Model

The final model involves the development of a comprehensive audiologic program within the LEA. In this model, services are provided by a coordinating audiologist and associated staff. This model provides the LEA with complete centralized control of audiologic services. Identification, assessment, and management are all under the jurisdiction of the coordinating school audiologist. The advantage to such a model is that the audiologist is where the children are—in the schools. Individualized educational programs (IEPs) for the hearing-impaired students can be developed and implemented in the schools. Effective input to these plans would be difficult for professionals outside the system. Other advantages of this model include immediate access to diagnostic information, development of evaluation data tailored to the educational setting, greater control over follow-up, good communication between the LEA staff and the school audiologist, and better potential for ongoing in-service education. The limitations of the model are the high costs of equipping a complete audiologic facility and employing the needed personnel and the problems that arise from duplicating services that are already available within the community. Now that we have reviewed three of the models used for delivering services to the schools, let us briefly examine some of the responsibilities of the school audiologist.

Responsibilities of Audiologists in the Schools

The duties of the audiologist in the school setting are numerous and require highly specialized skills and knowledge. These responsibilities include identification, assessment, audiologic management, educational admission and placement, and in-service training.

Identification

Ideally, the educational audiologist should have primary responsibility for the identification of preschool and school-age children with hearing loss or middle ear disease. Even if identification services are not offered directly by the school program, the educational audiologist should coordinate the screening program. Techniques for setting up screening programs are discussed in Chapter 6.

Assessment

A major responsibility of the educational audiologist is to assess the communicative efficiency of hearing-impaired children in the schools. The assessment battery should include traditional measurements of auditory function (pure-tone audiometry, speech audiometry, and immittance measures) as well as the evaluation of auditory processing and communication skills. Assessment protocols have been addressed in Chapter 4.

Audiologic Management

The school audiologist plays an important role in the audiologic management of the hearing-impaired child. The associated responsibilities might include selection and evaluation of amplification and assistive listening devices, maintenance of amplification devices, monitoring classroom noise, coordination of habilitation/rehabilitation activities, and parent counseling.

The selection and evaluation of amplification is a fundamental concern to the audiologist in education and warrants additional comment at this point. After the hearing aid has been selected, periodic reevaluations of the child's performance with amplification are essential. Occasionally, it becomes necessary to make minor modifications in the electroacoustic parameters of the hearing aid as more is learned about the child's hearing or as changes occur in hearing sensitivity. The educational audiologist is responsible not only for the selection and evaluation of the personal hearing aid but also for the classroom amplification system. The audiologist spends considerable time and effort in the selection and evaluation of a personal hearing aid for a hearing-impaired child; however, this is not always true regarding the selection and evaluation of classroom systems. Whatever is appropriate in the selection and evaluation of the child's personal aid should also be important in the selection and evaluation of the child's classroom system. The educational audiologist should make sure that the characteristics of both the personal and classroom hearing aids of a child are comparable and provide consistency in auditory input.

Far too often, hearing aids in the school do not function properly. To help eliminate these problems, a well-organized amplification maintenance program should be implemented in the schools. A maintenance program should contain the following essential elements: (a) education of parents and teachers on the use and care of a hearing aid, (b) a daily visual and listening examination, (c) monthly electroacoustic checks, and (d) comprehensive physical inspections of the hearing aid. At the outset, both the parents and the teachers should be taught how to troubleshoot a hearing aid and should be given a kit that permits simple inspection of a hearing aid. A traditional troubleshooting kit would include a drying agent for removing moisture, pipe cleaners, a battery tester, a hearing aid stethoscope, spare batteries, and an extra receiver. The parent should be instructed to examine their child's hearing aid each day prior to leaving for school, and the teacher or an assistant should recheck the instrument once each morning. It is important for teachers to have a supply of batteries in the classroom. A good maintenance program should also include an adequate stock of loaner aids (aids used as substitutes for personal hearing aids that are in need of repair).

Educational Admission and Placement

The audiologist should be an active member of the staff that reviews a child's school status for the purpose of deciding placement or admission. The audiologist's input should be evident in the IEP of PL 94–142 or the Individual Family Service Plan (IFSP) of PL 99–457 as it relates to amplification needs, the amount and type of language and speech intervention required, the classroom acoustic environment, parent and child counseling, and support systems for the classroom teacher. Recall from the beginning of this chapter that IEPs are written statements that detail the educational management of a given child and meet the unique needs of the family. These statements are generated because the child's handicapping condition precludes the use of a standard school curriculum. The IEP details special educational needs and special services the child will need on a daily basis. Hence, the IEP basically provides the child with an individualized and appropriate education in the least restrictive environment possible. It is critical that the child's audiologic needs be built into the IEP; otherwise, the local LEA will have no obligation to include such services in the child's educational management plan. Hence, the audiologist must become an advocate for the child and his or her parents from an audiologic standpoint.

In general, the IEP should include the following components: (a) statement of the child's educational performance, (b) statement of goals, including short-term and instructional objectives, (c) statement of the specific special education and related services to be provided to the child to enable him or her to participate in regular educational programs, (d) projected date for initiation and anticipated duration of such services, and (e) appropriate objective criteria and evaluation procedures and schedules for determining (at least annually) whether short-term instructional objectives are being achieved and whether placement is appropriate. The following information should be included in the IFSP: (a) child's current status and present levels of development as determined by objective criteria, (b) family information needed for facilitating the development of the baby/child, (c) expected outcomes of the early intervention program, (d) details of the specific plan for the delivery, location, and method of payment for early intervention, (e) other services not required by law but that are needed by the child (e.g., medical services), (f) duration and dates of the specific early intervention services, (g) designation of the case manager to ensure proper implementation of the IFSP, and (h) plans for transition into the school system. Unfortunately, the audiologist is generally not included in the development of the IEP/IFSP unless specifically requested by the parent or teacher.

In-Service Education

An important responsibility of the audiologist in the schools is the development of in-service education programs for school personnel who come in frequent contact with hearing-impaired children. In addition to providing in-service training to speech-language pathologists and teachers of the hearing-impaired, more generalized in-service programs should be developed for regular teachers, psychologists, administrators, and support personnel. Teachers of the hearing-impaired whose previous experience was confined to the self-contained classroom are now being asked to service children with hearing impairment either in a resource room or as an itinerant teacher. In addition, support personnel who previously only encountered children with mild-to-moderate hearing loss are now faced with the task of mainstreaming children with severe-to-profound hearing impairment. Many educators find themselves needing to upgrade and broaden their skills in order to meet the demands of children with hearing impairment and comply with the provisions of Public Laws 94–142 and 99–457.

Teachers and support personnel say that they lack the knowledge to provide adequate programs for children with hearing loss. Even after special training, they often do not recognize basic malfunctions in equipment or programs. It is generally recognized that teachers of children with hearing impairment receive little training in classroom amplification systems and other assistive devices. Other teachers have expressed concern about dealing with language and speech development and in training children with hearing loss to use their residual hearing.

In-service education for speech-language pathologists and teachers of children with hearing impairment should concentrate on six general areas: (a) the relationship between hearing loss and educational communicative skills, (b) the behavior of children with hearing loss, (*c*) principles of personal and classroom amplification, including other assistive devices, (*d*) the importance of the classroom environment and its effects on speech understanding, (e) the use of audition in training children with hearing loss, (*f*) the development of language skills in children with hearing impairment, and (*g*) the development of speech in children with hearing loss.

Summary

This chapter reviewed various aspects of education for the hearing-impaired child. It is clear that the changes in federal educational provisions for the hearing-impaired child have challenged today's audiologists. The emphasis is now on the early identification and management of hearing impairment, preferably prior to 2 years of age. Nevertheless, we find that hearing loss poses a significant threat to educational achievement. Even the milder forms of hearing loss have been shown to inhibit educational progress. These ever-increasing changes in the field of education for the hearing-impaired result in expanding responsibilities for both the speech-language pathologist and the audiologist working in a school setting.

References

1. United States House of Representatives 99th Congress, 2nd Session. Report 99–860. Report Accompanying the Education of the Handicapped Act Amendments of 1986.

2. Padden C, Humphries T. *Deaf in America: Voices from a Culture.* Cambridge, MA: Harvard University Press, 1988, p 1.

3. Davis JM, Elfenbein J, Scum R, Bundler RA: Effects of mild and moderate hearing impairments on language, educational and psychosocial behavior of children. *Journal of Speech and Hearing Disorders* 51:60, 61, 1986.

Suggested Readings

Alpiner, JG, McCarthy, PA (eds): *Rehabilitative Audiology: Children and Adults*, ed 2. Baltimore: Williams & Wilkins, 1993.

The Commission on Education of the Deaf: *Toward Equality: Education of the Deaf. A Report to the Congress of the United States.* Washington, DC, U.S. Department of Health, Education, and Welfare, 1988.

Bess FH, McConnell FE: *Audiology, Education, and the Hearing-Impaired Child.* St. Louis, CV Mosby, 1981.

Bess FH: Unilateral sensorineural hearing loss in children. *Ear and Hearing* 7:1–54, 1986.

Bornstein H: *Manual Communication—Implications for Deafness.* Washington, DC: Gallaudet University Press, 1990.

Davis J, Shephard N, Stelmachowicz P, Gorga M: Characteristics of hearing impaired children in the public schools. Part II. Psychoeducational data. *Journal of Speech and Hearing Disorders* 46:130–137, 1981.

Davis JM, Elfenbein J, Schum R, Bentler RA: Effects of mild and moderate hearing impairments on language, educational and psychosocial behavior of children. *Journal of Speech and Hearing Disorders* 51:53–62, 1986.

Feagans L: Otitis media: a model for long term effects with implications for intervention. *In* Kavanuagh JF (ed): *Otitis Media and Child Development.* Parkton, MD, York Press, 1986.

Moores DF: *Educating the Deaf—Psychology, Principles and Practices,* ed 3. Boston, Houghton Mifflin, 1987.

Moores DF, Meadow-Orlans KP (eds): *Educational and Developmental Aspects of Deafness.* Washington, DC, Gallaudet University Press, 1990.

Quigley SP, Thomure FE: *Some Effects of Hearing Impairment upon School Performance.* Springfield, IL, Office of Education, 1968.

Ross M (ed): *Hearing-Impaired Children in the Mainstream.* Parkton, MD, York Press, 1990.

Schien JD, Delk MT: *The Deaf Population of the United States.* Silver Spring, MD, National Association of the Deaf, 1974.

GLOSSARY

acute otitis media Middle ear disease of rapid onset and rapid resolution characterized by a reddish or yellowish bulging tympanic membrane, obliteration of ossicular landmarks, and conductive hearing loss.

adhesive otitis media Otitis media that results in adhesions between the tympanic membrane and the bony walls of the middle ear or the ossicles.

admittance Ease of flow of energy through a system; reciprocal of impedance.

afferent Centripetal; conveying nerve impulses toward a center.

American sign language Sign language used in the United States to differentiate from some of the more recent modifications devised to make signs more like the English language.

atresia Absence or closure of a normal body opening; in hearing it most often refers to the external acoustic meatus.

audiogram Graph used to display hearing sensitivity of a person. Intensity (in dB) is plotted on the ordinate and frequency is shown on the abscissa.

audioscope Hand-held otoscope with a built-in audiometer.

bilirubin A red bile pigment, sometimes found in urine, that is present in the blood tissues during jaundice.

broadband (white) noise An acoustic signal that contains energy of equal intensity at all frequencies.

Carhart Father of the profession of audiology.

cholesteatoma Accumulation of debris developed from perforations of the eardrum; sometimes referred to as a pseudotumor.

chromosome One of several small rod-shaped bodies, easily stained, that appear in the nucleus of a cell at the time of cell division. They contain the genes, or hereditary factors, and are constant in number in each species.

chronic otitis media Otitis media that is slow in its onset, tends to be persistent, and often can produce other complications. The most common symptoms are hearing loss, perforation of the tympanic membrane, and fluid discharge.

cilium (plural: cilia) Minute, vibratile, hairlike process attached to the free surface of a cell.

collapsed canal A canal that collapses as the result of pressure caused by earphone placement.

congenital Before birth, but usually prior to the 28th week of gestation.

cytomegalovirus infection Congenital viral infection that, in its more severe forms, produces symptoms similar to rubella and may cause hearing loss as well as other abnormalities.

decibel The logarithm of the ratio between two sound intensities, powers or sound pressures. The decibel (one tenth of a bel) was named in honor of Alexander Graham Bell.

effusion Collection of fluid, especially in middle ear.

electroacoustic Refers to the conversion of acoustic energy to electrical energy, or vice versa, for the purpose of sound generation or measurement.

electromagnetic field Field of energy produced by electrical current flowing through a coil of wire.

epithelium The covering over the internal and external surfaces of the body, including the lining of vessels and other small cavities.

endogenous Hereditary forms of hearing impairment—literally means "within the genes."

epidemiology Branch of medicine that studies epidemic diseases.

exogenous Acquired forms of hearing impairment—literally means "outside the genes."

gene The biologic unit of heredity, self-reproducing and located in a definite position on a particular chromosome.

gestational age Time between mother's last menstrual period and time of baby's birth.

helicotrema Passage that connects the scala tympani and the scala vestibuli at the apex of the cochlea.

high risk register Conditions for which children are at greater-than-average risk for hearing impairment.

impedance Opposition to the flow of energy through a system; reciprocal of admittance.

lesion Wound or injury; area of pathologic change in tissue.

Meniere's disease Disease of the membranous inner ear characterized by sensorineural hearing loss, vertigo (dizziness), and usually tinnitus (ringing in ears).

microtia A term that implies a small deformed pinna (or auricle).

myringotomy Surgical procedure that involves making an incision in the eardrum to release pressure, remove fluid, and restore hearing sensitivity.

narrow-band noise Band of noise limited to a restricted frequency region by filtering.

nasopharynx The part of the pharynx (throat) behind and above the soft palate, directly continuous with the nasal passages.

negative predictive value Probability that a person who has passed a hearing screening test truly has normal hearing.

nephritis Inflammation of the kidney.

otitic Pertaining to otitis.

otitis Inflammation of the ear.

otitis media Inflammation of the cleft or middle ear.

otolaryngology   Medical specialty associated with diseases of the ear and larynx.

otologist   A physician concerned exclusively with diseases of the ear.

otosclerosis   Formation of spongy bone in the labrynthine capsule and the stapes footplate. The most common site of the formation is just in front of the oval window. The disease produces impaired stapedial mobility and a gradual conductive hearing loss. Sometimes referred to as otospongiosis.

perinatal   Pertains to a condition that occurs in the period shortly before or after birth (from 8 weeks prior to birth to 4 weeks after).

periosteum   Specialized connective tissue covering all bones of the body, consisting of a dense, fibrous outer layer and a more delicate inner layer capable of forming bone.

petrous   Denoting or pertaining to the hard, dense portion of the temporal bone containing the internal auditory organs.

pneumatic otoscope   Hand-held instrument used to examine visually the external acoustic meatus and the tympanic membrane. A pneumatic bulb connected to the otoscope allows the examiner to vary air pressure in the canal while examining the mobility of the eardrum.

positive predictive value   Probability that a person who has failed a hearing screening test is truly hearing impaired.

postnatal   A condition acquired later in life.

prenatal   Something that occurs to the fetus before birth.

presbycusis   Hearing loss associated with aging.

prevalence   The number of cases of hearing impairment in a given population at a given point in time.

public law 94-142   A federal law designed to assure all handicapped school-age children a free and appropriate public school education.

public law 99-447   A new law designed to extend public law 94-142 to infants and toddlers.

real-ear gain   The gain of a hearing aid measured in the patient's ear in a sound-field setting.

reflectometer   Hand-held instrument designed to detect middle ear disease with effusion.

reticular lamina   Netlike layer extending over the surface of the organ of Corti.

sensitivity   Regarding test accuracy, proportion of truly hearing impaired persons in a screened population correctly identified by a screening test.

serous   A clear fluid free of debris and bacteria.

sickle cell anemia   Hereditary disease of the blood that occurs almost exclusively in blacks.

sound-field   An area (usually a room) into which sound is introduced (usually by a loudspeaker).

specificity Regarding test accuracy, proportion of truly normal hearing persons in a screened population correctly identified by a screening test.

spectrum (plural: spectra) Display of a sound's amplitude (amplitude spectrum) or phase (phase spectrum) as a function of frequency.

spiral ganglion Group of nerve cell bodies located in the modiolus of the cochlea, from which nerve fibers extend into the spiral organ.

stigmata Findings or landmarks indicative of a specific disorder.

synapse Region of contact between processes of two adjacent neurons where a nervous impulse is transmitted from one neuron to another.

syndrome A group of symptoms that are characteristic of a specific condition or disease.

temporary threshold shift (TTS) Temporary elevation of an auditory threshold following exposure to noise; frequently used to predict the potential danger of a noise environment.

time compression Process whereby speech is recorded and then played back in less time than the original recording; commonly expressed as a percentage. For example, speech that originally was recorded in 1 second and played back in $\frac{1}{2}$ second would be 50% time-compressed.

toxoplasmosis Organism that is transmitted to the child via the placenta. Infection is typically contracted by eating uncooked meat or making contact with the feces of cats. Possible cause of hearing loss.

uncomfortable loudness level Intensity level (in dB) at which audio signals (pure tones, noise, or speech) become uncomfortably loud.

warble tone Sound characterized by a continuous fluctuation in frequency of predetermined amount both above and below a central frequency.

waveform Display of an acoustic (or electrical) signal with amplitude along the y-axis and time along the x-axis.

FIGURE AND TABLE CREDITS

FIGURE 1.1. Adapted from Demographic Profile of ASHA Membership. American Speech-Language-Hearing Association, Research Division, 1993.

FIGURE 1.2. Adapted from Kirkwood DH. The economy + FDA + the media add up to an off year for hearing aid sales. *The Hearing Journal*, 46:7–14, 1993.

FIGURE 2.5. Adapted from Durrant JD, Lovrinic JH: Bases of Hearing Science, ed 2. Baltimore, Williams & Wilkins, 1986, p 41.

FIGURE 3.1. Adapted from Kessel RG, Kardon RH: *Tissues and Organs: A Text-Atlas of Scanning Electron Microscopy*. San Franciso, WH Freeman, 1979.

FIGURE 3.2. Adapted from Shaw EAG: The external ear. *In* Keidel WD, Neff WD (eds): *Handbook of Sensory Physiology*, vol 5(1). New York, Springer Veriag, 1974, p 463.

FIGURE 3.3. Adapted from Durrant JD, Lovrinic JH: *Bases of Hearing Science*, ed 2. Baltimore, Williams & Wilkins, 1984, p 98.

FIGURE 3.4. Adapted from Zemlin WR: *Speech and Hearing Science: Anatomy and Physiology*, ed 2. Englewood Cliffs, NJ, Prentice-Hall, 1988, p 464.

FIGURE 3.5. Adapted from von Bekesy G: *Experiments in Hearing*. New York, McGraw-Hill, 1960, p 462.

FIGURE 3.6. Adapted from von Bekesy G: *Experiments in Hearing*. New York, McGraw-Hill, 1960, p 448.

FIGURE 3.7. Adapted from Pickles JO: *An Introduction to the Physiology of Hearing*, ed 2. London, Academic Press, 1988, p 29.

FIGURE 3.8. Adapted from Zemlin WR: *Speech and Hearing Science: Anatomy and Physiology*, ed 2. Englewood Cliffs, NJ, Prentice-Hall, p 484.

FIGURE 3.13. Adapted from Yost WA: Nielsen DW: *Fundamentals of Hearing: An Introduction*, ed 2. New York, Holt, Reinhart, & Winston, 1985, p 98.

FIGURE 3.16. Adapted from Sivian LJ, White SD: Minimum audible pressure and minimum audible field. *Journal of the Acoustical Society of America* 4:288–321, 1933.

FIGURE 3.17. Adapted from Hawkins JE Jr, Stevens SS: The masking of pure tones and of speech by white noise. *Journal of the Acoustical Society of America* 22:6–13, 1950.

FIGURE 3.19. Adapted from Fletcher H, Munson WN: Loudness, its definition, measurement, and calculation. *Journal of the Acoustical Society of America* 5:82–108, 1933.

TABLE 4.1 Adapted from Northern J, Downs M: *Hearing in Children*, ed. 3. Baltimore, Williams & Wilkins, 1984.

VIGNETTE 4.4. From Northern JL: Acoustic impedance in the pediatric population. *In* Bess FH (ed): *Childhood Deafness: Causation, Assessment and Management*. New York, Grune & Stratton, 1977.

VIGNETTE 5.4. Adapted from Moody DB, Stebbins WC, Hawkins JE Jr, Johnsson L-G: Hearing loss and cochlear pathology in the monkey (macaca) following exposure to high levels of noise. *Archives of Oto-Rhino-Laryngology* 220:47–72, 1978.

FIGURE 5.4. From English GM: *Otolaryngology*. Hagerstown, MD, Harper & Row, 1976.

FIGURE 5.8. From English GM: *Otolaryngology*. Hagerstown, MD, Harper & Row, 1976.

FIGURE 5.9. From English GM: *Otolaryngology*. Hagerstown, MD, Harper & Row, 1976.

FIGURE 5.10. From English GM: *Otolaryngology*. Hagerstown, MD, Harper & Row, 1976.

FIGURE 5.13. From Goodhill V (ed): *Ear Diseases, Deafness and Dizziness*. Hagerstown, MD, Harper & Row, 1979.)

FIGURE 5.19. Adapted from Lebo CP, Reddell RC: The presbycusis component in occupational hearing loss. *Laryngoscope* 82:1399–1409, 1972.

FIGURE 6.3. From Roush J: Screening school-age children. In Bess FH, Hall JW (cds): *Screening for Auditory Function*. Nashville: Bill Wilkerson Center Press, 1992.

FIGURE 6.4. From Lichtenstein MJ, Bess FH, Logan SA: Validation of screening tools for identifying hearing impaired elderly in primary care. *JAMA* 259:2875–2878, 1988.

FIGURE 6.5. From American Speech-Language-Hearing Association: Guidelines for screening for hearing impairment and middle ear disorders. *ASHA* 32:17–24, 1990.

TABLE 6.1. Adapted from the American Speech-Language-Hearing Association Joint Committee of Infant Hearing 1993 Position Statement—Draft, 1993.

TABLE 6.2. Adapted from the American Speech-Language-Hearing Association Joint Committee of Infant Hearing 1993 Position Statement—Draft, 1993.

TABLE 6.3. From Matkin ND: Early recognition and referral of hearing-impaired children. *Pediatrics in Review* 6:151–156, 1984.

TABLE 6.8. Adapted from Ventry IM, Weinstein BE: Identification of elderly people with hearing problems. *ASHA* 25:37–42, 1983; and from Lichtenstein MN, Bess FH, Logan SA: Validation of screening tools for identifying hearing impaired elderly in primary care. *JAMA* 259:2875–2878, 1988.

TABLE 6.10. Adapted from Schow RL, Nerbonne MA: Communication screening profile: use with elderly clients. *Ear and Hearing* 3:135–147, 1982.

TABLE 6.11. From ASHA 1990. Reprinted with the permission of the American Speech-Language-Hearing Association.

TABLE 7.1. Adapted from Mueller HG, Grimes A: Amplification systems for the hearing impaired. *In* Alpiner JG, McCarthy PA (eds): *Rehabilitative Audiology: Children and Adults* Baltimore, Williams & Wilkins, 1987, p 119.

TABLE 7.2. Adapted from Finitzo-Hieber T, Tillman TW: Room acoustic effects on monosyllabic word discrimination ability for normal and hearing impaired children. *Journal of Speech and Hearing Research* 21:440–448, 1978.

TABLE 7.3. From Alpiner JG: Evaluation of adult communication function. *In* Alpiner JG, McCarthy PA (eds): *Rehabilitative Audiology: Children and Adults*. Baltimore, Williams & Wilkins, 1987.

TABLE 8.1. From Quigley SP: *Some Effects of Hearing Impairment upon School Performance*. Springfield, IL, Division of Special Education Services, Department of Special Education Development and Education, 1968.

FIGURE 8.1. From Quigley SP, Paul PV: *Language and Deafness*. San Diego, College-Hill Press, 1984.

FIGURE 8.2. From Schleper D: *Communicating with Deaf People: An Introduction*. Washington, DC, National Information Center on Deafness, Gallaudet University, 1987.

FIGURE 8.3. From Schleper D: *Communicating with Deaf People: An Introduction*. Washington, DC, National Information Center on Deafness, Gallaudet University, 1987.

FIGURE 8.4. From deVilliers, PA: Educational implications of deafness: language and literacy. In Eavey RD, Klein JO (eds): *Hearing Loss in Childhood: A Primer, Report of the 102nd Ross Conference on Pediatric Research*. Columbus, OH, Ross Laboratories, 1992.

FIGURE 8.5. From Feagans L: Otitis media: a model for long term effects with implications for intervention. *In* Kavanaugh JF (ed): *Otitis Media and Child Development*. Parkton, MD: York Press, 1986.

INDEX

Page numbers in *italics* denote figures; those followed by "t" denote tables.